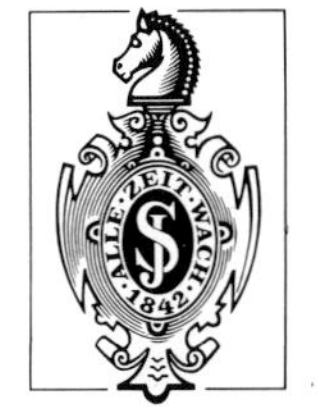

H. G. Beger   M. Büchler
R. A. Reisfeld   G. Schulz (Eds.)

Cancer Therapy

Monoclonal Antibodies, Lymphokines

New Developments in Surgical Oncology and Chemo- and Hormonal Therapy

With the Editorial Collaboration of
B. Greifenberg, Marburg and K. H. Link, Ulm

With 94 Figures and 92 Tables

Springer-Verlag
Berlin Heidelberg New York
London Paris Tokyo

Dr. Hans G. Beger, FACS
Professor of Surgery
Dr. Markus Büchler
Lecturer in Surgery
Department of General Surgery
University of Ulm
Steinhövelstraße 9, 7900 Ulm, FRG

Dr. Ralph A. Reisfeld
Division of Tumor Cell Biology
Scripps Clinic & Research Foundation
10666 North Torrey Pines Road, La Jolla, CA 92037, USA

Priv. Doz. Dr. Gregor Schulz
Clinical Research
Behringwerke AG Marburg
P.O. Box 1140, 3550 Marburg, FRG

ISBN 3-540-19293-X Springer-Verlag Berlin Heidelberg New York
ISBN 0-387-19293-X Springer-Verlag New York Berlin Heidelberg

Library of Congress Cataloging-in-Publication Data
Cancer therapy : monoclonal antibodies, lymphokines : new developments in surgical oncology and chemo- and hormonal therapy / H.G. Beger ... [et al.], (eds.) ; in collaboration with B. Greifenberg. p. cm. Includes bibliographies and index.
ISBN 0-387-19293-X (U.S.)
1. Cancer--Treatment. 2. Antibodies, Monoclonal--Therapeutic use. 3. Lymphokines--Therapeutic use. 4. Cancer--Surgery. 5. Cancer--Hormone therapy. 6. Cancer--Chemotherapy.
7. Beger, H.G. (Hans G.) I. Greifenberg, B.
[DNLM: 1. Antibodies, Monoclonal--therapeutic use. 2. Antineoplastic Agents--therapeutic use. 3. Hormones-therapeutic use. 4. Lymphokines--therapeutic use. 5. Neoplasms--drug therapy. 6. Neoplasms--surgery. QZ 266 C2172] RC270.8.C373 1988
616.99'406--dc19 DNLM/DLC 88-29509

Typesetting, printing, and binding: Appl, Wemding
2125/3140-543210 - Printed on acid-free paper.

Preface

The recent development of new strategies in cancer therapy was the main topic of an international meeting which took place at Reisensburg Castle in February, 1988. Here, experts in the field of tumor immunology, surgical oncology, and cancer chemotherapy discussed future directions in cancer treatment.

In 1975, Köhler and Milstein first described the technique of cell hybridization, which is used to produce monoclonal antibody (MoAb) reagents for the detection of tumor markers in sera, the in vitro analysis of leukemia or the histologic differential diagnosis of malignancies as opposed to chronic infectious diseases. Recently, it has been demonstrated that radiolabelled murine MoAbs are excellent tools for the in vivo localization of tumors. Meanwhile, initial clinical experience with the therapeutical use of MoAbs has been gained which shows that the latter either mediate cytotoxic functions, such as antibody-dependent cellular cytotoxicity or complement-dependent cytotoxicity, or are effective in conjugation with radionuclides, cytostatics, or toxins. New modifications, such as the "humanization" of murine antibodies, which will improve the efficacy of the above-mentioned therapy, are discussed in this volume.

Recent advances in DNA technology have resulted in the production of a number of recombinant glycoproteins, for example, interferons or tumor necrosis factor, which directly inhibit tumor growth. Other immune response modifiers, such as interleukin-2 (IL-2) or the colony-stimulating factors (CSFs), which are able to enhance proliferation and activity of T-lymphocytes or other hematopoietic cells, are now clinically available. Stimulated "killer lymphocytes" or macrophages are powerful "tumor killers", as has been demonstrated by clinical studies using recombinant IL-2, GM-CSF, or G-CSF. In addition, hematopoietic growth factors are able to accelerate regeneration of blood cells following chemotherapy. Initial clinical experience with GM-CSF and G-CSF has shown that severe neutropenia may be prevented or at least decelerated, which then results in a reduced number of severe infections. Other CSFs, such as interleukin 3 or erythropoietin, induce speedier reconstitution of platelets or erythrocytes. Thus, the clinical application of recombinant hematopoietic growth factors will

not only improve tolerability of chemotherapy, but may also allow the administration of higher doses of cytostatics, thus resulting in better response rates.
The approach of regional chemotherapy combined with new techniques of surgical oncology, including isolated regional hyperthermal perfusion and chemoembolization of tumors, presents a new concept of cancer treatment. Several randomized trials now exist which demonstrate a higher response rate following intrahepatic infusion rather than systemic infusion in the treatment of hepatic metastases from colorectal carcinoma. The results of regional chemotherapy of the liver from different research institutions are presented in this volume, the success rates pointing to the promising role of regional cancer treatment in the future.
In some malignancies, e.g., lymphoblastic leukemia, testicular cancer, and Hodgkin's disease, a high frequency of long-term cure rates has been achieved by the introduction of new chemotherapeutic regimens. However, patients with some of the most common cancers, for instance, lung cancer, colorectal cancer, or pancreatic cancer, still have a poor chance of survival if the tumor cannot be removed by surgery.
We hope that the various new strategies in cancer treatment presented in this book will help to point out that only combined research efforts in various fields of cancer treatment will result in improved therapy of malignancies.

December 1988

H. G. Beger M. Büchler
R. A. Reisfeld G. Schulz

Contents

Monoclonal Antibodies 1

R. A. REISFELD, B. MULLER, and H.-M. YANG
Immunochemotherapy of Cancer: A Perspective 3

K. BOSSLET, A. STEINSTRÄSSER, A. SCHWARZ, H. P. HARTHUS, G. LÜBEN, L. KUHLMANN, and H. H. SEDLACEK
Quantitative Considerations Supporting the Irrelevance of Circulating Serum Carcinoembryonic Antigen for the Immunoscintigraphic Visualization of Carcinoembryonic Antigen-Expressing Carcinomas 10

H. KALOFONOS and A. A. EPENETOS
Radioimmunotherapy with Iodine 131-Labelled Antibodies in Ovarian, Colonic and Brain Tumours 18

A. PLANTING, J. VERWEIJ, P. COX, M. PILLAY, and G. STOTER
Radioimmunodetection and Radioimmunotherapy in Myosarcoma 27

M. BÜCHLER, R. KÜBEL, R. KLAPDOR, K.-H. MUHRER, H. FRIESS, B. LORENZ, G. SCHULZ, K. BOSSLET, and H. G. BEGER
Immunotherapy of Pancreatic Cancer with Monoclonal Antibody BW 494: Results from a Multicentric Phase I–II Trial 32

H. MELLSTEDT, J.-E. FRÖDIN, G. MASUCCI, C. LINDEMALM, C. WEDELIN, B. CHRISTENSSON, J. SHETYE, P. BIBERFELD, A.-K. LEFVERT, P. PIHLSTEDT, J. MAKOWER, U. HARMENBERG, B. WAHREN, B. AHLMAN, B. CEDERMARK, R. ERWALD, I. MAGNUSSON, J. NATHANSSON, and A. RIEGER
Mab 17-1 A Used for Therapy of Patients with Metastatic Colorectal Carcinomas 42

W. G. DIPPOLD and K.-H. MEYER ZUM BÜSCHENFELDE
Immunotherapy of Malignant Melanomas 51

R. KLAPDOR
Interaction of Monoclonal Antibodies with Biological Response Modifiers and Cytostatics 56

Lymphokines 71

A. LINDEMANN, F. HERRMANN, H. GAMM, W. OSTER, and R. MERTELSMANN
Cancer Treatment with Cytokines: Concepts and First Clinical Experience 73

M. S. MITCHELL
Low-dose Cyclophosphamide and IL-2 in the Treatment of Advanced Melanoma 85

A. GANSER, B. VÖLKERS, J. GREHER, F. WALTHER, and D. HOELZER
Application of Granulocyte-Macrophage Colony-Stimulating Factor in Patients with Malignant Hematological Diseases . . 90

H. LINK, M. FREUND, H. KIRCHNER, M. STOLL, H. SCHMID, P. BUCSKY, J. SEIDEL, G. SCHULZ, R. E. SCHMIDT, H. RIEHM, H. POLIWODA, and K. WELTE
Enhancement of Autologous Bone Marrow Transplantation with Recombinant Human Granulocyte-Macrophage Colony-Stimulating Factor (rhGM-CSF) 96

R. G. STEIS, J. CLARK, D. L. LONGO, J. SMITH, R. MILLER, F. RUSCETTI, J. HURSEY, and W. URBA
A Phase Ib Evaluation of Recombinant Human Granulocyte-Macrophage Colony-Stimulating Factor 103

N. NIEDERLE and G. KUMMER
The Role of Interferon in the Management of Patients with Hairy Cell Leukemia and Multiple Myeloma 112

F. PORZSOLT, W. DIGEL, C. BUCK, A. RAGHAVACHAR, M. STEFANIC, and W. SCHÖNIGER
Possible Mechanism of Interferon Action in Hairy Cell Leukemia 124

R. SCHIESSEL
Tumor Vaccination in the Treatment of Colorectal Cancer . . . 132

New Approaches in Surgical Oncology 141

R. BITTNER and H. G. BEGER
New Developments in Surgical Oncology 143

P. SCHLAG
Cancer Surgery – Conservative or Radical? 154

S. BENGMARK
Regional Chemotherapy of the Liver and Hepatic Artery Occlusion 163

N. KEMENY
Regional Chemotherapy of Hepatic Metastases 169

F. SAFI, R. BITTNER, R. ROSCHER, K. SCHUMACHER, W. GAUS, and H. G. BEGER
Regional Chemotherapy in Hepatic Metastases of Colorectal Carcinoma: Continuous Intra-arterial Versus Continuous Intra-arterial/Intravenous Therapy 176

K.-H. MUHRER and H. GRIMM
Isolated Regional Hyperthermal Liver Perfusion: Indications, Technique and Results 190

K.-H. SCHULTHEIS, M. PLIESS, H.-H. GENTSCH, H. BÖDEKER, C. GEBHARDT, and K. SCHWEMMLE
Chemoembolization of Liver Tumors 201

S. G. BOWN
New Cancer Treatment with Lasers – Photodynamic Therapy and Interstitial Hyperthermia 216

E. KRAAS, E. LÖHDE, O. ABRI, H. SCHLICKER, S. MATZKU, H. KALTHOFF, and W. H. SCHMIEGEL
Specificity, Kinetics, and Distribution of Monoclonal Antibodies to Carcinoembryonic Antigen in Human Colorectal Carcinoma by Ex Vivo Human Tumor Perfusion . . 223

Chemotherapy and Hormonal Therapy 233

G. FALKSON
Chemotherapy: Benefits and Limits 235

H. P. KRAEMER and H. H. SEDLACEK
The Human Tumor Clonogenic Assay for the Prediction of Tumor Sensitivity 243

K. H. LINK
Chemosensitivity: Directed Regional Chemotherapy of Liver Metastases 249

I. H. KRAKOFF
Clinical Development of New Anthracyclines 259

J. VERWEIJ, E. SALEWSKI, and G. STOTER
First Clinical Experience with Cytorhodin S – The First Compound of a New Class of Anthracyclines 263

B. GREIFENBERG
Pirarubicin: A New Drug in the Treatment of Malignant Diseases 270

H.-H. FIEBIG, H. HENSS and H. ARNOLD
Pirarubicin – A New Anthracycline with High Activity in Untreated Patients with Small-Cell Cancer of the Lung 280

K. HÖFFKEN
New Approaches in the Hormonal Therapy of Breast Cancer . 284

E. D. KREUSER, W. D. HETZEL, F. PORZSOLT, and R. HAUTMANN
Reproductive Toxicity with and Without Administration of Luteinizing-Hormone-Releasing Hormone Agonist During Adjuvant Chemotherapy in Patients with Germ Cell Tumors . 292

Subject Index 303

List of Contributors*

Abri, O. 223[1]
Ahlman, B. 42
Arnold, H. 280
Beger, H.G. 32, 143, 176
Bengmark, S. 163
Biberfeld, P. 42
Bittner, R. 143, 176
Bödeker, H. 201
Bosslet, K. 10, 32
Bown, S.G. 216
Buck, C. 124
Bucsky, P. 96
Büchler, M. 32
Cedermark, B. 42
Christensson, B. 42
Clark, J. 103
Cox, P. 27
Digel, W. 124
Dippold, W.G. 51
Epenetos, A.A. 18
Erwald, R. 42
Falkson, G. 235
Fiebig, H.-H. 280
Freund, M. 96
Friess, H. 32
Frödin, J.-E. 42
Gamm, H. 73
Gaus, W. 176
Ganser, A. 90
Gebhardt, C. 201
Gentsch, H.-H. 201
Greher, J. 90
Greifenberg, B. 270
Grimm, H. 190
Harmenberg, U. 42
Hautmann, R. 292
Harthus, H.P. 10
Herrmann, F. 73
Hetzel, W.D. 292
Henss, H. 280
Höffken, K. 284
Hoelzer, D. 90
Hursey, J. 103
Kalofonos, H. 18
Kalthoff, H. 223
Kemeny, N. 169
Kirchner, H. 96
Klapdor, R. 32, 56
Kraas, E. 223
Kraemer, H.P. 243
Krakoff, I.H. 259
Kreuser, E.D. 292
Kübel, R. 32
Kuhlmann, L. 10
Kummer, G. 112
Lefvert, A.-K. 42
Lindemalm, C. 42
Lindemann, A. 73
Link, H. 96
Link, K.H. 249
Löhde, E. 223
Longo, D.L. 103
Lorenz, B. 32
Lüben, G. 10
Magnusson, I. 42
Makower, J. 42
Masucci, G. 42
Matzku, S. 223

* You will find the addresses at the beginning of the respective contribution.
[1] Page on which contribution begins.

Mellstedt, H. 42
Mertelsmann, R. 73
Meyer zum Büschenfelde, K.-H. 51
Miller, R. 103
Mitchell, M.S. 85
Muhrer, K.-H. 32, 190
Muller, B. 3
Nathansson, J. 42
Niederle, N. 112
Oster, W. 73
Pihlstedt, P. 42
Pillay, M. 27
Planting, A. 27
Pliess, M. 201
Poliwoda, H. 96
Porzsolt, F. 124, 292
Raghavachar, A. 124
Rieger, A. 42
Riehm, H. 96
Reisfeld, R.A. 3
Ruscetti, F. 103
Roscher, R. 176
Safi, F. 176
Salewski, E. 263
Schiessel, R. 132
Schlag, P. 154
Schlicker, H. 223
Schmid, H. 96
Schmidt, R.E. 96
Schmiegel, W.H. 223
Schöniger, W. 124
Schultheis, K.-H. 201
Schulz, G. 32, 96
Schumacher, K. 176
Schwarz, A. 10
Schwemmle, K. 201
Sedlacek, H.H. 10, 243
Seidel, J. 96
Shetye, J. 42
Smith, J. 103
Stefanic, M. 124
Steinsträsser, A. 10
Steis, R.G. 103
Stoll, M. 96
Stoter, G. 27, 263
Urba, W. 103
Verweij, J. 27, 263
Völkers, B. 90
Wahren, B. 42
Walther, F. 90
Wedelin, C. 42
Welte, K. 96
Yang, H.-M. 3

MONOCLONAL ANTIBODIES

Immunochemotherapy of Cancer: A Perspective

R. A. REISFELD,[1] B. MULLER,[1] and H.-M. YANG[1]

Introduction

Considerable advances in biomedical research during the last 20 years have led to an increased interest in human tumor-associated antigens as potential targets for the diagnosis and therapy of cancer. Research efforts in this area have intensified during the last decade because of the availability of monoclonal antibodies and the rapid emergence of increasingly sophisticated technologies of gene cloning. The relatively slow progress in the clinical treatment of solid tumors has provided further impetus to increased efforts to render immunological approaches useful for cancer therapy, particularly by applying immunoconjugates. Among these conjugates, those made between monoclonal antibodies and either chemotherapeutic drugs, radionuclides, or plant toxins represent the three major categories.

The idea of using antibodies as carriers for drugs and toxins was originally suggested by Paul Ehrlich in 1906 [4]. However, it was not until 1958 that chemoimmunotherapy really surfaced, when reasonably promising results were obtained in mice, using methotrexate conjugated to antibodies against L1210 leukemia cells [9]. There was a considerable lag until the mid-1970s, when some of the more commonly used chemotherapeutic drugs, such as doxorubicin (Adriamycin), daunomycin [8], and bleomycin [5] were conjugated to polyclonal antitumor antibodies and tested in mouse model systems. Some of these early results actually led to preliminary clinical investigations of chlorambucil-antibody conjugates, although with somewhat ambiguous results [6]. Since this brief article is not intended as a review of the field of chemoimmunoconjugates, the interested reader is referred to a recent review on the subject matter [12].

This article focuses mainly on the promises offered as well as on the problems posed by chemoimmunoconjugates involving monoclonal antibodies. Specifically, a human melanoma model in athymic (nu/nu) mice serves to illustrate those promises and problems that became apparent when doxorubicin was covalently conjugated to monoclonal antibody (Mab) 9.2.27, directed against a human melanoma-associated chondroitin sulfate proteoglycan [14].

[1] Department of Immunology, Scripps Clinic and Research Foundation, 10666 North Torrey Pines Road, La Jolla, CA 92037, USA.

H. G. Beger et al. (Eds.), Cancer Therapy

The Promise of Chemoimmunoconjugates for Cancer Therapy

The potential usefulness of monoclonal antibodies in delivering chemotherapeutic drugs to tumor sites in vivo is a contention that can be tested experimentally. Thus, monoclonal antibodies directed against well-characterized, tumor-associated antigens make ist possible to critically evaluate their suitabilities as carriers for cytotoxic molecules. The use of such chemoimmunoconjugates for receptor-mediated delievery of lethal agents to human tumor targets promises to create a new generation of treatment modalities that may reduce side effects, facilitate more selective tumor targeting, result in improved therapeutic indices, and decrease lethal doses, thus creating a wider therapeutic window. In addition, drugs bound to antibody may be protected from enzymatic degradation, thereby preventing their rapid excretion, possibly decreasing the formation of drug metabolites in the circulation, and increasing drug half-life.

To test this contention, doxorubicin (DXR) was covalently conjugated to Mab 9.2.27 via a cis-aconitic anhydride linker. Briefly, immunoconjugates were prepared with a molar ratio of DXR to monoclonal antibodies ranging from 2:1 to 10:1. The immunoreactivity of Mab 9.2.27 was well retained after conjugation. DXR-Mab 9.2.27 conjugates were found to be 2 logs more potent in killing tumor cells in vitro ($IC_{50} = 10^{-7} M$) than free drug.

Mab 9.2.27 was chosen as a drug-targeting device for these studies because it has several important characteristics. First, as observed in phase I clinical trials, it targets melanoma cells most effectively [10]. Second, the antibody has a very high affinity for melanoma cells ($K_A = 8 \times 10^9 M^{-1}$). Third, Mab 9.2.27 does not cause antigen modulation in vivo, and expression of the proteoglycan antigen recognized by it is not cell cycle-dependent. The most significant results of these phase I clinical trials indicate that Mab 9.2.27, administered i.v. in excess of 250 mg to melanoma patients, effectively covered all skin lesions, although these tumors usually have relatively poor blood circulation [10]. These properties of Mab 9.2.27 are particularly critical for effective tumor targeting of DXR-Mab conjugates. Finally, recent results indicate that DXR-Mab 9.2.27 conjugates are stable in the circulation of nude mice for up to 48 h, as revealed by sodium dedecyl sulfate and polyacrylamide gel electrophoresis (PAGE) analysis of ^{14}C-labeled DXR-Mab 9.2.27 conjugates [14].

Another significant finding made recently indicates that 30 days after tumor cell inoculation, four nude mice in the experimental group treated with DXR-Mab 9.2.27 conjugates still remained tumor free; the remaining eight animals developed only small lesions - at a much slower rate than control animals. The DXR-Mab 9.2.27 conjugate had an additional benefit, as mice treated with it showed an 81% increase in life span over a 120-day period. This was considerably greater than the improvement of 27% observed with animals treated with DXR alone. These data clearly indicate that the growth of an established tumor can be markedly suppressed by a DXR-Mab 9.2.27 conjugate. Results of biodistribution studies further demonstrate that Mab 9.2.27 is able to deliver at least fourfold more drug (3.7% injected dose per gram of tumor) to the tumor target than DXR in free drug form (0.8% injected dose per gram of tumor). Moreover, only free DXR, but not DXR-Mab 9.2.27 conjugates show a significant accumulation in bone. Therefore, conjugated DXR has overall a far better localization index than free DXR. These data are consistent with the specific tumor suppression and increased life span observed in the group of nude mice treated with DXR-Mab 9.2.27. Thus, DXR-Mab 9.2.27 conjugates effectively increase selective toxicity of free DXR [14].

A toxicity study in nude mice indicated that 400 μg free DXR (two injection of 200 μg (each) at 3-day interval) will kill 100% of the animals within 6 days. In addition, the dose is accumulative in nude mice; i.e. four doses of 100 μg free DXR will kill the mice within 14 days. Therefore, the dose used in this study, a total equivalent dose of 75 μg of DXR per mouse, can be significantly increased without toxicity. These data suggest that our present drug delivery, although effective, is still quite suboptimal and that even better results may be achieved under more optimal conditions.

Efforts were made to understand possible mechanism(s) of action by which DXR-Mab 9.2.27 conjugates suppress the growth of established tumors. To this end, studies were conducted that measured initial binding, internalization, processing, and degradation of such Mab-drug conjugates. An initial finding of these studies indicates that an excess amount of native Mab 9.2.27 can reverse growth inhibition caused by the DXR-Mab 9.2.27 conjugate, suggesting that the latter may actually enter some of the tumor target cells via an antigen-antibody complex rather than by diffusion, as observed by others in the case of free drug [3].

This hypothesis is further supported by a binding study in which ^{14}C-labeled DXR-Mab 9.2.27 conjugates bound to M21 but not to control NMB-7 neuroblastoma cells that do not express the 9.2.27 epitope [14]. Taken together, these data suggest that DXR-Mab conjugates are likely to be most effective once they are internalized. To this end, the intracellular localization of DXR-Mab conjugates was monitored with an anchored cell analysis and sorting (ACAS) work station. In an initial study, free DXR was localized in the nuclei of M21 cells after 30 min incubation at 37 °C. The nuclei-associated fluorescence in these cells was resistant to ribonuclease but sensitive to deoxyribonuclease treatment, indicating that DXR was bound to nuclear DNA. Under identical conditions (30 min at 37 °C), DXR-Mab 9.2.27 conjugates were predominantly oberved in the cytoplasm. However, after a 2-h incubation at 37 °C, the majority of fluorescence was found in the nucleus. This time lag required for the conjugate to enter the nucleus prompted an examination of the possible involvement of a lysosomal degradation of DXR-Mab conjugates during this process. As expected, when the pH of the lysosomal compartment of M21 cells was increased by treatment with 25 μm chloroquine, the majority of fluorescence was localized in a perinuclear region of these cells after a 2-h incubation with DXR-Mab 9.2.27 at 37 °C. In a control experiment, chloroquine treatment (25 μ *M*) alone did not affect either the transport or DNA binding ability of free DXR [14]. The results from these experiments suggest that DXR-Mab 9.2.27 conjugate and free DXR follow different routes of degradation. Thus, free DXR bound to DNA within 30 min, whereas the DXR-Mab 9.2.27 conjugates remained in the cytoplasm, most likely in the endosomal or lysosomal compartments, as previously suggested, since chloroquine is known to selectively increase the intracellular pH of lysosomes and endosomes [11]. Passive uptake of drug through membranes of binding to drug receptors appears to be less likely, especially since DXR per se is ineffective in our system.

In summary, although still suboptimal, conjugates of antimelanoma Mab 9.2.27 with DXR proved quite effective in specifically suppressing growth of established human melanoma xenografts in athymic (nu/nu) mice while markedly increasing the life span of these animals. These results are remarkable since neither Mab 9.2.27 nor DXR alone can achieve such results and also because it is well known that human melanoma cells are resistant to DXR. In fact, previous phase I clinical trials with Mab 9.2.27 alone demonstrated excellent tumor targeting but showed no effect at all on suppression of tumor growth [10]. Also, in prior studies of athymic (nu/nu) mice bearing human melanoma xenografts, Mab 9.2.27 did not supress growth of established tumors [1].

Possible Solutions to Problems Posed by Chemoimmunoconjugates

The promising results of our initial studies not withstanding, a considerable number of problems remain to be solved before chemoimmunoconjugates become optimal for tumor therapy. What becomes quite apparent ist that attempts to covalently bind generally hydrophobic drugs to relatively hydrophilic antibody molecules face immediate serious problems. A case in point is the fact that the most abundant drug linkage groups on antibodies, i.e., ε-amino groups on lysine residues, cannot be optimally utilized without losing conjugate solubility. For example, Mab 9.2.27 contains a total of 52 ε-amino groups per molecule, yet only 15 of them can be conjugated with DXR without substantial losses in antibody binding affinity and solubility. The number of actual ε-amino groups available under these criteria can be even less. Thus, another monoclonal antibody, 14G2a, directed against Gd2 ganglioside and, like Mab 9.2.27, also of IgG2a isotope, shows only five available ε-amino groups from a total of 63 such binding sites. It is therefore quite obvious that the drug pay load of monoclonal antibodies is often severely restricted. Earlier attempts by others to overcome this stricture by using linkers, such a soluble dextran, polynucleotides, or serum albumin have increased the number of drug molecules bound but have not shown real, clear-cut advantages in therapeutic efficacy. This may be because of losses in antibody activity and the sheer bulk of such conjugates [12].

The design of new, more hydrophilic antineoplastic drugs specifically suitable for linkage to monoclonal antibodies is, of course, another necessity to optimize chemoimmunoconjugates for cancer therapy. Furthermore, the availability of monoclonal antibodies targeted to suitable tumor antigen targets makes it possible to reexamine extremely cytotoxic substances that were previously not considered suitable for chemoterapy. In fact, it is the very essence of monoclonal antibody targeting to critically evaluate the use of such substances and thereby substantiate the very rationale for using chemoimmunoconjugates. This rationale is based on the ability of chemoimmunoconjugates to allow for more specific targeting of more effective drugs to tumor cells while diminishing many of the serious side effects previously observed with increased use of many chemotherapeutic drugs. One example of such an extremely cytotoxic drug is cyano-morpholino doxorubicin, which is at least 3 logs more cytotoxic than doxorubicin. In collaboration with Dr. W. Wrasidlo (Brunswick Biotechnetics, San Diego, California), we were able to

effectively couple this drug to Mab 9.2.27 by means of novel linker technologies and still retain full activity of both drug and monoclonal antibody.
Another example ist the use of trichothecenes, a class of mycotoxins produced by soil fungi of the class *Fungi imperfectii.* These relatively small molecules (mol. wt. 500–800) act at the level of the ribosome as inhibitors of protein synthesis. An advantage of these highly potent mycotoxins is that they are reported to lack nonspecific, receptor-mediated uptake by the liver. This property, as well as their very small molecular weight, distinguishes them favorably from the various plant toxins presently used in immunoconjugates, which are glycoproteins with molecular weights > 25000 that bind to the liver, unless carefully modified, and usually elicit a foreign protein response by the host. A further advantage of the trichothecenes is that one of their macrocylic species, i.e., *Verrucarin A,* is tenfold more potent than actinomycin D, one of the most potent chemotherapeutic drugs. In addition, it was reported that the toxicity of trichothecenes can be reduced by conjugation to Mab NRML-0.5, which, similar to Mab 9.2.27, also detects a specific epitope on a melanoma-associated chondroitin sulfate proteoglycan. In fact, this conjugate has an ID_{50} of 10 ng/ml (drug content) against cultured, human melanoma cells. This conjugate was found to localize to tumors to the same degree as unconjugated antibody, does not accumulate in the liver, and has a serum half-life equal to unconjugated antibody [13]. Obviously, mycotoxins such as the trichothecenes provide a most suitable class of substances for preparing additional, highly potent chemoimmunoconjugates. Of course, it remains to be determined whether resistance will develop to mycotoxins as it does to chemotherapeutic drugs after repeated use.
The key to the preparation of effective chemoimmunoconjugates is the development of novel reagents to link cytotoxic agents to monoclonal antibodies. In this case, one of the main objectives is to develop linkers that remain stable while the chemoimmunoconjugate is in the circulation but quickly release the drug once the conjugate reaches the tumor cell surface and/or is endocytosed into the lysozomal compartment. Novel biofunctional reagents, possibly with "biodegradable" linkages, such as nucleotides and suitable peptides, may serve this purpose. The development and application of these types of linkers is being actively pursued in a number of laboratories, including our own.
Finally, it is clear that ever more suitable monoclonal antibodies will be required to produce optimal chemoimmunoconjugates to achieve efficient cancer therapy. An obvious choice is offered by monoclonal antibodies directed to well-characterized receptor molecules that are expressed on the surface of tumor cells and are usually internalized by them. For example, monoclonal antibodies to the receptor of epidermal growth factor (EGF) fit this description and are presently under active investigation as drug carriers in the author's laboratory. Other drug carrier molecules that may prove highly effective to construct effective chemoimmunoconjugates are monoclonal antibodies directed against RGD-adhesion receptors, i.e., molecules with a critical functional role in cell adhesion and motility that may play an important role in tumor invasion and metastasis. In this regard, Mab LM609 [2] is presently under intensive investigation in the author's laboratory as a carrier for chemotherapeutic drugs in animal model systems involving spontaneous metastasis of human melanoma.

It should be pointed out that once optimal chemoimmunoconjugates have been produced, it is absolutely essential that they be critically evaluated in vivo in suitable animal model systems. Spontaneous metastatic systems in athymic (nu/nu) mice offer a good choice, and several of these, representing human malignant melanoma, are presently under active investigation in the author's laboratory. Another important point needs to be made regarding optimal delivery of chemoimmunoconjugates to tumor sites. The critical issue of delivering sufficient chemoimmunoconjugate to the tumor has been viewed with scepticism because data from tumor imaging in patients are often cited which indicate that only a fraction of one percent of radiolabeled antibody usually reaches a given tumor site in patients with advanced disease. However, in all imaging experiments, usually only 2-3 mg of labeled antibody is injected a single time. Consequently, a large percentage can not be expected to reach the tumor, considering the dilution in the circulation. An alternative might be a rather constant, slow infusion of chemoimmunoconjugates, using Alzet osmotic minipumps in laboratory animals, as performed previously with monoclonal antibodies per se [7]. This approach may be better than delivering repeated injections at various time intervals and may actually insure a greater concentration of chemoimmunoconjugates at tumor sites. This may have a positive effect by ultimately delivering greater concentrations of drugs to their intracellular target sites. It is certainly possible to critically evaluate the efficacy of such an approach in suitable animal model systems and to compare its effect on tumor growth with that achieved by repeated single injections of chemoimmunoconjugates over a given time period.
Chemoimmunoconjugates for ultimate clinical use should have a far better and more rapid "turn around time" between the preclinical and clinical components. New chemoimmunoconjugates that were critically evaluated and found effective at the preclinical level must receive prompt and critical evaluation in a suitable clinical setting. Once the safety or such compounds has been established, they should be given as fair a test in appropriately selected patients as that given chemotherapeutic drugs received over the course of the last 45 years. Although much is expected of chemoimmunoconjugates, they are nevertheless real, untried newcomers in chemotherapy, a field which has required many years to evolve and to progress. One can anticipate that, given a proper start, chemoimmunoconjugates will eventually become useful for adjuvant therapy and provide an improvement in the treatment of human cancer.

References

1. Bumol TF, Wang OC, Reisfeld RA, Kaplan NO (1983) Monoclonal antibody and an antibody-toxin conjugate to a cell surface proteoglycan of melanoma cells suppress in vivo tumor growth. Proc Natl Acad Sci USA 80: 529-533
2. Cheresh DA (1987) Human endothelial cells synthesize and express an Arg-Gly-Asp-directed adhesion receptor involved in attachment to fibrinogen and von Willebrand factor. Proc Natl Acad Sci USA 84: 6471-6475
3. Durand RE, Olive PL (1981) Flow cytometry studies of intracellular adriamycin in single cells in vitro. Cancer Res 41: 3489-3494
4. Ehrlich P (1906) In: Collected studies on immunity, vol II. John Wiley, New York

5. Ghose T, Guclu A, Tai J (1975) Suppression of an AKR lymphoma by antibody and chlorambucil. J Nat Cancer Inst 55: 1353–1357
6. Ghose T, Norvell ST, Guclu A, Bodurtha A, MacDonald AS (1977) Immunochemotherapy of malignant melanoma with chlorambucil-bound antimelanoma globulins: Preliminary results on patients with disseminated disease. J Nat Cancer Inst 58: 845–852
7. Herlyn AM, Steplewski Z, Herlyn MF, Koprowski H (1980) Inhibition of growth of colorectal carcinoma in nude mice by monoclonal antibody. Cancer Res 40: 717–721
8. Hurwitz E, Levy R, Maron R, Wilcheck M, Arnon R, Sela M (1975) The covalent binding of daunomycin and adriamycin to antibodies with retention of both drug and antibody activities. Cancer Res 35: 1175–1181
9. Mathe G, Loc TB, Bernard J (1958) Effet sur la Leucémie 1210 de la souris d'une combinaison par diazotation d'A-methopterine et de γ-globulins de hamsters porteurs de celle leucémie par hétérogreffe. CR Acad Sci Paris 246: 1626–1628
10. Oldham RK, Foon KA, Morgan AC, Woodhouse GA, Schroff RW, Abrams PG, Feer MF, Farrell MM, Kinball ES, Sherwin SA (1984) Monoclonal antibody therapy of malignant melanoma: In vivo localization in cutaneous metastasis after intravenous administration. J Clin Oncol 2: 1235–1244
11. Pastan I, Willingham MC (1983) Receptor-mediated endocytosis-coated pits, receptosomes and the Golgi. Trend Briochem Sci 8: 250–254
12. Pietersz GA, Kanellos J, Smyth MJ, Zalcberg J, McKenzie LFC (1987) The use of monoclonal antibody conjugates for the diagnosis and treatment of cancer. Immunol and Cell Biol 65: 111–125
13. Sivam GP, Comezoglu T, Jarvis BB, Morgan AC (1988) Immunoconjugates of ribosomal inhibiting drugs and monoclonal antibody. Abstract 34, meeting on immunoconjugates, San Diego, California 4–6 Feb 1988
14. Yang HM, Reisfeld RA (1988) Doxorubicin conjugated with a monoclonal antibody to a human melanoma-associated proteoglycan suppresses the growth of established term on xenografts in nude mice. Proc Natl Acad Sci USA 85: 1189–1193

Quantitative Considerations Supporting the Irrelevance of Circulating Serum Carcinoembryonic Antigen for the Immunoscintigraphic Visualization of Carcinoembryonic Antigen-Expressing Carcinomas

K. BOSSLET,[1] A. STEINSTRÄSSER,[2] A. SCHWARZ,[2] H. P. HARTHUS,[1] G. LÜBEN,[1] L. KUHLMANN,[2] and H. H. SEDLACEK[1]

Introduction

Since the first description of the carcinoembryonic antigen (CEA) in 1965 [14, 15] up to today, when the primary structure of CEA has been deduced from the cDNA sequence [22], CEA has become important as a tumor marker for the control of colorectal carcinomas [9, 13], as well as for the immunoscintigraphic visualization of CEA-expressing carcinomas [19]. In particular, the relatively new method of immunoscintigraphy requires the binding of monoclonal antibodies (MAb) to epitopes on CEA that are not detectable on the various nonspecific cross-reacting antigens (NCA) expressed on normal tissues [16, 24]. A so-called anti-CEA antibody with strong cross-reactivity to human granulocytes and erythrocytes (NCA) was not able to localize human colorectal carcinomas in vivo, but induced fever, rigors, emesis, and a short-term granulocytopenia [8]. Even those MAbs that are selective for protein epitopes on CEA [3, 6] and not cross-reactive with epitopes on NCAs or Y- or X-type carbohydrate moieties on CEA [21] are primarily confronted with high amounts of circulating CEA after their i.v. injection into the patient. The following in vitro experiments were conducted to explain why successful immunoscintigraphic localization of colorectal carcinomas using MAb binding to CEA are possible with a sensitivity of up to 90%, as shown in a multicenter study (100 patients) in the Federal Republic of Germany using the MAb BW 431/31 coupled via diethylene triamine penta-acetic acid (DTPA) to ^{111}In [5].

Materials and Methods

Tumor Cell Lines

The LoVo adenocarcinoma cell line of the colon was obtained from the American Type Culture Collection (ATCC, 12301 Parklawn Drive, Rockville, MD 20852, USA/ATCC-No.: CCL 229). It was routinely passaged in RPMI-1540 with 10% fetal bovine serum (FBS). Confluent cultures were treated for 3 min with a solution of 0.25% trypsin and 0.02 *M* (ethylene diamine tetra-acetate (EDTA) and subcultured at a ratio of 1:5.

[1] Department of Experimental Medicine, Behringwerke AG Marburg, P.O. Box 1140, 3550 Marburg/Lahn, FRG.
[2] Radiochemical Laboratory, Hoechst AG Frankfurt, Stroofstraße, 6230 Frankfurt/Main 80, FRG.

H. G. Beger et al. (Eds.), Cancer Therapy

Monoclonal Antibodies

The MAbs BW 374/14, BW 250/183, BW 431/31, and BW 431/26 (all of the IgG_1 isotype) recognize different epitopes on CEA [3, 5]. Briefly, the MAbs BW 431/31 and BW 431/26 are selective for CEA, whereas the MAbs BW 374/14 or BW 250/183 bind to NCA55, NCA95, and CEA or to NCA95 and CEA respectively. MAb BW 494 binds to a pancreatic and colonic carcinoma-associated mucin-molecule different from CEA [4]. MAb BW 575 is selective for small-cell lung carcinomas and does not show any significant binding to carcinomas of the gastrointestinal tract [2].

Radiolabelling of MAbs

Purified MAbs [11] were radiolabelled with ^{125}I using the iodogen method [12, 20]. The specific activities obtained for the different MAbs were:

BW 374/14: 3.9 μCi/μg
BW 431/31: 3.9 μCi/μg
BW 494: 4.03 μCi/μg
BW 250/183: 3.5 μCi/μg
BW 431/26: 2.9 μCi/μg
BW 575: 2.59 μCi/μg

Blocking Assay

^{125}I-labelled MAb protein (100 μl) was mixed with CEA-containing serum (100 μl) or purified CEA, which had been isolated from CEA-expressing human colon carcinomas and incubated for 90 min at 37 °C in round-bottom 96-well microtiter plates (Nunc: 1-63320). Thereafter, 10^6 LoVo cells in 25 μl phosphate-buffered solution/bovine serum albumin (PBS-BSA), which were detached from plastic by incubation with 0.02% EDTA for 5 min, were added to the MAb-serum or the MAb-CEA mixture. After 1 h incubation at 37 °C, the microtiter plates were spun, and the pellets were washed three times with PBS. The washed cell pellet was resuspended in 125 μl PBS-BSA and 100 μl thereof were counted in a well-type γ-counter to determine the cell-bound radioactivity.

Western Blotting Analysis

The methodology was performed essentially as described in [28]. Instead of radiolabelled second antibody, the ABC-vector-kit (Vector Burlingname) was used.

Scatchard Analysis

The affinity of the MAbs to tumor cells was evaluated according to Walker [29], based on the original papers of Scatchard [25] and Berson and Yalow [1]. As antigenic material, collagenized and formaldehyde-fixed cells derived from nude mouse xenografts transplanted with the CEA-expressing CoCa2 colonic carcinoma were used. A constant amount of these cells was added to each vial of a dilution series of the respective MAb. This mixture was incubated for 4 h at room temperature, the cells were spun down, washed, and the cell-bound activity was determined. The bound-to-free ratio was plotted against the concentration of cell-bound antibody molecules using the following corrections [27]:

1. The unspecific part (U) of the antibodies (determined with irrelevant cells or by an iterative procedure during the evaluation) was subracted.
2. The "free" part of antibodies (F) consisted only of immune-reactive molecules using the formula $F = r \cdot T - (B - U)$, where T is the total activity and r the immune-reactive fraction of the preparation, determined separately according to Steinsträsser and Schwarz [26]. The inverse of the slope of the described plot gives the affinity constant (l/mol).

CEA Assay

The amount of CEA present in the patient's sera was evaluated using the commercially available Behring Enzygnost CEA assay.

Results

Binding Inhibition Experiments on LoVo Cells

Incubation of 10^6 CEA-expressing living LoVo colonic carcinoma cells with 2-3 ng (10000 cpm) of the various MAb proteins for 60 min at 37 °C results in the binding of 0.2-0.3 ng (1000 cpm) to the cell membranes. Preincubation of the various MAbs ($\approx$ 10000 cpm) for 90 min at 37 °C with sera from patients with colonic carcinomas (Fig. 1) containing high levels (a-d), medium levels (e-f), or low levels (g-j) of CEA affected MAb binding to the cells as shown in Fig. 1. The binding of MAbs BW 431/26 and BW 431/31 to the LoVo cells is only weakly inhibited despite a 20-fold molar excess of soluble CEA (a-d). In contrast, the binding of MAbs BW 250/183 and BW 374/14 to the LoVo cells is efficiently inhibited under identical conditions (a-d). Marginal binding inhibition was observed with all anti-CEA MAbs with sera containing medium (e-f) or low amounts of CEA (g-j).
Purified CEA [17] isolated from primary carcinoma of the colon, did not inhibit the binding of MAbs BW 431/26 and BW 431/31 to the LoVo cells as efficiently as it inhibited the binding of MAbs BW 374/14 and Bw 250/183 (k).
The positive control MAb BW 494 binding to a high-molecular-weight mucin-epitope [4] not detectable on CEA could not be inhibited in its binding to the LoVo cells either by CEA-containing sera (a-j) or by purified CEA (k). The bind-

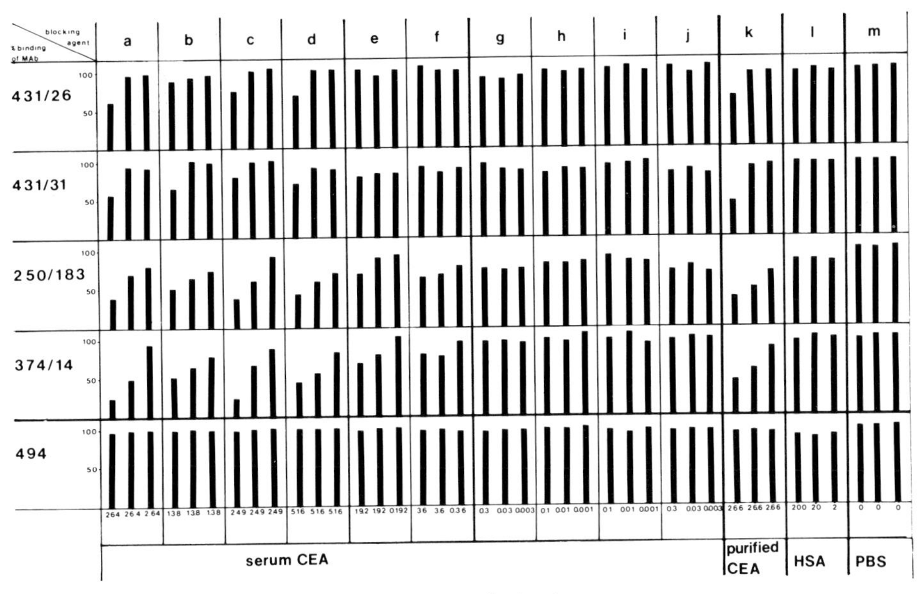

Fig. 1. Summary of results of a representative serum-blocking assay. Serum from various sources was incubated with radiolabelled MAbs 431/26, 431/31, 250/183, 374/14, and 494, and their binding to the epitope expressing LoVo colon carcinoma cell line was evaluated. *Black columns* represent percentage of binding of individual MAbs to the LoVo cell line after preincubation (blocking) with the corresponding CEA-containing serum, HSA, or PBS (100%)

ing of the anti-small-cell lung carcinoma MAb BW 575 [2] was in the range of 1%–3% of the binding obtained with the anti-CEA MAbs or MAb BW 494 (data not shown). Purified human serum albumin (l) as well as phosphate-buffered saline (m) showed no inhibition of binding with any MAb.

In summary, the binding of the anti-CEA-NCA MAbs 374/14 and BW 250/183 is inhibited equally effectively by CEA-containing sera and by purified CEA, whereas the binding of the anti-CEA MAbs BW 431/26 and BW 431/31 is neither inhibited by the purified CEA, isolated from a primary colonic carcinoma, nor by the CEA-containing sera.

Western Blotting Analysis of Patient's Sera Containing CEA

To investigate whether the reduced inhibition mediated by the CEA-containing sera on the binding of the CEA-specific MAbs BW 431/26 and BW 431/31 to the LoVo colonic carcinoma cell line is due to the absence of intact CEA in the sera, we performed Western blotting analysis after perchloric acid (PCA) extraction with the same sera and CEA preparation, as used in the inhibition experiments just described. The data presented in Fig. 2A–D show that all four MAbs bound to purified CEA (1 μg) to a similar extent, visualizing a 180-kdalton band (lane k, Fig. 2A–D). The CEA-specific MAbs BW 431/26 and BW 431/31 did not bind to

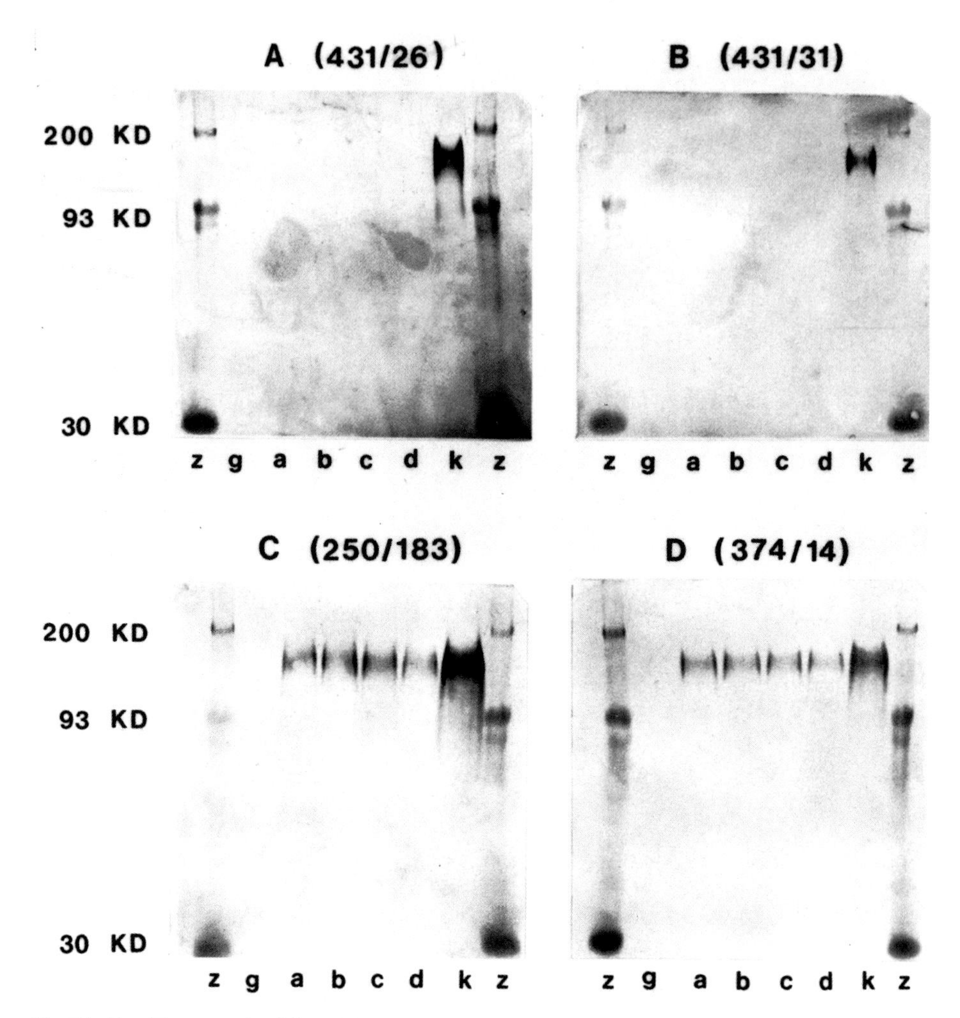

Fig. 2 A–D. Photograph of four blots independently blotted by means of 10% sodium dodecyl sulphate polyacrylamide gel electrophoresis and immunostained with: **A** MAb BW 431/26, **B** MAb BW 431/31, **C** MAb BW 250/183, **D** MAb BW 374/14. *Lanes a–d* represent PCA extracts of patient's sera containing CEA (compare Fig. 1); *lane g* represents control serum; *lane k* represents purified CEA; *lane z* visualizes the rainbow protein molecular weight markers (Amersham). *MAb*, monoclonal antibodies; *CEA*, carcinoembryonic antigen; *PCA*, perchloric acid; *HSA*, human serum albumin; *PBS*, phosphate-buffered solution

PCA extracts from the sera of patients with colonic carcinomas (Fig. 2 A, B; lanes a–d), whereas the CEA-NCA cross-reactive MAbs visualize the 180-Kd CEA band (Fig. 2 C, D; lanes a–d). Neither MAb bound to PCA extracts of a control serum (Fig. 2 A–D, lane g).

In summary, these data indicate that the sera of patients with colonic carcinomas contained intact 180 Kd CEA, which was detected by the CEA-NCA cross-reactive MAbs, but not by the CEA-specific MAbs. Purified CEA from a primary colonic carcinoma was detected to a similar extent by the four specific MAbs used.

The irrelevant MAbs, BW 494 and BW 575, did not show any binding to purified CEA or to patient's sera containing CEA (data not shown).

Estimation of the In Vitro Binding Affinity of MAbs to Cell-Membrane-Bound CEA

To verify that simple differences in the affinity of the various MAbs to CEA were not responsible for the results observed in the binding inhibition and Western blotting experiments, the affinity constants of the MAbs to tissue-associated CEA were determined, as detailed in "Material and Methods". Collagenized, formaldehyde-fixed cells from colonic carcinoma nude mouse xenografts were used as an antigen source. The affinity constants calculated were:

MAb BW 431/26 = 9×10^9 l/mol
MAb BW 431/31 = 3×10^8 l/mol
MAb BW 250/183 = 2×10^9 l/mol
MAb BW 374/14 = (not determined)

Discussion

This paper deals with the unexplained phenomenon that CEA-specific MAbs are able to localize CEA-expressing tumors in the patient, despite significant amounts of circulating CEA in the blood. In the binding inhibition experiments, we demonstrated that MAbs directed to CEA-specific epitopes on CEA (MAb BW 431/26 and BW 431/31) are only marginally blocked by CEA-containing sera. The CEA content of these sera was in 20fold molar excess (500 ng CEA ↔ 2 ng MAb) compared with the radiolabelled MAbs used in the binding assays.

In contrast, it was possible to block the CEA-NCA cross-reactive MAbs more efficiently under identical conditions. These findings could be explained (a) by the presence of NCA in the CEA-containing sera mediating the more efficient blocking of the CEA-NCA cross-reactive MAbs, or (b) by higher affinities of the CEA-NCA MAbs to *circulating CEA*. The Western blotting analysis performed thereafter showed that the CEA-containing sera did not contain detectable amounts of NCA, a finding that undermines the first explanation. Furthermore, the Western blot data indicated that both the CEA-specific MAbs (BW 431/26 and BW 431/31) and the CEA-NCA cross-reactive MAbs (BW 250/183 and BW 374/14) were able to detect CEA purified from primary tumors to a similar extent.

Therefore, the second explanation i.e. that the CEA-NCA cross-reactive MAbs have a higher affinity to circulating CEA than the CEA-specific ones, is probably correct. The Scatchard plot data showed that the CEA-specific MAb BW 431/26 had the highest affinity (range of 10^{10} l/mol) if *cell-bound CEA* is used as an epitope-bearing antigen. The reduced binding, especially of this MAb to circulating CEA as evinced by the binding inhibition experiments, could be explained by differences in the conformation between *cell-bound* and *circulating CEA*. Especially the class 5 epitopes [18], which are unique to CEA, are known to be weakly immunogenic if purified CEA is used as an immunogen. Furthermore, the affinity of those MAbs to CEA is mostly in the range of 10^8 l/mol. However, MAb BW 431/26, with an affinity constant of 9×10^9 l/mol, is an exception allowing

successful immunoscintigrams of colorectal carcinomas 4–6 h after i.v. application of the MAb-^{99m}Tc immunoconjugate in the patient (A. Scharz et al., manuscript in preparation). The success of the immunoscintigraphic evaluation is independent of the CEA content in the patient's serum, as revealed in a multicenter study performed with MAb BW 431/31 [5].
This clinical finding coincides with our in vitro binding-inhibition model. We confronted our radiolabelled MAbs for 90 min with up to 500 ng (1.6×10^{12} molecules) of CEA extracted via PCA from CEA-containing sera. This is a 20fold molar excess compared with the 2 ng of MAb (8×10^{10} molecules). Thereafter, 10^6 LoVo cells bearing between 10^{10}–10^{11} CEA epitopes (10^4–10^5 epitopes per cell) were added to this mixture and incubated for another hour. The binding data showed that especially the CEA-specific MAbs, BW 431/26 and BW 431/31, bound very efficiently to the CEA-expressing cells, suggesting a preferential binding of these MAbs to cell-bound CEA. For scintigraphic purposes with anti-CEA MAbs, patients received 2 mg purified MAb, resulting in a concentration of $\approx$ 670 ng MAb/ml (2.7×10^{12} molecules/ml). The serum CEA concentrations in patients with colonic carcinomas are mostly in the range of 1 ng–3000 ng CEA/ml (maximally 1×10^{13} molecules/ml), yielding maximally a 4fold molar excess of CEA compard with the MAb in the serum. This molar excess of circulating CEA does not seem adequate to block the binding of the MAb to the tumor-associated CEA epitopes. Despite our detailed knowledge about CEA (i.e., the cDNA sequence [22], the immunoglobulin domain-like structure [23], the *N*-linked carbohydrate chains [7], and the NH_2-terminal amino acid sequence [10], both the exact structure of MAb-defined epitopes and the MAb-detected conformational differences between serum CEA and tumor-associated CEA remain to be elucidated.

Acknowledgement. The technical assistance of H. Schmidt and Norbert Döring, as well as the secretarial assistance of I. Gimbel and S. Lehnert, are greatly appreciated.

References

1. Berson SA, Yalow RS (1959) Quantitative aspects of the reaction between insulin-binding antibody. J Clin Invest 38: 1996–2016
2. Bosslet K (1987) Monoclonal antibodies suited for the immunoscintigraphic differential diagnosis of human lung cancer. Abstract of the 3rd international congress on hormones and cancer, September 1987, Hamburg, FRG
3. Bosslet K, Lüben G, Schwarz A, Hundt E, Harthus HP, Seiler FR, Muhrer C, Klöppel G, Kayser K, Sedlacek HH (1985) Immunohistochemical localization and molecular characteristics of three monoclonal antibody-defined epitopes on carcinoembryonic antigen (CEA). Int J Cancer 36: 75–84
4. Bosslet K, Kern HF, Kanzy EJ, Steinsträsser A, Schwarz A, Lüben G, Schorlemmer HU, Sedlacek HH (1986) A monoclonal antibody with binding and inhibiting activity towards human pancreatic carcinoma cells. Cancer Immunol Immunother 23: 185–191
5. Bosslet K, Schwarz A, Steinsträsser A, Kuhlmann L, Seidel L, Schulz G (1988) Immunszintigraphie kolorektaler Karzinome und spezifische Immuntherapie von Pankreaskarzinomen mittels monoklonaler Antikörper. Wien Med Wochenschr 11: 255–257
6. Buchegger F, Schreyer M, Carrel S, Mach JP (1984) Monoclonal antibodies identify a CEA cross-reacting antigen of 95 kD (NCA-95) distinct in antigenicity and tissue distribution from the previously described NCA of 55 kD. Int. J Cancer 33: 643–649
7. Chandrasekaran EV, Davila M, Nixon DW, Goldfarb M, Mendicino J (1983) Isolation and

structures of the oligosaccharide units of carcinoembryonic antigen. J Biol Chem 258: 7213-7222
8. Dillman RO, Beauregard JC, Sobol RE, Royston I, Bartholomew RM, Hagan PS, Halpern SE (1984) Lack of radioimmunodetection and complications associated with monoclonal anticarcinoembryonic antigen antibody. Cancer Res 44: 2213-2218
9. Egan ML, Engvall E, Ruoslahi EI, Todd CW (1977) Detection of circulating tumor antigens. Cancer Res 40: 458-466
10. Engvall E, Shively JE, Wrann M (1978) Isolation and characterization of the normal cross-reacting antigen: Homology of its NH_2-terminal amino acid sequence with that of carcinoembryonic antigen. Proc Natl Acad Sci USA 75: 1670-1674
11. Ey PL, Prowse SJ, Jenkin CR (1978) Isolation of pure IgG_1, IgG_{2a}, IgG_{2b} immunoglobulins from mouse serum using protein A-sepharose. Immunochemistry 15: 429-436
12. Fraker PJ, Speck JC (1978) Protein and cell membrane iodinations with a sparingly soluble chloroamide, 1,3,4,6,-tetra chloro-3,6-diphenyl glycoluril. Biochem biophys Res Comm 80: 849-857
13. Fuks A, Shuster J, Gold P (1980) Theoretical and practical considerations of the utility of the radioimmunoassay for carcinoembryonic antigen in clinical medicine. In: Sell S (ed) Cancer Markers. Human Press, Clifton, NJ, pp 315-327
14. Gold P, Freedman SO (1965a) Demonstration of tumor-specific antigens in human colonic carcinomata by immunological tolerance and absorption techniques. J exp Med 121: 439-462
15. Gold P, Freedman SO (1965 b) Specific carcinoembryonic antigens of the human digestive system. J exp Med 122: 467-480
16. Kleist S von, Chavanel G, Burtin P (1972) Identification of an antigen from normal human tissue that cross-reacts with the carcinoembryonic antigen. Proc Nat Acad Sci (Wash) 69: 2492-2494
17. Krupey J, Gold P, Freedman SO (1968) Physicochemical studies of the carcinoembryonic antigen of the human digestive system. J exp Med 128: 387-398
18. Kuroki M, Arakawa F, Higachi H, Matsunaga A, Okamoto N, Takakura K, Matsuoka Y (1987) Epitope mapping of the carcinoembryonic antigen by monoclonal antibodies and establishment of a new improved radioimmunoassay system. Jpn J Cancer Res 78: 386-396
19. Mach JP, Buchegger F, Forni M, Ritschard J, Berche C, Lumbroso J-D, Schreyer M, Girardet C, Accolla RC, Carrel S (1981) Use of radiolabelled monoclonal anti-CEA antibodies for the detection of human carcinomas by external photoscanning and tomoscintigraphy. Immunology today 2: 239-249
20. Markwell MAK, Fox CF (1978) Surface-specific iodination of membrane proteins of viruses and eucaryotic cells using 1,3,4,6-tetrachloro-3,6-diphenylglycoluril. Biochemistry 17: 4807-4817
21. Nichols EJ, Kannagi R, Hakomori SI, Krantz MJ, Fuks A (1985) Carbohydrate determinants associated with carcinoembryonic antigen (CEA). J Immunol 135: 1911-1913
22. Oikawa S, Nakazato H, Kosaki G (1987a) Primary structure of human carcinoembryonic antigen (CEA) deduced from cDNA sequence. Biochem biophys Res Commun 142: 511-518
23. Oikawa S, Imajo S, Noguchi T, Kosaki G, Nakazato H (1987b) The carcinoembryonic antigen (CEA) contains multiple immunoglobulin-like domains. Biochem biophys Res Commun 144: 634-642
24. Rogers GI (1983) Carcinoembryonic antigens and related glycoproteins. Molecular aspects and specificity. Biochim Biophys Acta 695: 227-249
25. Scatchard G (1949) The attractions of proteins for small molecules and ions. Ann NY Acad Sci 51: 660-672
26. Steinsträsser A, Schwarz A (1986) Quality control of iodinated monoclonal antibodies. Nucl Med 25: A75-76
27. Steinsträsser A, Schwarz A, Kuhlmann, L (1987) Monoclonal antibodies: Optimising of labelling procedures by quality control methods, In: Kristensen K, Dige-Peterson H, Marquersen I (eds) Abstract of the 3rd European Symposium on Radiopharmacy and Radiopharmaceuticals, 1-4 May 1987. Elsinore, Denmark: Isotope Pharmacy Bronshoj pp 68-69
28. Towbin T, Gordon J (1979) Electrophoretic transfer of proteins from polyacrylamide gels to nitrocellulose sheets: Procedure and some applications. Proc Nat Acad Sci USA 76: 4350-4354
29. Walker WHC (1977) The scatchard plot in immunometric assay. Clin Chem 23: 588-590

Radioimmunotherapy with Iodine 131-Labelled Antibodies in Ovarian, Colonic and Brain Tumours

H. KALOFONOS[1] and A. A. EPENETOS[1]

Introduction

Radiolabelled monoclonal antibodies have been shown to react preferentially to neoplastic cells and offer new approaches for targeted cancer treatment [1]. Monoclonal antibody technology [2] enables an antibody-producing lymphocyte to be fused with a cultured myeloma cell, thus producing a hybridoma that secretes a specific monoclonal antibody. It is now possible to manufacture large quantities of immunoglobulins with unique specificity. Monoclonal antibodies have been raised against tumor-associated antigens found in many types of cancer such as breast, lung, colonic, ovarian and bone cancer, as well as glioma, melanoma etc. Great effort has been directed towards the use of monoclonal antibodies to target potent cytotoxic or biologically active agents. Radiolabelled monoclonal antibodies have been utilised in patients for tumour localisation by external body scintigraphy, and encouraging clinical results have been reported by many workers [3-6]. Other potential uses of monoclonal antibodies include the delivery of chemotherapy [7], toxins [8] or radionuclides [9-13] to specifically destroy tumour cells.

However, certain practical limitations need to be overcome, and the main problem is the cross-reactivity of the antibody with antigens on normal tissue. This is seen, for instance, in the gut which expresses many of the common antigenic determinants, such as carcinoembryonic antigen (CEA). The aim now is to increase the concentration of the antibody in the tumour over time compared with the concentration in the normal tissues. The number of radiolabelled antibodies reaching the tumour after i.v. administration is insufficient in most cases to deliver a lethal dose. Therefore, we have investigated alternative routes of administering the radiolabelled monoclonal antibodies intraregionally for therapy with encouraging results. This form of therapy has been applied in the peritoneum for the treatment of ovarian cancer, where a high dose of radiation can be delivered to the whole peritoneal cavity without endangering some of the areas otherwise most at risk, such as the paracolic gutters and the diaphragm. Radiolabelled monoclonal antibodies can also be administered to the pleural cavity for palliation of malignant effusions [14] and intra-arterially for the treatment of gliomas [12] and liver metastases of colonic carcinoma [15].

[1] Royal Postgraduate Medical School and Imperial Cancer Research Group, Hammersmith Hospital, Du Cane Road, London W12 OHS, UK.

H. G. Beger et al. (Eds.), Cancer Therapy

Until recently, only iodine isotopes have been attached to monoclonal antibodies with serious limitations to the depth dose from the poorly penetrating beta particles. Recently, we started a phase I trial using ^{90}Y-labelled monoclonal antibodies, administered intraperitoneally in patients with stage III ovarian cancer and minimal residual disease. This report outlines our experience using radiolabelled monoclonal antibodies with ^{131}I given to patients with stage III ovarian cancer, recurrent brain gliomas resistent to conventional treatment and liver metastases of colonic cancer for palliation.

Patients

Ovarian Cancer

Since 1983, 34 patients with residual ovarian cancer following chemotherapy have been considered for intraperitoneal radiolabelled monoclonal antibody therapy. These patients were treated with ^{131}I-antibodies. A peritoneal catheter was inserted into the abdomen and the position verified by infusion of 1 mCi of technetium 99m (^{99m}Tc), which was evenly distributed throughout the peritoneal cavity. The labelled antibody was then infused with 1–2 litres 0.9% saline solution and the catheter removed. Patients treated with ^{131}I received potassium iodide to decrease the thyroid incorporation of ^{131}I.
Patients were classified according to the amount of tumour present in the peritoneal cavity at the time of treatment with radiolabelled monoclonal antibody. The classification was as follows: macroscopic disease, nodules of more than 2 cm in diameter and minimal residual disease nodules of less than 2 cm in diameter. Some patients had a second-look laparoscopy to monitor the response. Patients whose laparoscopy provided no evidence of disease were considered to be in complete remission. Patients who were not assessed by laparoscopy but were clinically free of disease were described as having "no evidence of disease". A 50% reduction in the tumour size was called "a partial response", and patients who did not respond were considered to have progressive disease. The dose given was increased from 20 to 150 mCi ^{131}I.

Glioma

Seven patients, aged 14–63 years (mean = 50 years) with recurrent grade III or IV glioma were treated with ^{131}I-labelled monoclonal antibodies delivered to the tumour area by infusion into the internal carotid artery ($n=4$) or by intravenous administration ($n=3$). The antibodies used were EGFR1, which were directed against epidermal growth factor receptors and H17E2 antiplacental alkaline phosphatase. ^{123}Iodine-labelled antibodies were used first for imaging studies, and then ^{131}I was administered for therapy. The dose given was increased from 40 mCi to 140 mCi of ^{131}I-labelled monoclonal antibodies; one patient was treated twice with 100 mCi each time.

Hepatic Metastases

Two patients, aged 36 and 70, with hepatic metastases secondary to carcinoma of the colon, were treated with ^{131}I-labelled anti-CEA monoclonal antibodies. The antibodies were administered via the hepatic artery concurrently with starch-degradable microspheres (SPHEREX, Pharmacia, Upsalla, Sweden). These microspheres simultaneously but irreversibly embolise the vessels, causing blood flow stasis. In this way, a high local concentration of the antibodies within the hepatic vasculature can be maintained for the period of embolisation, enabling antibodies to diffuse extravascularly and target onto tumour cells.

Materials and Methods

Monoclonal Antibodies

Production, characterisation and purification of antibodies have been described elsewhere [16-21].

HMFG1/HMFG2. These are mouse IgG1 directed against large, mucin-like molecules normally produced by the lactating breast. The antibodies react with similar components expressed by the majority (>90%) of ovarian, breast and other carcinomas [16, 17].

AUA1. This is a mouse IgG1 directed against an antigen expressed by carcinomas of the ovary. The antigen is a glycoprotein with a molecular weight of 40 Kd [18].

H17E2. This is mouse IgG1 directed against placental-like alkaline phosphatase [19]. It is expressed as a surface membrane antigen of many neoplasms, including ovarian carcinomas, gliomas, testicular tumours etc.

EGFR1. This is mouse IgG1 raised against the human and the rat epidermal growth factor receptors [20].

Anti-CEA Antibody. This is mouse IgG1 raised against the CEA antigen [21].

Radionuclides

Iodine 131. This isotope has been used extensively, both for scanning and radiotherapy [22, 23]. Its high-energy gamma rays (364 KeV) allow detection by gamma camera, and its beta emission makes it suitable for therapy. Disadvantages of using ^{131}I-labelled monoclonal antibodies for treatment are the in vivo dehalogenation, serious limitations to the depth dose from the poorly penetrating beta particles and the fact that, when a therapeutic dose of 30 mCi or more is given, hospitalisation of the patient is essential because the high-energy gamma emission presents a hazard to the public.

Radiolabelling

Monoclonal antibodies (10 mg/ml) were iodinated with ^{131}I (Amersham International, IBS30) using the iodogen method [24]. Free iodine was removed by gel filtration usine Sephadex G-50 in a sterile 20-ml syringe and eluted with phosphate buffered solution (PBS, pH 7.4). The specific activity was in the range of 5–10 mCi/mg. Radiolabelled antibody was diluted in 1% human serum albumin (HSA) and millipore filtered prior to patient administration.
The labelling procedure with ^{90}Y includes conjugation of the monoclonal antibody (10 mg/ml) with a bifunctional chelating agent, dethylene-triamine pentacetic acid (DTPA), using the cyclic anhydride form [25]. Coupled antibody was labelled with ^{90}Y, and free yttrium was separated through a column with Sephadex G-50 [26]. Specific activity was in the range of 5–15 mCi/mg. Aggregate formation, stability and immunoreactivity of the antibodies were satisfactory.

Immunoperoxidase Staining

All the patients had histologically proven epithelial tumours of the ovary, and fresh frozen sections from the original and subsequent biopsy specimens were examined for staining by a panel of monoclonal antibodies as well as by positive and negative control. Tumours that had more than 50% of the cells stained with these antibodies were considered positive.

Dosimetry

It is important to have information on the amount of radiation that can be delivered, to both the tumour and non-tumour sites. To carry out a dosimetry calculation effectively, all that is required in the way of data is the activity at the site, the time course of the activity and knowledge of the radiation emitted by the radionuclide involved. Those data can then be related to some standard formulation [27] to provide an answer that, although of limited accuracy, is of sufficient validity to judge whether the therapeutic procedure is worthwhile.
The measurement of activity at each site requires the combination of opposed computer-acquired, digital gamma-camera views with corrections for attenuation. These can be obtained using relatively simple phantoms [28]. Dosimetric studies in patients with small-volume disease (<2 cm in diameter) have shown that 150 mCi of ^{131}I-labelled antibody can deliver more than 80 Gy to tumour cells. Radiation doses in patients with large-volume disease would be less. These dosimetric calculations have been reported in detail elsewhere [29].

Table 1. Patient numbers and responses

Disease status	No.	Response	Local relapse	Deceased
Gross disease	7	0	7	7
Tumor nodules (less than 2 cm)	14	1 PR, 1 NED	12	9
Positive washings only	6	3 CR, 2 NED	1	1
Adjuvant	1	NED		

CR, complete response; *PR*, partial response; *NED*, no evidence of clinical response.

Clinical Results

Ovarian Cancer

Of 34 patients, 28 have been followed up for more than 3 months and are analyzed in this report. Details of patients treated are shown in Table 1. Patients with macroscopic disease (nodules >2 cm in diameter) did poorly following monoclonal antibody therapy and died from the tumour within 1-19 months after treatment. Patients with minimal residual disease did better, with 1 partial response and one patients free of disease at 12 months. However, all other patients followed up for more than 3 months have developed progressive disease, and the ultimate survival has been poor. Toxicity has been acceptable, and there have been no deaths from the procedure. One patients developed a subphrenic abscess, and another had a perforated sigmoid colon (caused by catheter insertion) requiring a temporary colostomy. Four patients developed unexplained pyrexias of short duration, six patients, nausea and vomiting and two patients, abdominal pain with temporary peritonism. Two patients complained of "flu-like" symptoms lasting for a week with myalgia following therapy. No bone marrow supression was noted at doses below 100 mCi ^{131}I-labelled monoclonal antibodies. Patients who received 150 mCi developed reversible thrombocytopenia (nadir at 30 days) and neutropenia (nadir at 42 days). The best survival rate was observed among patients with positive washings; of this group, only one patient relapsed.

Glioma

Four out of seven patients with glioma showed clinical improvement lasting from 6 months to 2 years. One patient, who was treated on two occasions with 100 mCi each time, continues in complete remission 2 years after therapy, but three out of four patients who responded initially relapsed and died 6-12 months after therapy. No acute toxicity was encountered in any of our patients. Furthermore, we did not observe any impairment in liver or renal function tests. The patients who received more than 100 mCi of ^{131}I subsequently developed thrombocytopenia and neutropenia (nadir at 4-6 weeks), recovering 10-14 days after the nadir. In one patient, we observed transient hemiparesis due to the insertion of the intra-arterial catheter into the internal carotid artery. This lasted for 5 min and was self-limiting.

Hepatic Metastases

Two patients with hepatic metastases underwent treatment. The patients responded clinically with increased appetite, weight gain and CEA levels falling to normal. Computed tomographic scans 1 month later showed some hepatic metastases to have decreased in size, but with no greater than a 50% reduction in diameter. Toxicity was acceptable; both patients complained of mild discomfort at the right hypochondrium which resolved spontaneously and was thought to be secondary to transient liver ischaemia. One patient developed a haematoma at the catheter insertion site and underwent laparotomy. Moderate reversible leukopenia and thrombocytopenia were noted 3 weeks after treatment and lasted for 1 week.

Discussion

In these phase I/II studies, we demonstrate that radiolabelled, tumour-associated monoclonal antibodies administered intraregionally can achieve therapeutic effect in patients with small-volume, stage III ovarian cancer, in recurrent grade III and IV brain gliomas resistant to conventional treatment and in liver metastases of primary colonic carcinoma. Cells in ascites have been shown to take up 0.2%-0.8% of the injected i.p. dose/g of tumour, which could deliver over 60 Gy to the tumour cells [30]. Up to 0.1% of the injected amount of radiolabelled antibodies is taken up per gram of tumour in tumours <2 cm in diameter [31]. However, the dose in solid tumours is less certain, especially using radionuclides such as ^{131}I with poorly penetrating beta particles. This is probably the explanation for the poor results seen in patients with large tumour nodules.
Despite the small number of patients with ovarian cancer studied, several points are already apparent. The lack of response in patients with bulky disease might be expected because of the problems of antibody diffusion and poor penetration of beta particles from ^{131}I. However, the patients with small tumour nodules also did poorly; only one patient remains free of disease. One other patient had a partial response with positive washings rather than nodules at laparoscopy. Finally, the patients with positive washings appeared to do optimally; five are clinically disease free, and only one has had a relapse. Whether these results can be improved using a pure beta emitter (^{90}Y) with more energetic beta rays and greater tissue penetration cannot yet be answered.
In previous studies [12], we showed that a radiolabelled, tumour-associated antibody, when given by an internal carotid artery infusion, (in a patient with grade IV glioma resistant to conventional treatment) resulted in tumour regression. This prompted us to perform a larger study to exame the reproducibility of that report using monoclonal antibodies against the epidermal growth factor receptors and placental alkaline phosphatase. Both of the latter, in addition to the increased expression on brain gliomas, may play a fundamental role in carcinogenesis and tumour promotion [32]. We were encouraged that four out seven patients treated showed a clinical response even after one therapeutic administration with acceptable toxicity. One patient, who was treated on two occasions, continues in complete remission 2 years after treatment. We were unable to treat the other six pa-

tients with repeated administrations because of the development of the human antimouse immunoglobulin response [33].

Dosimetric calculations based on our biopsy and imaging data indicated that a dose of 150 mCi ^{131}I-labelled antibody should deliver 50–100 Gy to 1–2 g tumour, with no significant radiation to normal brain and acceptable and reversible radiation toxicity to the whole body and single organs [34]. These doses are not sufficient on their own to sterilise brain gliomas, but they may make an important contribution if used in conjunction with radical external beam radiotherapy in patients with grade III or IV gliomas of poor prognosis. All these results may be improved if one could use smaller molecules, such as antibody fragments with a better extravasation fraction and deeper penetration in the tumour, as well as pure beta emitters, such as ^{90}Y. Biodegradable starch microspheres concurrently administered with radiolabelled anti-CEA monoclonal antibodies in the hepatic artery can achieve temporary embolisation, causing blood flow stasis. High local concentrations of antibody within the hepatic vasculature can thus be maintained, enabling antibodies to diffuse extravascularly and target onto tumour cells. We were encouraged that both patients treated showed a positive clinical response with acceptable toxicity. The rapid development of interventional radiological techniques means that alternative treatment to chemotherapy may be given to patients with inoperable malignant liver lesions for palliation. Arterial interventional techniques are effective because approximately 90% of the blood supply of malignant liver tumours derives from the hepatic artery.

In conclusion, we have shown that radiolabelled monoclonal antibodies locally administered to patients with stage III ovarian carcinoma and minimal residual disease, brain gliomas or liver metastases may play a role in eradicating microscopic disease following surgery or chemotherapy. Our studies have also demonstrated that antibody-guided irradiation is a minimally toxic form of therapy. Finally, further studies are required to establish conclusively the efficacy and the mode of action of this form of cancer treatment.

References

1. Epenetos AA, Britton KE, Mather S, Shepherd J, Geanovska M, Taylor-Papadimitriou J, Nimmon CC, Durbin H, Hawkins LR, Malpas JS, Bodmer WF (1982) Targetting of Iodine 123-labelled tumour associated monoclonal antibodies to ovarian, breast and gastrointestinal tumours. Lancet 2: 999–1005
2. Köhler G, Milstein C (1975) Continuous cultures of fused cells secreting antibody of predefined specificity. Nature 256: 495–497
3. Mach J-P, Buchegger F, Forni M, Ritschard J, Berche C, Lumbroso JD, Schreyer M, Girardet C, Accola R, Carrel S (1981) Use of radiolabelled monoclonal anti-CEA antibodies for the detection of human carcinomas by external photoscanning and tomoscintigraphy. Immunol Today 2: 239–249
4. Farrands PA, Perkins AC, Pimm MV, Hardy JD, Embleton MJ, Baldwin RW, Hardcastle JD (1982) Radioimmunodetection of human colorectal cancer by an antitumour monoclonal antibody. Lancet 2: 397–400
5. Larson SM, Brown JP, Wright PW, Carrasquillo JA, Hellstrom I, Hellstrom KE (1983) Imaging of melanomas with I 131-labelled monoclonal antibodies. J Nucl Med 23: 123–129
6. Buraggi GL, Callegaro L, Mariani G, Turrin A, Caseinelli N, Attili A, Bombardieri E, Terno G, Plassio G, Dovis M (1985) Imaging with ^{131}I-labelled monoclonal antibodies to a high-

molecular-weight melanoma-associated antigen in patients with melanoma: Efficacy of whole immunoglobulin and its $F(ab')_2$ fragments. Cancer Res 45: 3378-3387
7. Baldwin RW, Pimm V (1983) Antitumour monoclonal antibodies for radioimmunodetection of tumours and drug targetting. Cancer Metastasis Rev 2: 89-106
8. Thorpe RE, Ross WC (1982) The preparation and cytotoxic properties of antibody-toxin conjugates. Immunol Rev 62: 119
9. Order SE, Klein JL, Ettinger D, Alderson P, Siegelman S, Leichner P (1980) Use of isotopic immunoglobulin in therapy. Cancer Res 40: 3001
10. Epenetos AA, Courtenay-Luck N, Halnan KE, Hooker G, Hughes JMB, Krauz T, Lambert J, Lavender JP, MacGregor WG, McKenzie CG, Munro A, Myers MJ, Orr JS, Pearse EE, Snook D, Webb B, Burcell J, Durbin H, Kemshead J, Taylor-Papadimitriou J (1984) Antibody guided irradiation of malignant lesions. Lancet 30: 1441-1443
11. Carrasquilo JA, Krohn KA, Beaumier P, McGuffin RW, Brown JP, Hellstrom E, Hellstrom I, Larson SM (1984) Diagnosis of and therapy for solid tumour with radiolabelled antibodies and immune fragments. Cancer Treat Rep 68: 371-378
12. Epenetos AA, Courtenay-Luck N, Pickering D, Hooker G, Durbin H, Lavender JP, McKenzie CG (1985) Antibody-guided irradiation of brain glioma by arterial infusion of radioactive monoclonal antibody against epidermal growth factor receptor and blood group A antigen. Br Med J 290: 1463-1466
13. Epenetos AA, Munro AJ, Stewart S, Rampling R, Lambert HE, McKenzie CG, Soutter P, Rahemtulla A, Hooker G, Sivolapenko GB, Snook D, Courtenay-Luck N, Dhokia B, Krauz T, Taylor-Papadimitriou J, Durbin H, Bodmer WF (1987) Antibody-guided irradiation of advanced ovarian cancer with intraperitoneally administered radiolabelled monoclonal antibodies. J Clin Oncol 5: 1890-1899
14. Kalofonos HP, Epenetos AA (1987) Antibody-guided diagnosis and therapy of patients with breast cancer. In: Ceriani RL (ed) Immunological approaches to the diagnosis and therapy of breast cancer. Plenum, New York, pp 245-257
15. Wilson CB, Epenetos AA (1987) Use of monoclonal antibodies for diagnosis and treatment of liver tumours. Bailliere's Clinical Gastroenterology 1 (1): 115-130
16. Arklie J, Taylor-Papadimitriou J, Bodmer WF, Egan M, Millis R (1981) Differentiation antigens expressed by epithelial cells in the lactating breast are also detectable in breast cancers. Int J Cancer 28: 23-29
17. Burcell J, Durbin H, Taylor-Papadimitriou J (1983) Complexity of expression on antigenic determinants recognised by monoclonal antibodies HMFG1 and HMFG2 in normal and malignant tissue. J Immunol 131: 508-513
18. Epenetos AA, Nimmon CC, Arklie J, Elliot AT, Hawkins LA, Knowles RW, Britton KE, Bodmere WF (1982) Radioimmuno-diagnosis of human cancer in an animal model using labelled tumour associated monoclonal antibodies. Br J Cancer 46: 1-8
19. Travers P, Bodmer WF (1984) Preparation and characterization of monoclonal antibodies against placental alkaline phosphatase and other human trophoblast-associated determinants. Int J Cancer 33: 633-641
20. Waterfield MD, Mayes ELV, Stroonbard P, Bennet PL, Young G, Goodfellow PN, Banting GS, Ozone B (1982) A monoclonal antibody to the human epidermal growth factor receptor. J Cell Biochem 20: 148-161
21. Bosslet K, Luben G, Schwarz A, Hundt E, Harthus HP, Seiler TR, Muhrer C, Kloppel G, Kayser K, Sedlacek HH (1985) Immunohistochemical localisation and molecular characteristics of three monoclonal antibody-defined epitopes detectable on carcinoembryonic antigen (CEA). Int J Cancer 36: 75
22. Leichner PK, Klein JL, Garrison JB, Jenkins RE, Nickoloff EL (1981) Dosimetry of I 131-labelled anti-ferritin in hepatoma: a model for radio-immunoglobulin dosimetry. Int J Rad On Biol Phys 7: 323-333
23. Larson SM, Carrasquillo JA, McGuffin RW, Kohn KA, Ferens JM, Hill LD, Beaumier PL, Reynolds JC, Hellstrom KE, Hellstrom I (1985) Use of ^{131}I-labelled murine Fab against a high molecular weight antigen of human melanoma. Preliminary experience. Radiology 155: 487-492
24. Fraker PJ, Speck JC (1978) Protein and cell membrane iodination with a sparingly soluble chloramine 1,3,4,6,tetrachloro-5,6-diphenyl-glycoril. Biochem Biophys Res Commun 80: 849-854

25. Hnatowich DJ, Layne WW, Childs RL (1983) Radioactive labeling of antibody: a simple and efficient method. Science 220: 613-615
26. Hnatowich DJ, Virzi F, Doherty PW (1985) DTPA-coupled antibodies labelled with yttrium 90. J Nucl Med 5: 503-509
27. Snyder WS, Ford MR, Warner GG (1978) Estimates of specific absorbed fractions for photon sources uniformly distributed in various organs of a heterogeneous phantom. Medical International Radiation Dose (MIRD) pamphlet 5. Society of Nuclear Medicine, New York, pp 5-67
28. Myers MJ, Lavender JP, de Oliveira JB (1981) A simplified method of quantitating organ uptake using a gamma camera. Br J Radiol 54: 1062-1067
29. Myers MJ, Hooker GR, Epenetos AA (1986) Dosimetry of radiolabelled monoclonal antibodies used for therapy. In: Schlafke-Stelson AT, Watson EE (eds) Fourth International Radiopharmaceutical Dosimetry Symposium, 5-8 Nov 1985. Oak Ridge Associated Universities, Oak Ridge, Tennessee, pp 409-420
30. Ward BG, Mather SJ, Shepherd JH (1986) Prospects for antibody targetted radiotherapy of cancer. Lancet 2: 580-581
31. Malamitsi J, Skarlos D, Fotiou S, Valvaligiou A, Papakostas P, Aravantinos G, Taylor-Papadimitriou J, Epenetos AA, Koutoulidis K (in press). Pharmacokinetics and diagnostic contribution of I 131-labelled HMFG2 monoclonal antibody in pleural and peritoneal metastases from breast and ovarian carcinomas: Advantages of intracavitary administration. J Nucl Med (in press)
32. Stoscheck CM, King LE (1986) Role of epidermal growth factor in carcinogenesis. Cancer Res 4: 1030-1037
33. Courtenay-Luck N, Epenetos AA, Moore R, Larche M, Pectasides D, Dhokia B, Ritter MA (1986) Development of primary and secondary immune responses to mouse monoclonal antibodies used in the diagnosis and therapy of malignant neoplasms. Cancer Res 46: 6489-6493
34. Epenetos AA, Snook D, Durbin H, Johnson PM, Taylor-Papadimitriou J (1986) Limitations of radiolabelled monoclonal antibodies for the localisation of human neoplasms. Cancer Res 46: 3181-3191

Radioimmunodetection and Radioimmunotherapy in Myosarcoma

A. PLANTING,[1] J. VERWEIJ,[1] P. COX,[1] M. PILLAY,[1] and G. STOTER[1]

Introduction

Soft-tissue sarcomas account for approximately 1% of all malignancies. The treatment of choice is surgery, which is the only curative treatment for primary tumors of the trunk, head, and neck primaries. Initially, sarcomas of the limbs had to be treated with amputation, but since the discovery that adjuvant radiotherapy can prevent almost half of the local recurrence in sarcoma of the extremities [1, 2], limb-sparing surgery has become possible.

The role of adjuvant chemotherapy in soft-tissue sarcomas remains a matter for further discussion, and most randomized studies do not suggest a benefit for survival [3-5]. Many patients cannot be cured by local treatment modalities and develop a local recurrence and/or metastases. In this patient group, combination chemotherapy can yield a response rate of 30%-40%, with tendency among responders toward prolonged survival times [6-8]. However, at least 60% of the patients are resistant to any known type of chemotherapy, stressing the need for better drugs and other therapies.

With the introduction of the hybridoma technique by Köhler and Milstein in 1975 [9], it has become possible to produce monoclonal antibodies directed against cell surface and intracellular antigens. By means of labeling techniques, radiopharmacons can be coupled to these antibodies, and these complexes are known to be of some value in the diagnosis of several tumors, such as gastrointestinal and ovarian carcinomas [10]. In the Rotterdam Cancer Institute, we are studying an antimyosin antibody. Antigen-binding (Fab) fragments of R11 D10 antimyosin antibody were able to pass the cell membrane of damaged myocardial cells and to bind to the intracellular myosin [11]. Normal myocardial cells showed no uptake. Because cells of rhabdo- and leiomyosarcomas contain myosin and their cell membranes may be more permeable than those of normal cells, we initiated a diagnostic study with the antimyosin monoclonal antibody in this patient group.

Materials and Methods

Patients were considered eligible for the study if they had a histologically proven rhabdo- or leiomyosarcoma. Local recurrences or metastases were confirmed his-

[1] Department of Medical Oncology, Rotterdam Cancer Institute, Groene Hilledijk 301, 3075 EA Rotterdam, The Netherlands

H. G. Beger et al. (Eds.), Cancer Therapy

tologically or cytologically. The tumor extent was staged with available conventional techniques, such as X-ray films, ultrasound, or computed tomography. Diagnostic scanning was performed with Fab fragments of the R11 D10 antimyosin monoclonal antibody (Centocor) coupled with diethylene triamine penta-acetic acid (DTPA) and labeled with Indium 111. A dose of 74 MBeq of this indium antimyosin monoclonal antibody complex (IAMAC) was administered by slow intravenous injection. Total body scanning was performed by a gamma-camera at 4, 24, and 48 h.

Results

In all patients it was possible to evaluate the tumor localizations by X-ray films, ultrasound, or computed tomography with the exception of two patients with rhabdomyosarcoma, where the scan was performed after surgery. The characteristics of the patients studied and the results of their scans are presented in the Table 1.

Table 1. Indium antimyosin monoclonal antibody complex *(IAMAC)* scan: characteristics of patients studied

Patient	Histology	Primary tumor localization	Localization of metastases	Previous therapy	IAMAC uptake
1. m 53 y	R	left thigh	lung	chemotherapy	+
2. f 18 y	R	uterus		surgery	– [a]
3. m 33 y	L	vesicula seminalis	pelvic/liver	chemotherapy	+
4. f 60 y	R	uterus	local recurrence	chemotherapy	+
5. m 35 y	L	stomach	local recurrence	chemotherapy	+
6. m 48 y	L	stomach	local recurrence	chemotherapy	–
7. f 60 y	L	vulva	local recurrence/liver	chemotherapy	+
8. m 64 y	L	leg	lung	chemotherapy	+
9. f 21 y	R	neck		–	+
10. f 38 y	L	uterus	lymph nodes	chemotherapy	+/– [b]
11. m 43 y	L	retroperitoneum	liver	chemotherapy	–
12. m 43 y	L	pancreas/mediastinum		chemotherapy	–
13. f 44 y	L	lung	bone	MIBG	+
14. m 50 y	L	stomach	liver		+
15. m 55 y	L	axilla	liver		+
16. f 55 y	L	uterus	lung		–
17. m 1 y	R	cerebrum			+
18. m 71 y	L	prostate	lung		–
19. m 2 y	R	orbita			– [c]
20. f 58 y	L	trunk			+

m, male; *f*, female; *R*, rhabdomyosarcoma; *L*, leiomyosarcoma; *MIBG*, [I 131]-meta-jodo-benzyl-guanidine; +, uptake of IAMAC in known tumor site(s); –, no uptake of IAMAC in known tumor site(s).

[a] True-negative scan; at second-look laparotomy, no tumor residue was found.

[b] False positive in skull (bone) but false negative in para-aortic lymph nodes.

[c] Probably true negative after extended local surgery.

Four patients with rhabdomyosarcoma had a true-positive scan. Their scans showed an uptake of IAMAC at all known tumor sites. The other two patients' scans were considered to be true-negative. In a woman with rhabdomyosarcoma of the uterus (patient 2), a scan after primary surgery was negative, while at second-look laparotomy no tumor could be detected, and all biopsies were negative. The second true-negative scan concerns a boy with rhabdomyosarcoma of the orbita, where scanning was done following extensive surgery. The boy is still well, but the follow-up is short.
Of 14 patients with a leiomyosarcoma, eight had a true-positive scan, while a false-negative scan was found in five. One patient had IAMAC uptake at the base of the skull, although no tumor deposit could be confirmed there by other methods. In the same patient, a known tumor deposit in the para-aortic lymph nodes did

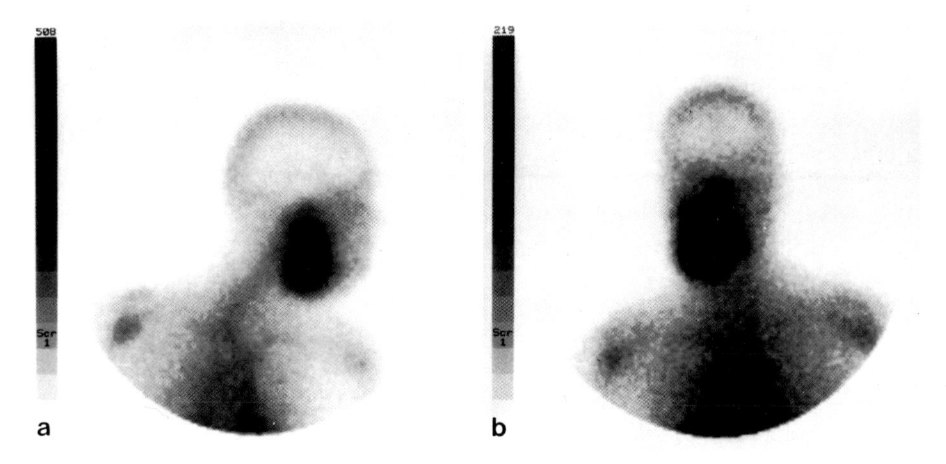

Fig. 1. **a** Uptake if indium antimyosin monoclonal antibody complex in a rhabdomyosarcoma of the floor of the mouth (lateral view). **b** Same patient (anteroposterior view)

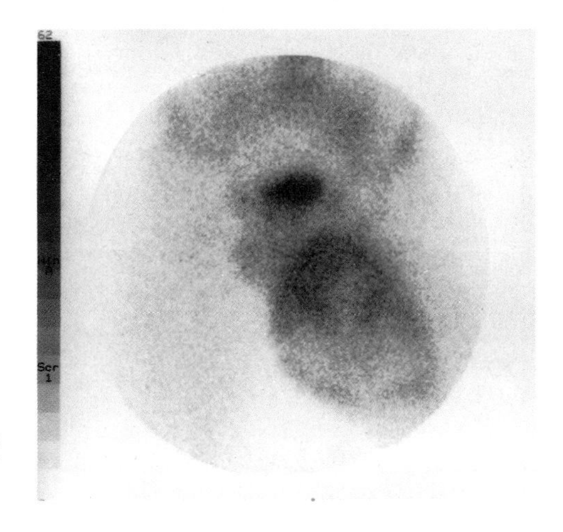

Fig. 2. Uptake of indium antimyosin monoclonal antibody complex in a patient with a rhabdomyosarcoma of the left thigh showing areas of high uptake and areas of necrosis (patient 1)

not show IAMAC uptake. We consider this scan to present combined false-positive and false-negative results.
Optimal results of the scans were found at 24 and at 48 h IAMAC uptake was insufficient at 4 h. Two examples of scans are given in Figs. 1 and 2. Dosimetric calculations indicated that the tumor:background uptake ratio can be as high as 10:1, but a high concentration of IAMAC was also observed in the bone marrow, liver, spleen, and kidneys. No side effects of the diagnostic IAMAC scanning were observed.

Discussion

By labeling monoclonal antibodies with radiopharmacons, tumor deposits and metastases can be detected in several tumors. Interest is now focusing on treatment with these complexes, e.g., in gastrointestinal and ovarian cancer [10]. In most of these cancers, monoclonal antibodies are directed against cell surface antigens. The monoclonal antibody we used is directed against an intracellular antigen. The disadvantage of such an antigen is that it has to cross cell membranes; in tumor cells, the cell membranes appear to be more permeable for these monoclonal antibody-radiopharmacon complexes in comparison to cells in healthy tissue. This results in a tumor:background ratio that can be as high as 10:1; this ratio is higher than that observed with most antibodies directed against cell surface antigens.
For rhabdomyosarcoma we expect the IAMAC to be a useful diagnostic tool, but the number of patients we studied is too small to draw definite conclusions. The observed high rate of false-negative scans in patients with leiomyosarcoma is difficult to explain. A possible cause may be the fact that most patients were pretreated with chemotherapy because, in a rhabdomyosarcoma patient with high uptake of IAMAC before chemotherapy (patient 9, Fig. 1), a second scan after several cycles of chemotherapy was negative, although residual tumor was known to be present. To clarify this observation, we plan to study patients before and after chemotherapy.
Because the IAMAC uptake in several patients was very high and no toxicity was observed in this study, treatment with monoclonal antibodies labeled with radiopharmacons in patients with leiomyo- and rhabdomyosarcoma may be feasible. The IAMAC used in this study is not appropriate for treatment. For therapy, the whole immunoglobulin is more suitable because of higher affinity and longer binding to the antigen than Fab fragments [12]. Furthermore, iodine 131 has better radiation characteristics than indium.
The disadvantage of using whole immunoglobulin monoclonal antibodies is the higher binding rate to cells of the reticuloendothelial system. Also antibodies against the antibody complexes may develop and cause a dangerous accumulation of radioactivity in the bone marrow, liver, spleen, and kidneys. This possibility exists especially when repeated dosages are required, as can be expected in sarcoma, where only high irradiation dosages are effective. In the near future, we shall start a phase-I-II study in patients with advanced rhabdo- and leiomyosarcoma, where special attention will be focused on organ toxicity and the development of anti-antibodies.

References

1. Abbatucci JS, Boulier N, de Ranier J, Mandard AM, Tanguy A, Busson A (1984) Radiotherapy as an integrated part of the treatment of soft tissue sarcomas. Radiother Oncol 2: 115-121
2. Rosenberg SA, Tepper J, Glatstein E, Costa J, Baker A, Brennan M, DeMoss EV, Seipp C, Sindelar WF, Sugarbaker P, Wesley R (1982) The treatment of soft tissue sarcomas of the extremities. Prospective randomized evaluation of (1) limb sparing surgery plus radiation therapy compared with amputation and (2) the role of adjuvant chemotherapy. Ann Surg 196: 305-315
3. Rosenberg SA, Chang E, Glatstein E (1985) Adjuvant chemotherapy of extremity soft tissue sarcomas: review of National Cancer Institute experience. Cancer Treat Symp 3: 83-88
4. Edmonson JH, Fleming TR, Vins JCI, Omer Burgert E, Soule EH, O'Connell MJ, Sim FH, Ahmann DL (1984) Randomized study of systemic chemotherapy following complete excision of non-osseous sarcomas. J Clin Oncol 2: 1390-1396
5. Bramwell VHC (1986) Adjuvant chemotherapy for soft tissue sarcomas. In: Pinedo HM, Verweij J (eds) Clinical management of soft tissue sarcomas. Martinus Nijhoff, Boston, pp 89-101
6. Yap BS, Sinkovics JG, Burgess MA, Benjamin RS, Bodey CP (1983) The curability of advanced soft tissue sarcomas in adults with chemotherapy. Proc ASCO abstr C-937, p 239
7. Pinedo HM, Bramwell VHC, Mouridsen HT, Somers R, Vendrik CPJ, Santoro A, Buesa J, Wagener T, v Oosterom AT, v Unnik JAM, Sylvester R, de Pauw M, Thomas D, Bonadonna G (1984) CYVADIC in advanced soft tissue sarcoma: a randomized study comparing two schedules. Cancer 53: 1852-1832
8. Verweij J, Pinedo HM (1986) Chemotherapy in advanced soft tissue sarcomas. In: Pinedo HM, Verweij J (eds) Clinical management of soft tissue sarcomas. Martinus Nijhoff, Boston, pp 81-88
9. Köhler G, Milstein G (1975) Continuous cultures of fused cells secreting antibody of predefined specificity. Nature 256: 495-497
10. Kalofonos HP, Epenetos AA (1986) The role of monoclonal antibodies in tumor diagnosis. Cancer Treat Rev 13: 243-252
11. Cox PH, Verweij J, Pillay M, Stoter G, Schönfeld D (1988) Indium-111 antimyosin for the detection of leiomyosarcoma and rhabdomyosarcoma. Eur J Nucl Med 14: 50-52
12. Lowder JN (1986) The current status of monoclonal antibodies in the diagnosis and therapy of cancer. Current problems in cancer 10: 502-507

Immunotherapy of Pancreatic Cancer with Monoclonal Antibody BW 494: Results from a Multicentric Phase I-II Trial

M. BÜCHLER,[1] R. KÜBEL,[1] R. KLAPDOR,[2] K.-H. MUHRER,[3] H. FRIESS,[1] B. LORENZ,[1] G. SCHULZ,[4] K. BOSSLET,[4] and H. G. BEGER[1]

Introduction

In this age of modern diagnostic procedures and highly developed conservative and surgical therapeutic strategies in oncology, pancreatic carcinoma of ductal origin is still almost invariably an incurable disease [1, 2]. A characteristic tumor biology with regard to growth behavior, metastatic mode, and unspecific symptoms in the initial stage are responsible for this poor prognosis [3-5]. The incurability of pancreatic cancer is duly emphasized by the evaluation of data collected from 15000 patients. These statistics show that after 5 years, independent of the type of therapy, a total of 60 patients (0.4% with 5-year survival) were still alive [2]. Only about 10%-20% of the patients are able to undergo a potentially curative operation in the form of a partial or total pancreatoduodenectomy [1, 2, 6-9]. The therapeutic dilemma is further characterized by the lack of response to chemo- or radiotherapy [10-15].

The development and characterization of a sensitive monoclonal antibody (BW 494) directed against a membrane and cytoplasma antigen associated with pancreatic carcinoma [16, 17] and the partial success in the use of monoclonal antibodies in the treatment of gastrointestinal tumors and malignant melanomas in clinical trials [18, 19], provided the indication for intravenous immunotherapy of ductal pancreatic cancer in the context of a phase I-II study. The following positions were considered for this first clinical trial of a monoclonal antibody against pancreatic carcinoma:

1. The antibody (BW 494) shows a strong binding capacity to human pancreatic carcinoma cells of grades I and II both in vitro and in vivo [16, 20, 21].
2. The antibody mediates what is known as antibody-dependent cellular cytotoxicity (ADCC) against pancreatic carcinoma cells in vitro when human mononuclear cells are coincubated as effector cells [16].
3. In vitro, the antibody inhibits specific functions of pancreatic cancer cells, like endocytosis or the release of lysosomal enzymes [17, 22].
4. The ^{131}I-labelled antibody suppresses the growth of pancreatic tumors transferred to nude mice [23].

[1] Department of General Surgery, University of Ulm, Steinhövelstraße 9, 7900 Ulm, FRG.
[2] Department of Internal Medicine, University Hospital Eppendorf, Martinistraße 52, 2000 Hamburg 20, FRG.
[3] Department of General and Thoracic Surgery, Justus Liebig University Clinic, Klinikstraße 29, 6300 Gießen, FRG.
[4] Clinical Research, Behringwerke AG Marburg, 3550 Marburg, FRG.

H. G. Beger et al. (Eds.), Cancer Therapy

Material and Methods

Patients

A total of 39 patients have entered the study since April 1986. Inclusion criteria were advanced tumor stage (locally infiltrating growth corresponding to a stage T_3 according to the Union Internationale Contre le Cancer (UICC) classification of 1987 or lymph node or systemic metastases) and a Karnofsky index [24] of over 30%. There were 18 patients from the Department of Surgery, University of Ulm; 15 patients from the Department of Internal Medicine, University of Hamburg, and 6 patients from the Department of Surgery, University of Gießen. The personal data of the patients who were treated in Ulm with tumor staging and grading, as well as the type of surgical therapy, are summarized in Table 1.

The Monoclonal Antibody BW 494

The development of BW 494 by Bosslet and coworkers is described elsewhere [16, 17]. The antibody is a murine immunoglobulin (IgG 1). It recognizes a membrane and cytoplasma-specific epitope on a 200-kD glycoprotein antigen. The immunohistochemically established sensitivity is 92% for pancreatic carcinoma of ductal origin [25].

Table 1. Personal data, pancreatic tumor location, stage, grade, and type of surgical treatment in 18 patients of the Ulm study group

Patient	Sex	Age (years)	Pancreas tumor localisation	Stage	Grade	Therapy
1 W.R.	f	51	Head	$T_3N_1M_0$	II	Biliary bypass
2 O.H.	m	49	Head	$T_3N_0M_0$	II	Bilioenteral bypass
3 W.H.	m	75	Head	$T_3N_1M_1$	II	Biliary bypass
4 S.J.	m	65	Body, tail	$T_3N_1M_1$	II	Left resection
5 M.I.	f	56	Local recurrence after Whipple	$T^*N_1M_1$	II	Gastric bypass
6 A.G.	f	75	Head, tail	$T_2N_1M_0$	III	Exploratory laparotomy
7 S.C.	m	45	Head	$T_3N_1M_1$	III	Bilioenteral bypass
8 R.E.	f	75	Body	$T_2N_0M_1$	III	Exploratory laparotomy
9 D.H.	m	72	Body, tail	$T_2N_1M_1$	II	Exploratory laparotomy
10 B.E.	m	68	Local recurrence after Whipple operation	$T^*N_1M_1$	II	Exploratory laparotomy
11 H.C.	m	50	Body, tail	$T_3N_1M_1$	I	Exploratory laparotomy
12 S.F.	f	67	Body	$T_3N_0M_0$	I	Exploratory laparotomy
13 W.E.	m	56	Body, tail	$T_2N_1M_1$	II	Exploratory laparotomy
14 F.G.	m	48	Head, tail	$T_2N_xM_1$	II	Exploratory laparotomy
15 S.H.	m	66	Head, tail	$T_3N_1M_0$	II	Biliary bypass
16 K.T.	f	46	Head	$T_2N_1M_0$	II	Whipple operation
17 S.H.	f	50	Head	$T_3N_0M_0$	II	Whipple operation
18 S.H.	m	53	Head	$T_3N_1M_0$	II	Whipple operation

* Classification according to TNM scheme not possible.

Immunohistochemical Investigations

The intraoperatively obtained tumor samples were fixed in Bouin solution. The binding of the antibody BW 494 to the tumor cells was immunohistochemically analyzed [26, 27] in 14 of 18 patients from the Ulm University Hospital.

Immunoscintigraphy

In 5 cases, the tumor was localized immunoscintigraphically after the operation following the application of 5 mg BW 494 radioactively labelled with 3 mCi indium-111 Planar scintigrams were performed 24, 28, and 72 h after the initial antibody injection.

Determination of In Vitro ADCC

The antibody-dependent cellular cytotoxicity (ADCC) [28, 29] was determined in 11 patients with pancreatic carcinoma prior to immunotherapy to exclude effector cell insufficiency. The peripheral blood leukocytes of the patients were used as effector cells; the target cells were from the commercially available pancreatic carcinoma cell line PaTu1. A constant in vitro ratio of effector to target cells of between 25:1 and 100:1 was maintained.

Intravenous Antibody Therapy

After acquiring informed consent of the patients, immunotherapy was usually instituted in the third postoperative week. In keeping with the design of a phase I study, three different protocols were used. Patients 1-5 from Ulm were treated on 5 successive days, beginning with an initial dose of 20 mg with a daily increase of 20 mg up to a total dose of 180-300 mg. After an initial dose of 50 mg, patients 6-10 from Ulm were given a constant dose of 30 mg in 3-day intervals up to a total dose of 150-230 mg (total treatment time: 21 days). Patients 11-18 were treated with an initial dose of 100 mg and subsequent infusions of a constant dose of 30 mg, increasing to a total dose of 250-340 mg in a period of 2 weeks.
The antibody was always administered in 250 ml sodium chloride solution (0.9%) via a peripheral vein over a period of 30-60 min. The patients were carefully monitored for general and cardiovascular status during the infusions to control possible allergic reactions. The administration protocol of the patients treated in Ulm is given in Table 2.

Post-therapeutic Monitoring

As a rule, the patients were examined every 4 weeks either on an outpatient basis or in the hospital. They were checked for general clinical status, for morphologic tumor growth by means of computed tomography and/or ultrasound, and for the

Table 2. Phase I application regimes of monoclonal antibody BW 494 in the Ulm patients

Patients 1–5:	20-40-60-80-100 = 300 mg (1 week)
Patients 6–10:	50-30-30-30-30-30-30 = 230 mg (3 weeks)
Patients 11–18:	100-30-30-30-30-30-30-30-30 = 340 mg (2 weeks)

Table 3. Immunohistochemical results with monoclonal antibody BW 494 in 14 patients

Grade		I ($n=1$)	II ($n=9$)	III ($n=4$)
	0			2
	+		2	2
Reaction	++	1	3	
	+++		4	

0, no reaction; +, weak reaction in single cells; ++, moderate or strong reaction in up to 50% of tumor mass; +++, moderate or strong reaction in more than 50% of tumor mass.

serum tumor markers, carcinoembryonic antigen (CEA) and CA 19-9. Two patients additionally required a second-look operation. A pharmacokinetic study with determination of the half-life of the monoclonal antibody [30] was conducted on one patient. A total of 16 blood specimens were taken within 240 h after the initial administration of 100 mg antibody protein to analyze the murine IgG in the serum. Human antimouse antibody (HAMA) response in the serum was also measured in eight patients by means of an indirect immunoassay [31].

Results

Immunohistochemistry

The tumor tissue of 14 patients was immunohistochemically examined for a reaction to monoclonal antibody BW 494. The results are summarized in Table 3. All tumors of grades I–II showed a medium to strong reaction. Only 50% of the preparations from patients with undifferentiated grade III pancreatic carcinoma showed an antigen-antibody reaction.

Immunoscintigraphy

Following prior sensitivity testing, five patients underwent planar whole-body scintigraphy after a radioactively labelled antibody was administered (an average of 150 mBc ^{111}In). Only patient 1, with a $T_3N_1M_0$ pancreatic tumor, grade II, showed a definite accumulation of activity in the carcinoma and the lymph node metastases. In the remaining four patients, the accumulation in the reticuloendothelial system of the liver was so pronounced that an objective evaluation of the pancreas head and peripancreatic regions proved impossible. Owing to this poor result, no further immunoscintigrams were performed.

In vitro ADCC

Leukocytes from the peripheral blood were obtained from 11 patients in order to establish the in vitro, antibody-dependent cellular cytotoxicty. The percentage of the specific cytolysis mediated by BW 494 was between 10% and 34% (median: 17%). This in vitro ADCC corresponded to that of 23 healthy controls, who were also examined and found to have a median ADCC of 17% (range: 12%-38%).

Pharmacokinetics and HAMA-induction

The pharmacokinetics of monoclonal antibody BW 494 were determined in a patient following bolus administration of 100 mg antibody protein. The elimination kinetics presented in Fig. 1 resulted in a calculated primary half-life of 0.2 h and a terminal half-life of 47.8 h.
Eight patients of the study group were tested for development of serum antimouse antibodies. All eight patients were found to have positive serum HAMA titers 4 weeks after therapy had been initiated. These primarily anti-isotypical IgG antibodies developed between the 1st and 14th day after infusion. Figure 2 depicts the development of IgG antimouse antibodies in a female patient.

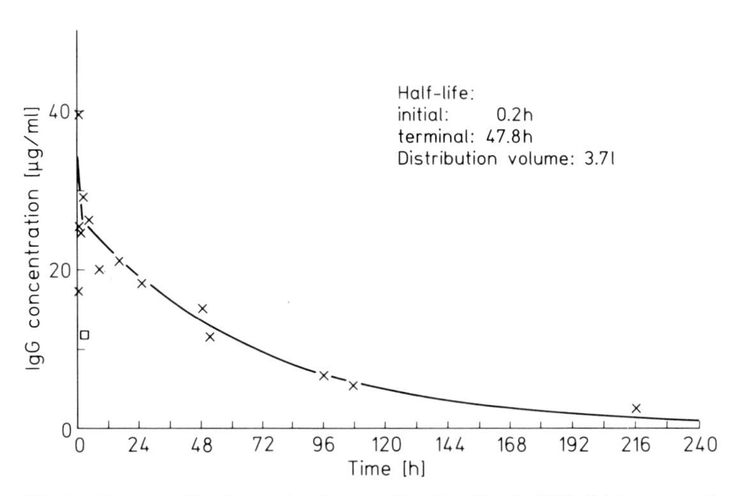

Fig. 1. Pharmacokinetic study of monoclonal antibody BW 494 in one patient after a single dose of 100 mg

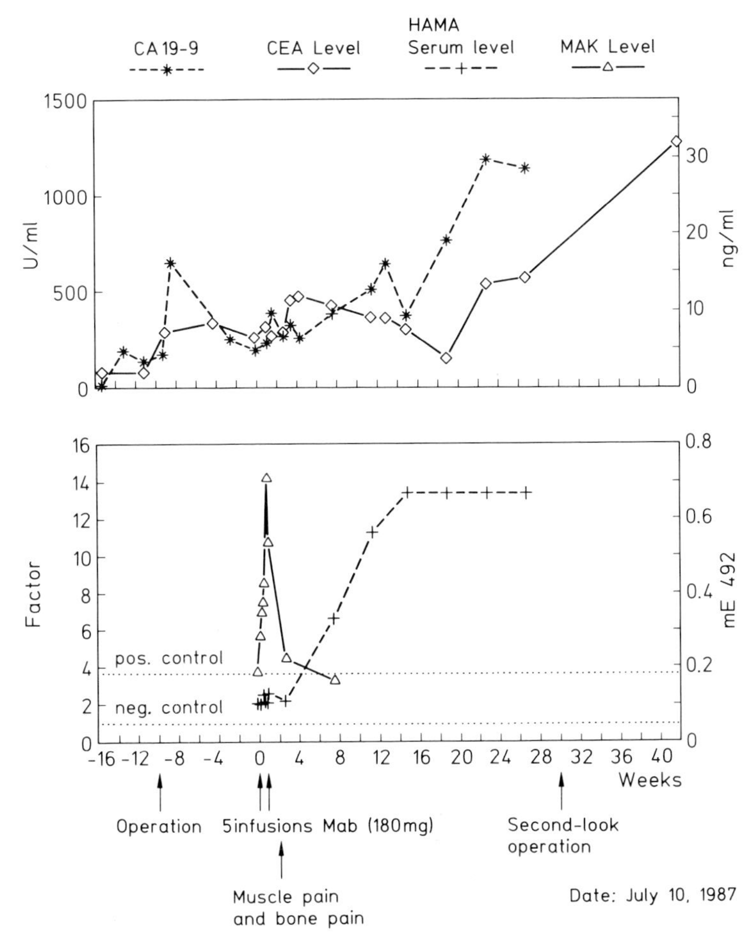

Fig. 2. *Upper curves:* serum tumor markers CA 19-9 and carcinoembryonic antigen *(CEA)* in one female patient with stable disease over 5 months. *Lower curves:* serum levels of monoclonal antibody *(MAK) (triangles)* after five repeated infusions and development of serum human antimouse antibody *(HAMA)* levels *(crosses)* after treatment

Side Effects of Immunotherapy

There were no side effects or untoward reactions to immunotherapy in the majority of the patients. Patients 1 and 2 (Ulm) developed diffuse muscular aches in the lower extremities and in the lumber region 14 and 20 days after the beginning of therapy, without objective neurologic impairment. These symptoms, which must be considered as side effects of therapy, since they occurred in two patients in a very similar form, subsided after 48 h without specific therapy. Patients 10 and 13 (Ulm) experienced anaphylactic reactions during the ninths antibody application on day 19 (patient 10) and during the fifth application on day 12 (patient 13), developing acute back pain and hypotension. Those reactions were immediately controlled without further complications by stopping the infusion and administering

analgetics, steroids and epinephrine. Subsequent serum analysis showed highly positive HAMA titers at the time of the infusion, which might explain the anaphylactoid reactions.
In the context of the phase I study, a repeated dose was administered to patient 2 of the Ulm population 3 months after the primary antibody therapy. This led to a comparable anaphylactoid reaction after only 5 mg BW 494 had been administered intravenously. The reaction was controlled by the appropriate measures. In both cases, the allergic reaction was due to high serum levels of HAMA. This experience ruled out the application of further secondary therapy to the patients treated subsequently.

Response Rate and Clinical Results

Clinical results and response rates are summarized in Table 4. The course of the disease was evaluated primarily on the basis of general clinical status, subjective status, the serum tumor markers CA 19-9 and CEA, and tumor expansion as determined by CT and ultrasonography. According to these criteria, one patient from the Hamburg population had a partial remission (3%), and the disease of nine patients' (23%) remained stable for at least 3 months after therapy. Twenty-nine patients (74%) showed continued tumor progression.

Discussion

The main rationale for the first clinical use of monoclonal antibodies in the treatment of pancreatic cancer was the fact that the monoclonal antibody BW 494 induces ADCC [16]. The effector cells for ADCC could be macrophages, as well as lymphocytes with natural killer cell activity [32, 33]. Numerous studies on tumors transferred to nude mice have shown that tumor growth can, indeed, be inhibited by antibodies that induce ADCC [32–34].
Therapeutic effects were also demonstrated in clinical studies using ADCC-producing antibodies. A further advantage of monoclonal antibody BW 494 was the in vitro inhibition of the specific functions of human pancreatic carcinoma cells [17, 22]. Although no in vivo reduction of tumor cells could be expected from this

Table 4. Clinical results and response rates of 39 patients treated with monoclonal antibody BW 494 in a pilot study in Ulm, Hamburg, and Gießen

Study center	Patients (*n*)	Clinical results		
		Partial remission *n* (%)	Stable disease >3 months *n* (%)	Disease progression *n* (%)
ULM	(18)		6	12
Hamburg	(15)	1	1	13
Gießen	(6)		2	4
		1 (3%)	9 (23%)	29 (74%)

effect, there was a justified expectation of growth suppression due to the inhibition of endocytosis and enzyme release [17].

Only one partial and no complete remission was achieved in the 39 patients in the study by the intravenous administration of the monoclonal antibody. Although the results of this phase I-II study are preliminary, the clinical evaluation shows that 9 patients with advanced pancreatic cancer reacted to the antibody with a stabilization of their disease course. The clinical and subjective status, tumor expansion, and serum tumor markers CA 19-9 and CEA remained unchanged in these patients for at least 3 months after therapy. A 51-year-old female patient in the primary tumor stage $T_3N_1M_0$ has been alive for 20 months, maintaining a constant body weight and working full time.

The majority of the patients were able to tolerate intravenous monoclonal antibody treatment in a total dosage of 180-340 mg given in 5-9 individual doses without side effects. Two patients developed muscular and back aches, which subsided without further therapy. Two further patients experienced anaphylactoid reactions on day 12 and on day 19, respectively, necessitating the discontinuation of the treatment. These patients already showed HAMA in the serum at the time of the allergic reaction, which explains these incidents. The relatively early development of HAMA within 14-21 days following infusion of the IgG 1 mouse antibody resulted in a change of the study design. Patients 11-19 from the Ulm population were given the total quantity of infused antibody within 10 days, i.e., prior to the rise of serum HAMA. All eight of the patients tested for serum HAMA after therapy showed a rise in serum HAMA levels within 4 weeks after therapy. This finding does not agree with the study by Sears and coworkers [19], who found HAMA in only half of the patients previously treated with the monoclonal antibody 17-1A (an IgG 2A). The 100% induction of HAMA by monoclonal antibody BW 494 raises questions as to the direct antitumor action of the antibody. Further, the interesting hypothesis that the induction of anti-idiotypical antibodies in the human organism results in a modulated immunogenic response directed against the tumor, which can lead to tumor cell destruction [35] also remains open.

A terminal half-life of 47.8 h was calculated after administration of 100 mg of monoclonal antibody BW 494. These pharmacokinetics correspond to an open, two-compartment model, and the half-life times are comparable to the other murine antibodies in the human organism [36]. The immunohistochemical results obtained in the course of this study confirmed the high sensitivity of over 90% of monoclonal antibody BW 494 for pancreatic cancer of ductal origin [20, 25] because all tumor tissue grades I-II showed medium-to-strong immunoreactions, and 50% of the undifferentiated pancreatic carcinomas could be stained.

This first experience with immunotherapy for pancreatic cancer of ductal origin justifies the use of monoclonal antibody BW 494 in larger controlled studies. Since June 1987, we have started three further multicentric trials with monoclonal antibody BW 494: one further phase I trial to evaluate the effect of high-dose therapy of up to 1000 mg antibody protein, a second uncontrolled phase II study with monoclonal antibody BW 494 in unresectable pancreatic tumors, and a third randomized phase II study in resectable pancreatic tumors.

Therapeutic success from these recently initiated trials may be expected primarily for less advanced tumor stages. In the future, the combination with immune response modifiers like interleukin 2 or colony-stimulating factors may form the basis for new strategies in the oncologic therapy of pancreatic cancer. In particular, pancreatic cancer of ductal origin, as a prototype of the generally incurable tumor at the time of its diagnosis, should be included in future clinical trials with the combination of monoclonal antibodies and immunomodulators.

References

1. Beger HG, Bittner R (1985) Die operative Therapie beim Pankreaskopfkarzinom. Eine chirurgische Standortbestimmung. Z Gastroenterol 23: 240
2. Gudjonsson B, Livstone EM, Spiro HM (1978) Cancer of pancreas. Cancer 42: 2494
3. Hermanek P (1984) Pathologie der Pankreastumoren. In: Gebhardt C (ed) Chirurgie des exokrinen Pankreas. Thieme, Stuttgart, p 192
4. Kümmerle F, Mangold G, Rückert K (1979) Chirurgie des Pankreas. Internist 20: 399
5 Moossa AR, Levin B (1981) The diagnosis of "early" pancreatic cancer. Cancer 47: 1688
6. Beger HG, Bittner R (1986) Das Pankreaskarzinom. Springer-Verlag, Berlin Heidelberg New York Tokyo
7. Knight RW, Scarborough JP, Goss JC (1978) Adenocarcinoma of the pancreas. A 10-year experience. Arch Surg 113: 1401
8. Malt RA (1983) Treatment of pancreatic cancer. JAMA 250: 1433
9. Moossa AR (1982) Pancreatic cancer. Approach to diagnosis, selection for surgery and choice of operation. Cancer 50: 2689
10. Dobelbower RR Jr (1981) Current radiotherapeutic approaches to pancreatic cancer. Cancer 47: 1729
11. Frey C, Twomey P, Keehn R, Elliot D, Higgens E (1981) Randomized study of 5-FU and CCNU in pancreatic cancer. Cancer 47: 27
12. Gall FP, Zirngibl H (1984) Chirurgische Therapie der Pankreastumoren. In: Gebhardt C (ed) Chirurgie des exokrinen Pankreas. Thieme, Stuttgart, p 235
13. Klapdor R, Lehmann U, v Ackeren H, Schreiber HW, Klöppel G, Greten H (1986) Chemotherapy des inoperablen Pankreaskarzinoms. In: Beger HG, Bittner R (eds) Das Pankreaskarzinom. Springer-Verlag, Berlin Heidelberg New York Tokyo
14. Mallinson CN, Rake MO, Cocking JB, Fox CA, Cwynarski MT, Diffey BL, Jackson GA, Hanley J, Wass VJ (1980) Chemotherapy in pancreatic cancer. Br Med J 281: 1589
15. Tepper J, Nardi G, Suit H (1976) Carcinoma of the pancreas. Analysis of surgical failure and implications for radiation therapy. Cancer 37: 1519
16. Bosslet K, Kern HF, Kanzy EJ, Steinsträsser A, Schwarz A, Lüben E, Schorlemmer HU, Sedlaczek HH (1986) A monoclonal antibody with binding and inhibiting activity towards human pancreatic carcinoma cells. Cancer Immunol Immunother 23: 185
17. Schorlemmer HU, Bosslet K, Kern HF, Sedlaczek HH (1988 in press) A monoclonal antibody with binding and inhibiting activity towards human pancreatic carcinoma cells. Cancer Immunol Immunother
18. Houghton AN, Mintzer D, Cordon-Cardo C, Welt S, Fliegel B, Vadhan S, Carswell E, Melamed MR, Oettgen HF, Old RJ (1985) Mouse monoclonal IgG3 antibody detecting G D3 ganglioside: A phase I trial in patients with malignant melanoma. Proc Nat Acad Sci USA 82: 1242
19. Sears HF, Herlyn D, Steplewsky Z, Koprowski H (1985) Phase II clinical trial of a murine monoclonal antibody cytotoxic for gastrointestinal adenocarcinoma. Cancer Res 45: 5910
20. Kübel R, Büchler M, Baczako K, Beger HG (1986) Immunohistochemical analysis of new monoclonal antibodies for pancreatic carcinoma associated antigens. In: Greten H, Klapdor R (eds) Tumor markers. Thieme, Stuttgart, p 76
21. Montz R, Klapdor R, Rothe B, Heller M (1986) Immunoscintigraphy and radioimmunotherapy patients with pancreatic carcinoma. Nuklearmedizin 25: 239
22. Kern HF, Bosslet K, Sedlaczek HH, Schorlemmer HU (1986) Monocyte specific functions expressed in cell lines from human pancreatic adenocarcinoma. Dig Dis Sci 31: 1136

23. Klapdor R, Lander S, Balo M, Montz R (1986) Radioimmunotherapy of xenografts of human pancreatic carcinomas. Nucl Med 25: 235
24. Karnofsky DA, Abelmann WH, Craver LF, Burdenal JH (1948) The use of the nitrogen mustards in the palliative treatment of carcinoma. Cancer 1: 634
25. Kübel R, Büchler M, Baczako K, Beger HG (1987) Immunhistochemie beim Pankreaskarzinom mit dem monoklonalen Antikörper BW 494. Lang Arch Chir 371: 5-9
26. Hsu SM, Raine L, Fanger H (1981) The use of avidin-biotin peroxidase complex in immunoperoxidase techniques. Cytochem 29: 577
27. Sternberger LA (1974) Immunohistochemistry. Prentice-Hall, Englewood Cliffs, NJ
28. Kübel R, Büchler M, Bosslet K, Beger HG (1987) Antibody dependent cellular cytotoxicity (ADCC) in patients with gastrointestinal cancer. Cancer Res Clin Oncol 113: 41
29. Sears HF, Matthys J, Herlyn D, Häyry P, Atkinson B, Ernst C, Steplewski Z, Koprowski H (1982) Phase I clinical trial of monoclonal antibody in treatment of gastrointestinal tumours. Lancet I: 762
30. Watts DG (1981) An introduction to nonlinear least squares. In: Endrenyi L (ed) Kinetic data analysis. Raven, New York, pp 1-37
31. Madry N, Harthus HP (1987) Anwendung von monoklonalen Antikörpern in-vivo: Messung der Maus-Antikörper und der Anti-Maus-Antikörper-Serumspiegel. Lab Med 10: 161
32. Herlyn D, Koprowsky H (1982) IgG2a monoclonal antibodies inhibit tumor growth through interaction with effector cells. Proc Natl Acad Sci USA 79: 4761
33. Schulz G, Staffileno LK, Reisfeld RA, Dennert G (1985) Eradication of established human melanoma tumors by antibody directed effector cells. J Exp Med 161: 1315
34. Schulz G, Bumol TF, Reisfeld RA (1983) Monoclonal antibody directed effector cells selectively lyse human melanoma cells in vitro and in vivo. Proc Natl Acad Sci USA 80: 5407
35. Koprowsky H, Herlyn D, Lubeck M, De Freitas E, Sears H (1984) Human anti-idiotype antibodies in cancer patients: is the modulation of the immune response beneficial for the patient? Proc Natl Acad Sci USA 81: 216
36. Goldstein G, Fuccello AJ, Norman DJ (1986) OKT3 monoclonal antibody plasma levels during therapy and the subsequent development of host antibodies to OKT3. Transplantation 42: 57

Mab 17-1A Used for Therapy of Patients with Metastatic Colorectal Carcinomas*

H. MELLSTEDT,[1,5] J.-E. FRÖDIN,[1,5] G. MASUCCI,[1,5] C. LINDEMALM,[1]
C. WEDELIN,[1] B. CHRISTENSSON,[2] J. SHETYE,[1,2,5] P. BIBERFELD,[2]
A.-K. LEFVERT,[5] P. PIHLSTEDT,[3] J. MAKOWER,[4] U. HARMENBERG,[6]
B. WAHREN,[6] B. AHLMAN,[7] B. CEDERMARK,[8] R. ERWALD,[9]
I. MAGNUSSON,[11] J. NATHANSSON,[10] and A. RIEGER[11]

Introduction

Tumor cells may express tumor-associated antigens (TAA). However, TAA are also present on normal cells during various stages of differentiation, especially on fetal cells. On normal mature cells, TAA might be detected only by highly sensitive techniques or after manipulation of the cell membrane. On malignant cells, TAA are often re-expressed in high concentrations. Such antigens can be exploited not only for diagnostic purposes, but also as targets for immunotherapy.
In colorectal carcinomas, the TAA CO17-1A, is expressed in practically all cases on the majority of the tumor cells (data to be published). The antigen is a non-secreted glycoprotein with a molecular weight of 37 kD. A mouse monoclonal antibody (MAb) (IgG_{2A}) has been raised against the antigen [5]. MAb 17-1A has been extensively used for therapy of patients with gastrointestinal tumors.
The in vivo mechanisms of tumor cell destruction mediated by MAb are not completely understood. In animal and in vitro experimental systems, it has been suggested that antibody-dependent cellular cytotoxicity (ADCC) is an important component of tumor cell lysis [4]. Cell subpopulations significant in this respect seem to be monocytes/macrophages and natural killer and killer cells [1, 10, data to be published]. Complement-mediated lysis is thought to play a minor role in the destruction of solid tumors, but there are indications that this mechanism might also be operating [data to be published, 8].

* This study was supported by grants from Cancer Society in Stockholm, the Swedish Cancer Society, the King Gustaf V Jubilee Fund, and the Karolinska Institute Foundations.

[1] Department of Oncology (Radiumhemmet), Karolinska Hospital, P.O. Box 60500, 10401 Stockholm, Sweden.
[2] Department of Pathology, Karolinska Hospital, P.O. Box 60500, 10401 Stockholm, Sweden.
[3] Department of Transfusion Medicine, Karolinska Hospital, P.O. Box 60500, 10401 Stockholm, Sweden.
[4] Department of Diagnostic Radiology, Karolinska Hospital, P.O. Box 60500, 10401 Stockholm, Sweden.
[5] Immunological Research Laboratory, Karolinska Hospital, P.O. Box 60500, 10401 Stockholm, Sweden.
[6] National Bacteriological Laboratory, 10401 Stockholm, Sweden.
[7] Department of Surgery, St. Göran Hospital, 10401 Stockholm, Sweden.
[8] Department of Surgery, Karolinska Hospital, P.O. Box 60500, 10401 Stockholm, Sweden.
[9] Department of Surgery, Danderyd Hospital, 10401 Stockholm, Sweden.
[10] Department of Surgery, Nacka Hospital, 10401 Stockholm, Sweden.
[11] Department of Surgery, South Hospital, 10401 Stockholm, Sweden.

H. G. Beger et al. (Eds.), Cancer Therapy

To date, metastatic colorectal carcinomas cannot be cured by cytostatic therapy or by any other treatment modalities. The median survival from the time of diagnosis of metastasis in untreated patients is about 6–8 months and for patients given chemotherapy, about 12 months [2, 3]. Thus, there is a clear need for other therapeutic approaches to improve the prognosis for these patients.
MAb against TAA on colorectal cells offers a new potential therapeutic strategy. Naked MAb alone can induce tumor regression. However, a lot of work is required before an effective treatment concept can be achieved using unconjugated MAb. In this article, we summarize some of our experience in the treatment of colorectal carcinoma patients and focus on a few factors which might be considered in the future planning of MAb therapy.

Methods

MAb 17-1A in Serum and Antimouse Antibodies

Mouse immunoglobulin (MAb 17-1A) and class-specific human antimouse antibodies were assayed by enzyme-linked immunosorbent assay (ELISA) using flat-bottomed microtiter ELISA plates (Dynatech) coated at 4 °C overnight with goat antimouse IgG (Nordic, Tilburg, The Netherlands) for mouse Ig determination and with mouse Ig (Nordic, Tilburg, The Netherlands) for human antimouse Ig analysis. After blocking with 0.5% bovine serum albumin in coating buffer for 1 h at 37 °C, diluted samples to be tested were added in triplicate for 2 h at 37 °C. Finally, the plates were reacted for 2 h at 37 °C with goat antimouse IgG peroxidase conjugate (Nordic, Tilburg, The Netherlands) or rabbit antihuman IgG or IgM peroxidase conjugates (DAKO A/S, Copenhagen, Denmark) respectively. After enzyme reaction for 20 min using 1,2-phenylen-diamindihydro-chlorid (0.55 mg/ml) in Tris-HC1 buffer (pH 7.6) containing 30 µl H_2O_2 per 100 ml of volume, the extinction at 492 nm was measured using an automatic ELISA reader (Titertec, Multiscan). Absorbance of normal control serum for antimouse IgG antibodies was 0.26 (±0.008) and for IgM antibodies 0.06 (±0.03). The background, determined by incubating the antigen-coated wells with medium alone, was subtracted.

Serum Immune Reactivity Against CO17-1A

The human colorectal cell line, SW948, expressing the antigen CO17-1A, was trypsinized with 0.1% trypsin (Flow Lab, Scotland) in PBS for 3–4 min and washed twice in phosphate-buffered solution (PBS). Fifty microliters of the diluted serum sample were added to 5×10^5 cells, incubated at 4 °C for 30 min, and washed twice in PBS. The cell pellet was further incubated at 4 °C for 30 min with 50 µl absorbed fluoresceinated goat antimouse IgG (Becton-Dickinson, Mountain View, California) and then washed twice in PBS. Five-thousand (5×10^3) cells were analyzed by flow cytometry (FACScan; Becton-Dickinson) at 480 nm with a flow rate of <300 cells/s. As a measurement of intact MAb 17-1A in serum, the immune reactivity of the patient serum against the cell line SW948 was expressed as the highest dilution staining ≥10% cells. The pretreatment serum and serum from healthy control donors did not stain SW948. Moreover, the patient serum containing MAb 17-1A did not stain unrelated cell lines, i.e., cells not expressing CO17-1A (K562, M5).

Criteria for Response

A clinically complete response (CCR) was defined as a complete disappearance of all clinical, radiological, and biochemical evidence of the disease. A partial response (PR) was attained when there was a decrease of at least 50% in the product of two perpendicular diameters of all measurable disease manifestations and a > 50% decrease in the serum concentrations of carcinoembryonic antigen (CEA), CA 19-9, and CA 50. A minor response (MR) was defined as a decrease of 25%–50% in the product of two perpendicular diameters of at least one tumor lesion and/or a >50% decrease in the serum concentrations of CEA, CA 19-9, and/or CA 50. Stable disease (SD) was defined as no significant change (<25%>) in the size of all measurable lesions and no significant change (<50%>) in the serum concentrations of CEA, CA 19-9, and CA 50. Progressive disease (PD) was defined as an increase of >25% in the size of at least one measurable lesion and a >50% increase in the serum concentration of CEA, CA 19-9, and/or CA 50.

Results

Patients

Nineteen patients (as of February 1988) with metastatic colorectal carcinomas were entered in the study. All patients had metastatic disease not accessible to surgery. The median age was 62 years (range: 32–81 years). There were 8 males and 11 females. The median time from primary surgery was 14 months (range: 1–75 months). One patient had received cytostatic therapy and another, radiation therapy for their metastases. All the others were untreated. No other treatment was given during therapy with MAb.

The tumors of all patients expressed CO17-1A, which is the epitope for MAb 17-1A reactivity. CO17-1A is mainly concentrated at the base of the tumor glands, where the blood supply is good. In all but one patient, practically all tumor cells expressed the antigen. In that particular patient, 50%–90% of the tumor cells of a thick needle biopsy were found to exhibit CO17-1A.

Dose Schedules of MAb 17-1A

An important question concerning the implementation of MAb alone is the optimal dose and time schedule. Experimental studies in animals with solid tumors have shown that a maximum of 8% of the administered MAb reached the tumor, in most cases about 1% [9]. To achieve maximal ADCC, optimal surface saturation should be pursued. Extrapolating from a human melanoma system, 100 mg MAb is required to optimally saturate 100–400 g of tumor tissue [6]. Thus, in patients with metastatic disease, depending on the tumor load, at least 5–15 g should be given. From a pharmacological point of view, it is preferable to maintain a constant level of MAb in the plasma for a long time. In experimental systems, it has also been suggested that MAb should be given every 2–4 days [9].

Based on these assumptions and our own results during the progress of the study, escalating dose schedules of MAb 17-1A have been used. The first 10 patients received 400 mg initially as a single infusion and then 200 mg three additional times, 6 weeks apart, for a total dose of 1000 mg MAb. After a single infusion of MAb 17-1A, the half-life ($T_{\beta 1/2}$) was approximately 24 h (Fig. 1).

After 70% of the total number of infusions, MAb 17-1A remained in the serum for 1 week, while in the remaining cases it was detected for 2 weeks. All patients developed IgM and IgG antimouse antibodies. The titers rose following each infusion. Immediately after an infusion of MAb 17-1A (within 1 h), there was a sharp decrease in the IgG antimouse antibody titers (Fig. 2). The most likely explanation is antigen-antibody complex formation with a rapid clearance by the reticuloendothelial system. Gradually (within a week), the IgG titers rose to an even higher level than before the infusion. However, the antigen-antibody complex formation did not change the pharmacokinetics of MAb 17-1A, indicating that the antigen (MAb 17-1A) excess was tremendous. Moreover, no signs of immune-complex related symptoms were registered (see below).

The following five patients received 400 mg MAb daily on days 1, 3, and 6. The course was repeated twice to a total dose of 3.6 g MAb 17-1A. With this dose

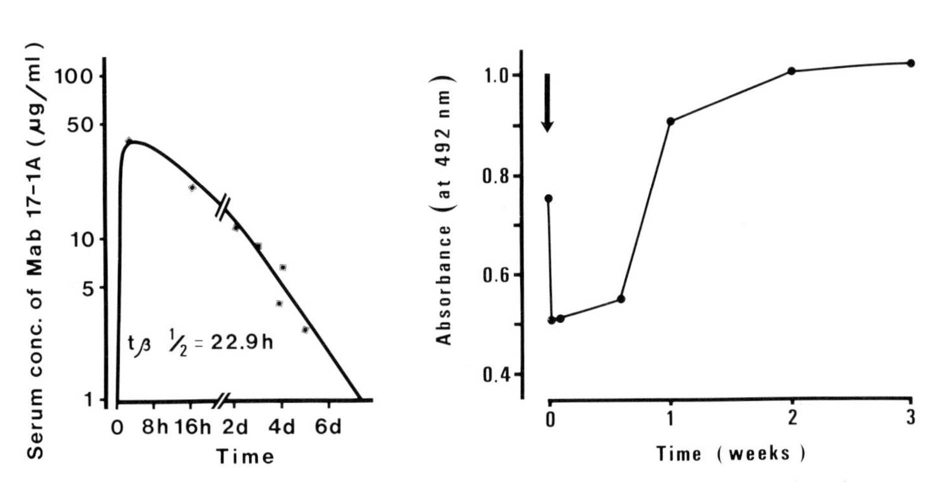

Fig. 1 *(left)*. Serum pharmacokinetics of a single infusion of 200 mg MAb 17-1A. The values represent the mean of ten individuals

Fig. 2 *(right)*. Serum antimouse IgG titers after a single infusion of 200 mg MAb 17-1A. The patients had received three infusions of MAb 17-1A previously. The values represent the mean of three individuals. *Arrow* represents infusion

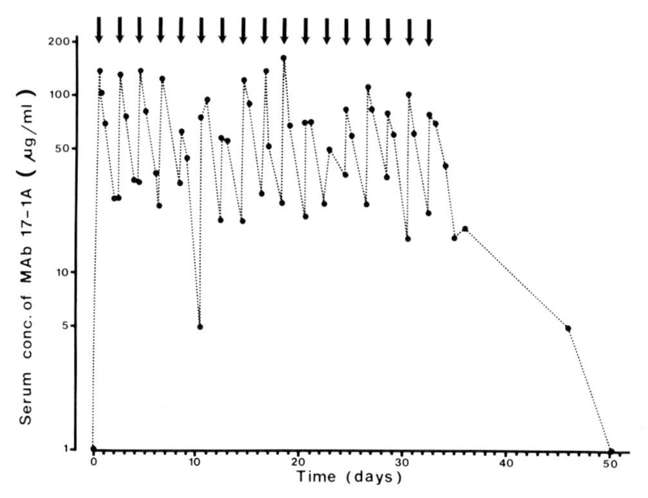

Fig. 3. Serum pharmacokinetics of MAb 17-1A in patient no. 17, who was treated with 400 mg MAb every second day. *Arrows* indicate infusions of MAb

schedule, a sustained plasma level of MAb 17-1A was present as long as the infusions were given, but 9–14 days following the first infusion, MAb 17-1A was no longer detectable.

In the ongoing study protocol, the patients receive higher doses on a continuous basis. MAb 17-1A is administered every second day. The first patient (No. 16) was given 200 mg daily, with a total dose of 4.8 g. The others receive 400 mg daily, with a total dose of 7.6 g. Seven patients will be treated by this route of administration, and four finished their treatment by February 1, 1988. With this mode of administration, it was possible to maintain a high constant level of MAb 17-1A (Fig. 3). The peak values, when administering 400 mg of MAb 17-1A every second day, varied between 60 and 160 µg/ml and the nadir values, between 10–40 µg/ml.

The method used to determine MAb 17-1A pharmacokinetics in serum was an ELISA technique detecting constant regions of mouse IgG. To ascertain the presence in serum of immune-reactive MAb 17-1A serum was used to stain the human colorectal carcinoma cell line SW 948 (see "Methods"). As can be seen in Fig. 4, the patient's serum stained the cell line as long as there was mouse IgG in the serum. The half-life profile of the immune reactivity was the same as for mouse IgG, indicating the presence of intact MAb 17-1A molecules. The staining for SW948 was specific.

Antimouse Antibodies

All patients developed both IgM and IgG antibodies against MAb 17-1A. The antibody titers increased after each infusion. Patients having received repeated infusions and analyzed for antimouse antibodies 1 year after the initiation of therapy still had high titers of IgG antibodies. There was no relation between serum antibody titers and side effects (see below).

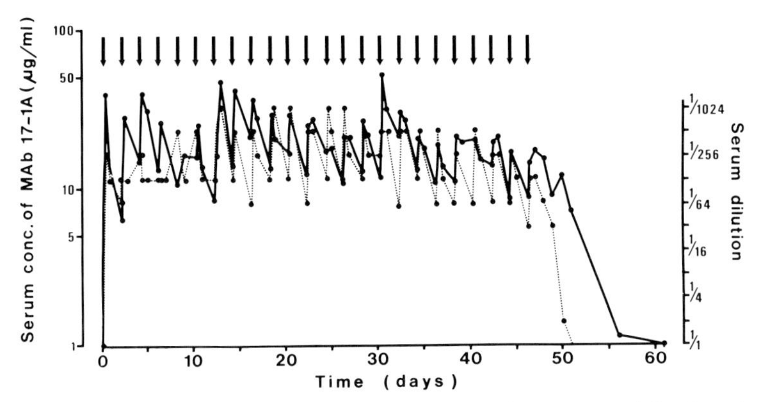

Fig. 4. Serum pharmacokinetics of mouse-IgG (———) and serum immune reactivity (·····) against SW948 in patient no. 16 after infusions of 200 mg MAb 17-1A every second day. The immune reactivity is expressed as the highest serum dilution staining 10% or more of the cells of the cell line SW948. *Arrows* indicate infusions of MAb

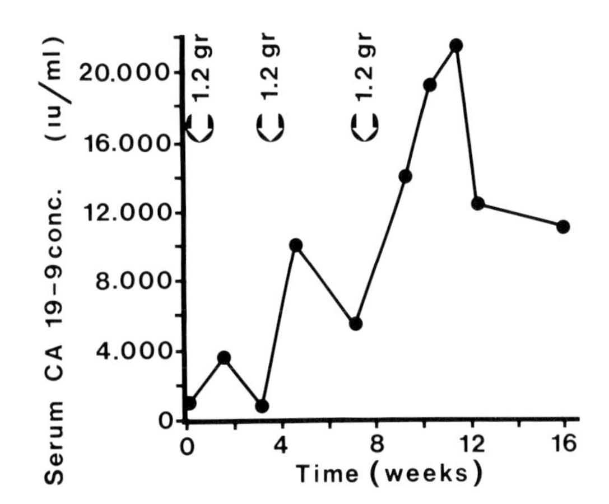

Fig. 5. Changes in serum CA 19-9 concentration during therapy with MAb 17-1A in patient no. 12. *Arrows* indicate infusions of MAb

Table 1. Therapeutic effects of MAb 17-1A in patients with metastatic colorectal carcinoma ($n = 17$)

Clinically complete response	Partial response	Minor response	Stable disease >3 months
1 (6%)	0	2 (12%)	2 (12%)

Therapeutic Effects

By February 1, 1988, 17 patients were evaluable for response. The therapeutic effects are shown in Table 1. One patient was considered to have a biological response, which means objective evidence of tumor cell lysis, but the patient could not be classified as having CR, PR, MR, or SD. This is illustrated in Fig. 5, which

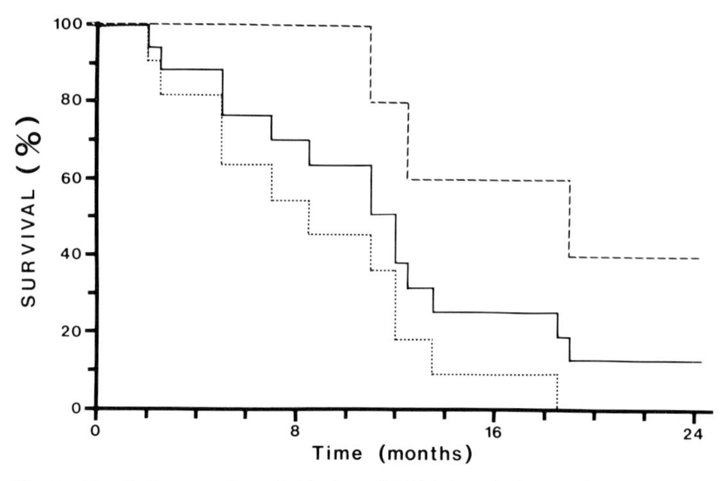

Fig. 6. Survival curves from initiation of MAb 17-1A therapy in patients with metastatic colorectal carcinomas. (———) all patients ($n = 17$); (- - - -) responders ($n = 6$); (· · · · · ·) nonresponders ($n = 11$)

Table 2. Side effects of MAb 17-1A in relation to dosage

Type	200 mg MAb 17-1A ($n = 46$)	400 mg MAb 17-1A ($n = 97$)
Diarrhea		35 (34%)
Slight abdominal pain	2 (4%)	24 (25%)
Nausea/vomiting		19 (20%)
Fever (37.5°-38.5 °C)	4 (9%)	10 (10%)
Moderate abdominal pain		6 (6%)
Shivering	3 (7%)	2 (2%)
Allergic reaction	3 (7%)	

shows that every infussion of MAb 17-1A induced a sharp temporary increase in the serum concentration of CA 19-9.

The survival curves of the patients are shown in Fig. 6. The total median survival from diagnosis of metastasis was 12 months. For responding patients ($n = 6$), the median survival was 19 months, and the corresponding figure for nonresponding patients was 8 months.

Side Effects

The types and frequencies of side effects are shown in Table 2. Altogether 143 infusions of MAb 17-1A have been given. Doses of 200 mg have been administered 46 times, and 400 mg MAb 17-1A has been infused 97 times. All the side effects were of short duration. Fever disappearaed within 72 h and diarrhea, within 24 h. All the other symptoms lasted for only a few hours. No medical intervention was necessary. Allergic reactions occurred three times. One patient experienced itchy palms after the second infusion. Two patients became hypotensive after the third and fifth infusions respectively. The infusions were stopped immediately, and hydrocortisone was given. Blood pressure normalized within 15 min. Our hand skin test seems to predict allergic reactions reliably, while no relation to serum IgM and IgG antibody titers were noted.

Discussion

Mouse MAb 17-1A alone can induce tumor regression in patients with colorectal carcinomas. Even complete remissions have been observed. More than 500 patients with metastatic colorectal carcinomas have received treatment with MAb 17-1A. The observed CR rate is about 5%. In the present study, 35% of the patients had an objective, measurable effect. Moreover, total survival was similar to that reported for patients treated with cytostatic therapy [2], and those patients responding to MAb 17-1A had a significantly better survival than the nonresponding patients. Thus, mouse monoclonal antibodies exert antitumoral effects in solid tumors. However, much remains to be done to improve this treatment modality.

An important factor is to find the optimal dose schedule for MAb 17-1A. In our therapeutic strategy, an escalation of the total dose administered is included. In a subsequent patient series, 12 g will be given during a period of 8 weeks. By this approach, we aim to optimize the tumor cell surface saturation and thereby try to create favorable conditions for ADCC.

The use of chimeric MAb (mouse-human) might be another way to increase the efficacy. The antibody response against the infusion MAb decreases, and only anti-idiotypic (ab_2) antibodies are induced, which might be of therapeutic benefit [7]. Moreover, chimeric antibodies seem to induce a stronger ADCC than the corresponding mouse MAb (data to be published), an effect which might also increase the therapeutic efficacy.

Activation of the effector cells mediating the tumor cell killing in ADCC may facilitate the use of MAb. Potential killer cell stimulators are interleukin-2 (IL-2), granulocyte-monocyte colony-stimulating factor (GM-CSF), monocyte colony-stimulating factor (M-CSF), gamma-interferon (γ-IFN), and tumor necrosis factor (TNF). Our own in vitro experiments have shown a strong augmentation of ADCC, using SW948 as target cells and MAb 17-1A, after preincubation of the effector cells with IL-2 (data to be published). Clinical trials are also in progress using a combination of MAb and IL-2. By combining MAb, IL-2, and lymphokin activated killer (LAK) cells, it may be possible to reduce the side effects from IL-2 by lowering the dose while maintaining therapeutic effect with a high tumor cell killing capacity.

In conclusion, treatment with MAb has been shown to induce tumor regression with virtually no side effects and may also prolong survival. However, much work has to be done to increase the therapeutic efficacy of the treatment by titrating out the optimal dose of MAb and finding the best combination of MAb with other biological response modifiers. Given time, research relating to this mode of treatment should have a major impact on oncologic practice.

Acknowledgement. We wish to express our sincere gratitude to Prof. H. Koprowski and Dr. Z. Steplewski for providing us with MAb 17-1A. For skillful technical assistance, we thank Miss Birgitta Hagström and Mrs. Harriet Grabö. The excellent secretarial help of Mrs. Gunilla Burén is gratefully acknowledged. For the drawings, we thank Mrs. Rivka Sundfeldt.

References

1. Adams DO, Hall T, Steplewski Z, Koprowski H (1984) Tumors undergoing rejection induced by monoclonal antibodies of the IgG_{2A} isotype contain increased numbers of macrophages activated for a distinctive form of antibody-dependent cytolysis. Proc Natl Acad Sci 81: 3506-3510
2. Beditian AY, Chen TT, Malaky MA, Patt YZ, Body GP (1984) Prognostic factors influencing survival of patients with advanced colorectal cancer: Hepatic artery infusion versus systemic intravenous chemotherapy for liver metastases. J Clin Oncol 2: 174-180
3. Bergmark S, Hafström LO (1969) The natural history of primary and secondary malignant tumors of the liver. I. The prognosis for patients with hepatic metastases from colonic and rectal carcinoma by laparotomy. Cancer 23: 198-202
4. Herlyn D, Steplewski Z, Herlyn M, Koprowski H (1980) Inhibition of growth of colorectal carcinoma in nude mice by monoclonal antibody. Cancer Res 40: 717-21
5. Herlyn D, Herlyn M, Ross AH, Ernst C, Atkinsson B, Koprowski H (1984) Efficient selection of human tumor growth-inhibiting monoclonal antibodies. J Immunol Methods 73: 157-167
6. Herlyn D, Powe J, Ross AK, Herlyn M, Koprowski H (1985) Inhibition of human tumor growth by IgG_{2A} monoclonal antibodies correlates with antibody density on tumor cells. J Immunol 134: 1300-1304
7. Koprowski H, Herlyn D, Lubeck M, DeFreitas E, Sears HF (1984) Human anti-idiotype antibodies in cancer patients: Is the modulation of the immune response beneficial for the patient? Proc Natl Acad Sci 81: 216-219
8. Mellstedt H, Frodin J-E, Christensson B, Shetye J, Biberfeld P, Lefvert A-K, Pihlstedt P, Sylvén M, Makower J, Wahren B, Ahlman B, Cedermark B, Erwald R, Klingenström P, Nathansson J, Rieger Å, Koprowski H (1988) Application of monoclonal antibodies (MAb 17-1A) in the treatment of colorectal carcinomas. In: Douillard JY, Carrano R (eds) Monoclonal antibodies in Oncology. Marcel Dekker, New York
9. Pimm MV, Baldwin RW (1985) Localization of an antitumor monoclonal antibody in human tumor xenografts: Kinetic and quantitative studies with the 791T/36 antibody. In: Baldwin RW, Byers VS (eds) Monoclonal antibodies for cancer detection and therapy. Academic, New York, pp 97-128
10. Schulz G, Stafficeno LK, Reisfeld RA, Dennent G (1985) Erradication of established human melanoma tumor in nude mice by antibody-directed effector cells. J Exp Med 161: 1315-1325

Immunotherapy of Malignant Melanomas

W. G. DIPPOLD[1] and K.-H. MEYER ZUM BÜSCHENFELDE[1]

Introduction

A large number of antigens on human melanoma cells have been identified by means of monoclonal antibody technology [18, 21]. The availability of monoclonal antibodies has rapidly led to clinical investigations. Experience with monoclonal antibodies in the treatment of patients with melanoma is limited [4, 9, 10, 12, 13, 17, 19] because only small groups of patients have been treated so far. According to these studies, treatment with ganglioside antibodies appears most promising.

Evidence for the Importance of Gangliosides for Immunologic Effector Mechanisms

The importance of gangliosides as targets for immunologic effector mechanisms in neuroectodermal tumors is based on a number of recent findings. In particular, the gangliosides GD3 and GD2 represent tumor-restricted molecules [4, 8, 20]. Ganglioside antibodies interfere with cell attachment [2, 6] and mediate complement [23] and antibody-dependent cellular cytotoxicity [3, 16]. These effects, observed on cultured human melanoma and neuroblastoma cells, depend on the levels of gangliosides GD3 and GD2 expressed on the cell surface. Only tumor cells with high ganglioside levels are affected. In addition, monoclonal GD3-ganglioside antibody R-24 can stimulate T cells to proliferate [11, 25]. High levels of GD3-ganglioside antibody R-24 can block the function of cytotoxic T cells [15]. According to these findings, antibody levels may be very important in regard to the therapeutic effects we see with ganglioside antibodies used in patients.
Naturally occurring ganglioside antibodies have been found in patients with malignant melanoma [1, 14, 24], and we and others [4, 9, 12, 13] have demonstrated the efficacy of monoclonal mouse antibodies to gangliosides in inducing inflammatory responses and tumor regressions.

Treatment of Tumor Patients with Ganglioside Antibodies

In 1983 we reported the first administration of ganglioside antibody in patients with advanced malignant melanoma [7]. Following treatment with monoclonal antibody Mab R-24, inflammatory cutaneous responses around tumor nodules (blis-

[1] 1. Medical Clinic, University of Mainz, Langenbeckstraße 1, 6500 Mainz, FRG.

H. G. Beger et al. (Eds.), Cancer Therapy

ter formation and inflammatory perinodular halos) were observed. Local pain in bulky intestinal tumor sites occurred in all three patients about 3 h after onset of antibody infusion. Adverse side effects of antibody administration were not observed with single antibody doses of up to 200 mg and total dose of 440 mg [9]. Meanwhile, eight more patients with disseminated malignant melanoma (but with less advanced disease) were treated by administering 5 mg/m^2 Mab R-24 daily for 3 weeks. In two patients, regression of subcutaneous tumor nodules was observed, but no complete or partial responses were seen. In the other six patients, the tumor remained unchanged or progressed.

Houghton et al. [12] carried out a phase I study and observed a tumor response of greater than 50% in three out of 12 patients, treated every 2nd day for 2 weeks. In five patients, they saw a mixed response with some tumor nodules regressing and others progressing. Three patients showed no response to antibody therapy, and their tumors progressed. With higher antibody dose levels, a lower rate of tumor responses [26] was observed.

Irie and Morton and Cheung et al. also observed tumor responses using GD2 ganglioside antibodies [4, 13]. Irie and Morton reported on the regression of cutaneous metastatic melanoma by intralesional injection with human monoclonal antibody to ganglioside GD2. Cheung et al. treated 17 patients with a mouse monoclonal GD2 ganglioside antibody. Four dose levels (5, 20, 50, and 100 mg/m^2) were administered. Antitumor responses occurred in seven of 17 patients. These ranged from complete clinical remissions to mixed responses.

Here, we report on the first administration of a ganglioside antibody into the cerebrospinal fluid (CSF) of two patients with meningeosis melanotica. The aim of this study was not only to achieve tumor remission but also to monitor closely the immunologic effects induced by this antibody.

Intrathecal Application of GD3-Ganglioside Antibody to Patients with Cerebrospinal Fluid Melanosis

Two patients with melanosis of the meninges received Mab R-24 intrathecally. The first patient received 10 doses of Mab R-24 (dose 1: 2 mg; doses 2–10: 10 mg), the second patient, 8 doses of 1 mg Mab R-24 after incomplete removal of a malignant melanoma near the brain stem. Tumor cells and inflammatory cells in the CSF were monitored during and after treatment. Antibodies applied intrathecally were also detectable in the serum of both patients. Patient A developed anti-mouse antibodies; patient B did not. The administration of Mab R-24 caused an increase in the number of inflammatory cells in the CSF of both patients. GD3-ganglioside-negative tumor cells were found at high antibody levels in the CSF of patient A. Nevertheless, regressive changes of tumor cells were observed in the CSF of patient A 6 weeks after starting Mab therapy. No tumor cells were detected in the CSF of patient B after antibody therapy. Meanwhile, 13 months have passed, and no evidence of tumor has been obtained either by cytologic studies or by CAT, or NMR images of this patient. He is working again full time. Six weeks after the end of his treatment, CSF lymphocytes were cultured by limiting dilution and tested for tumor cell cytotoxicity. In 13 out of 96 wells plated, lymphocytes grew. All 13 different CSF lymphocyte cultures showed a high degree of cytotoxicity for malignant melanoma cells and the natural killer (NK) cell target K-562, but not for the corresponding Epstein-Barr virus (EBV)-transformed B cells. One highly cytotoxic CSF lymphocyte culture grew well enough for fluorescense-activated cell sorting (FACS) analysis to be performed. The cells expressed the antigens CD2 (99.6%), CD3 (53.5%), and CD8 (68%). In contrast, lymphocyte cultures established simultaneously from peripheral blood leukocytes (PBL) of patient B did not show this cytotoxic activity. Therefore, this treatment approach may induce a cellular response against the tumor.

Discussion

The tumor responses induced by ganglioside antibodies, which have been observed by several investigators in two different tumor systems, melanoma and neuroblastoma, are encouraging. However, experience with this form of therapy is still very limited. For example, dose levels or intervals of antibody administration are chosen arbitrarily. Ganglioside antibodies represent good tools for tumor treatment because they are immunologically "armed," being potent activators of human complement and mediators of antibody-dependent cellular cytotoxicity. In addition, GD3-ganglioside antibody R-24 induces an increase in the number of inflammatory cells at the tumor site, as shown in both patients with melanosis of the meninges. The mechanism of tumor regression, which occurs as late as 8–10 weeks after ganglioside antibody therapy, still remains to be elucidated. The occurrence of GD3-ganglioside-positive lymphocytes 6 weeks after the end of antibody administration in the CSF of patient B appears in this regard to be very interesting. We cannot claim that these cytotoxic lymphocytes were induced by Mab R-24 because lymphocyte cultures were not established from CSF cells before starting antibody treatment.

However, the generation of 13 highly cytotoxic lymphocyte cultures which all efficiently lysed melanoma and K-562 target cells is striking, in particular, because similar cytotoxic cells were not obtained in PBL cultures, which were established at the same time. The functional properties of these cells, as well as their antigenic phenotype, characterizes these cells as cytotoxic T cells with NK cell activity and without major histocompatibility complex (MHC) restriction. This phenotype does not characterize the major human NK effector cell, which is a non-T/non-B $CD3^-$ lymphocyte [22]. However, human cells with NK activity are heterogeneous in their antigenic phenotype, and cells that display a combination of T-cell markers (CD2, CD3, CD7, and CD8) have been described.

Tumor responses could be a sequence of events induced by Mab R-24. Complement is activated during treatment, as evidenced by decreases in serum complement levels and by the deposition of complement components at tumor sites [12]. Complement fixation, which leads to the production of histamine and other mediators of inflammation, may play a role in increasing blood flow, which in turn may permit better access of infiltrating lymphocytes into tumors. GD3-ganglioside-positive lymphocytes may then preferentially locate at the tumor site because Mab R-

24 may bring together GD3-ganglioside-positive tumor cells and GD3-positive lymphocytes.

The results of the studies published so far do not permit any conclusions about the efficacy of treatment or about factors that predict response. However, it is interesting to note that lower doses of antibody may be more effective than higher doses. Based on our own experience, daily treatment does not appear promising. The challenge now is to optimize dose and schedule and to evaluate methods to augment the antitumor effects of ganglioside antibodies in vivo. An obvious next step in the treatment of patients consists of combining monoclonal antibodies with different ganglioside molecules (GD3, GD2, GM2). An additional way of augmenting the observed responses may be to combine ganglioside antibodies with cytostatic drugs or with biological response modifiers. In the long term, well-characterized tumor-restricted monoclonal antibodies will gain more clinical application because selective tumor cell destruction will remain a central goal in cancer therapy.

Another conclusion that may be drawn from our present status of knowledge is that immunity against a group of ganglioside antigens should be inducible by active vaccination. The immunologic status of the individual patient may be one of the reasons for the unpredictable natural course of the disease that we regularly observe in patients with malignant melanoma.

References

1. Cahan LD, Irie RF, Singh R, Cassidenti A, Paulson JC (1982) Identification of a human neuroectodermal tumor antigen (OFA-12) as ganglioside GD2. Proc Natl Acad Sci USA 79: 7629-7633
2. Cheresh DA, Harper JR, Schulz G, Reisfeld RA (1984) Localization of the gangliosides GD2 and GD3 in adhesion plaques and on the surface of human melanoma cells. Proc Natl Acad Sci USA 81: 5767-5771
3. Cheresh DA, Honsik CJ, Staffileno LK, Jung G, Reisfeld RA (1985) Disialoganglioside GD3 on human melanoma serves as a relevant target antigen for monoclonal antibody-mediated tumor cytolysis. Proc Natl Acad Sci USA 82: 5155-5159
4. Cheung NK, Lazarus H, Miraldi FD, Abramowsky CR, Kallick S, Saarinen UM, Spitzer T, Strandjord SE, Coccia PF, Berger NA (1987) Ganglioside GD2 specific monoclonal antibody 3F8: a phase I study in patients with neuroblastoma and malignant melanoma. J Clin Oncol 5: 1430-1440
5. Dippold W, Lloyd KO, Li LTC, Ikeda H, Oettgen HF, Old LJ (1980) Cell surface antigens of human malignant melanoma: definition of six antigenic systems with monoclonal antibodies. Proc Natl Acad Sci USA 77: 6114-6118
6. Dippold WG, Knuth A, Meyer zum Büschenfelde KH (1984) Inhibition of human melanoma cell growth in vitro by monoclonal anti-GD3-ganglioside antibody. Cancer Res 44: 806-810
7. Dippold WG, Knuth A, Meyer zum Büschenfelde KH (1984) Melanoma antibodies: specificity and interaction with melanoma and cytotoxic T-cells. Behring Inst Mitt 74: 14-18
8. Dippold W, Dienes HP, Knuth A, Meyer zum Büschenfelde KH (1985) Immunohistochemical localization of ganglioside GD3 in human malignant melanoma, epithelial tumors, and normal tissues. Cancer Res 45: 3699-3705
9. Dippold WG, Knuth A, Meyer zum Büschenfelde KH (1985) Inflammatory tumor response to monoclonal antibody infusion. Eur J Cancer Clin Oncol 21: 907-912
10. Goodman GE, Beaumier P, Fernyhough B, Hellström I, Hellström KE (1985) Pilot trial of murine monoclonal antibodies in patients with advanced melanoma. J Clin Oncol 3: 340-352

11. Hersey P, Schibeci SD, Townsend P, Burns C, Cheresh DA (1986) Potentiation of lymphocyte responses by monoclonal antibodies to the ganglioside GD3. Cancer Res 46: 6083–6090
12. Houghton AN, Mintzer D, Cordon-Cardo C, Welt S, Fliegel B, Vadhan S, Carswell E, Melamed M, Oettgen HF, Old LJ (1985) Mouse monoclonal antibody detecting GD3 ganglioside: A phase I trial in patients with malignant melanoma. Proc Natl Acad Sci USA 82: 1242–1246
13. Irie RF, Morton DL (1986) Regression of cutaneous metastatic melanoma by intralesional injection with human monoclonal antibody to ganglioside GD2. Proc Natl Acad Sci USA 83: 8694–8698
14. Irie RF, Sze LL, Saxton RE (1982) Human antibody to OFA-1, a tumor antigen, produced in vitro by Epstein-Barr virus-transformed human B-lymphoid cell lines. Proc Natl Acad Sci USA 79: 5666–5670
15. Knuth A, Dippold W, Meyer zum Büschenfelde KH (1984) Target level blocking of T-cell cytotoxicity for human malignant melanoma by monoclonal antibodies. Cell Immunol 83: 398–403
16. Knuth A, Dippold WG, Meyer zum Büschenfelde KH (1985) Disialoganglioside GD3-specific monoclonal antibody in ADCC for human malignant melanoma. In: Gagnara J, Klaus SN, Paul E, Schartl M (eds) Biological, molecular and clinical aspects of pigmentation. University of Tokyo Press, Tokyo, pp 421–424
17. Larson SM, Carrasquillo JA, Krohn KA, Brown JP, McGruffin RW, Ferens JM, Graham MM, Hill LD, Beaumier PL, Hellström KE (1983) Localization of ^{131}I-labeled p97-specific Fab fragments in human melanoma as a basis for radiotherapy. J Clin Inves 72: 2101–2114
18. Lloyd KO (1983) Human tumor antigens: Detection and characterization with mouse monoclonal antibodies. In: Herberman RB (ed) Basic and clinical tumor immunology. Martinus Nijhoff, The Hague, pp 160–214
19. Oldham RK, Foon KA, Morgan AC, Woodhouse CS, Schroff RW, Abrahams PG, Fer M, Schoenberger CS, Farrell M, Kimball E (1984) Monoclonal antibody therapy of malignant melanoma: In vivo localization in cutaneous metastasis after intravenous administration. J Clin Oncol 2: 1235–1244
20. Real FX, Houghton A, Albino AP, Cordon-Cardo C, Melamed M, Oettgen HF, Old LJ (1985) Surface antigens of melanomas and melanocytes defined by mouse monoclonal antibodies: specificity analysis and comparison of antigen expression incultured cells and tissues. Cancer Res 45: 4401–4411
21. Reisfeld RA, Ferrone S (eds) (1982) Melanoma antigens and antibodies. Plenum, New York
22. Reynolds CW, Ortaldo JR (1987) Natural killer activity: the definition of a function rather than a cell type. Immunol Today 8: 172–174
23. Vogel CW, Welt SW, Carswell EA, Old LJ, Müller-Eberhard HJ (1983) A murine IgG3 monoclonal antibody to a melanoma antigen that activates complement in vitro and in vivo. Immunobiology 164: 309
24. Watanabe T, Pukel C, Takeyama H, Lloyd KO, Shiku H, Li LTC, Travassos LR, Oettgen HF, Old LJ (1982) Human melanoma antigen AH is an autoantigenic ganglioside related to GD2. J Exp Med 155: 1884–1889
25. Welte K, Miller G, Chapman PB, Yuasa H, Natoli E, Kunicka JE, Cordon-Cardo C, Buhrer C, Old LJ, Houghton AN (1987) Stimulation of T-lymphocyte proliferation by monoclonal antibodies against GD3 ganglioside. J Immunol 139: 1763–1771
26. Houghton A, Vadhans S et al. (1986) Clinical study of a mouse monoclonal antibody directed against GD3 ganglioside in patients with melanoma. Proc ASCO 906

Interaction of Monoclonal Antibodies with Biological Response Modifiers and Cytostatics

R. KLAPDOR[1]

Introduction

Palliative treatment may be of benefit for some patients suffering from carcinomas of the gastrointestinal tract and pancreas (Fig. 1) and may also result in prolonged survival compared with nonresponders. However, chemotherapy and irradiation do not allow cure of these patients. Palliative amelioration is reported in no more than 10%-30% of the patients, and we do not have a treatment modality of choice [19, 21, 22, 26, 29, 56]. With respect to gastrointestinal and pancreatic cancer, which is our main focus of interest, clinical experience indicates (a) that all the different single drugs or drug combinations tested result in similar response rates, (b) that second- or third-line therapy may be active even in the event of nonresponse in the first trial, and (c) that we do not have clinical parameters indicating tumor sensitivity or insensitivity before therapy is initiated.

One factor responsible for this situation seems to be the heterogeneity of these tumors. This concept represents the basis for pretherapeutic sensitivity tests in in vitro or in vivo studies involving cell cultures and nude mice [9, 11, 23, 24, 27]. At the same time, this heterogeneity stimulates gastroenterologists to focus their interest on new developments such as therapy with monoclonal antibodies (Mab) or cytokines.

Monotherapy with Monoclonal Antibodies and Cytokines

A number of studies investigating promising results after therapy of gastrointestinal and pancreatic carcinomas in cell cultures and with nude mice.

From our own studies on nude mice with human pancreatic and gastric/colorectal carcinomas, it was possible to confirm that "adjuvant" therapy with the Mab 17-1A [20] or BW 494/32 [7], which are characterized by antibody-dependent cell-mediated cytotoxicity (ADCC), is able significantly to inhibit the growth of responding xenografts [20, 30, 32, 33, 36]. In our use of the term, "adjuvant" therapy means that in the animal studies, treatment was started immediately after subcutaneous transplantation of the tumor material (slices 2×2 mm in size). Furthermore, we were also able to confirm that recombinant tumor necrosis factor-alpha (rTNF-α), recombinant interferon-gamma (rIFN-γ), and lymphokine-activated

[1] Department of Internal Medicine, University Hospital Eppendorf, Martinistraße 52, 2000 Hamburg 20, FRG.

H. G. Beger et al. (Eds.), Cancer Therapy

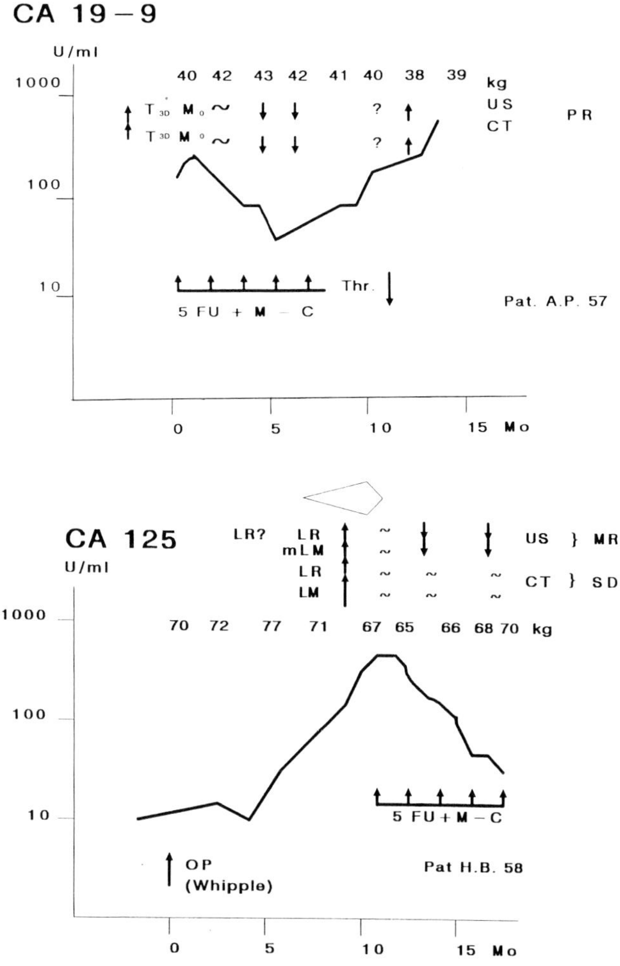

Fig. 1. Benefits of palliative chemotherapy for two patients suffering from pancreatic cancer. *Above: Curve* shows serum levels of CA 19-9 over course of therapy after diagnosis of unresectable disease for patient A. P. 57. Patient experienced relief of pain, weight gain *(kg)*, partial remission *(PR)* as revealed by ultrasound *(US)* and computerized tomography *(CT)*, as well as a temporary decrease in serum levels of CA 19-9. Treatment had to be discontinued because of therapy-induced thrombocytopenia (*Thr.* ↓). *Bottom:* Serum levels of CA 125 over course of therapy for patient H. B. 58 after diagnosis and Whipple resection. Patient experienced pain relief (◇), weight gain *(kg)*, decrease in CA 125 levels, and minor response *(MR)*, as shown by ultrasound *(US)* and stable disease *(SD)* as shown by computerized tomography *(CT)*. ↓ decrease; ↑ increase; *5-FU*, 5-fluorouracil; *M-C*, mitomycin C; *LR*, local recurrence; *mLM*, multiple liver metastases

killer (LAK) cells may have significant, mainly antiproliferative effects in cell cultures and in nude mice [27, 28, 37-40].

However, clinical phase I trials on patients suffering from advanced gastrointestinal tumor disease have been unable to produce convincing results in recent years [8, 12, 33, 36, 49, 52, 55, 57]. Clinical studies have shown that treatment with 17-1A

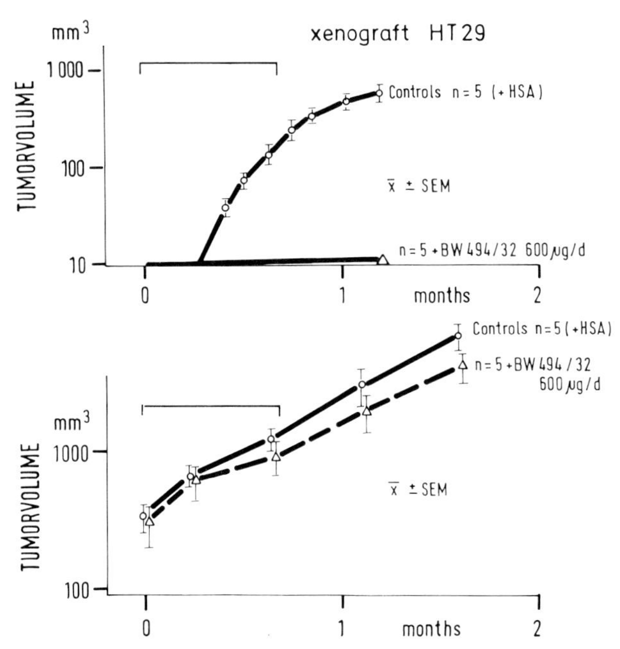

Fig. 2. Evidence for significant inhibition of tumor growth in the case of "adjuvant" treatment of xenografts of cell line HT 29 in nude mice *(above)* in contrast to only slight inhibition of tumor growth when treatment was administered with already established tumors *(below)*. Treatment: Mab BW 494/32, 600 µg/day i.p. for 21 days

or BW 494/32 have produced antitumor effects in no more than 20%–30% of the patients studied. Systemic treatment with rTNF-α, rIFN-γ, and rIFN-α has also shown disappointing results, with the exception of endocrine gastrointestinal-tract carcinomas [3, 13, 34, 45, 47, 51, 54].

There seem to be various reasons for these disappointing clinical data:

1. The phase I trials reported so far were performed on patients with advanced tumor disease. This seems to be a bad precondition if we consider animal experiments. One typical study involving Mab with ADCC is shown in Fig. 2. In contrast to significant inhibition of tumor growth with adjuvant therapy, we find only a slight inhibition of tumor growth in already established xenografts. In order to evaluate the potential efficacy of adjuvant Mab therapy, clinical trials have recently been started. In the Federal Republic of Germany, there are currently two studies involving patients suffering from gastrointestinal-tract or pancreatic carcinomas in which we are also taking part: an investigation of adjuvant therapy with Mab 17-1A after resection of C1/C2 tumors of the colon or resection of colorectal liver metastases (directed by Prof. Riethmüller, Institute of Immunology, University of Munich), and a study involving Mab BW 494/32 after resection of exocrine pancreatic carcinoma (organized by the Behring Werke, Marburg).
2. With systemic administration, the uptake of Mab into the tumor is too low for appreciable antitumoral activity. For example, insufficient Mab uptake into the tumor after systemic application explains differences in local antitumoral irradiation

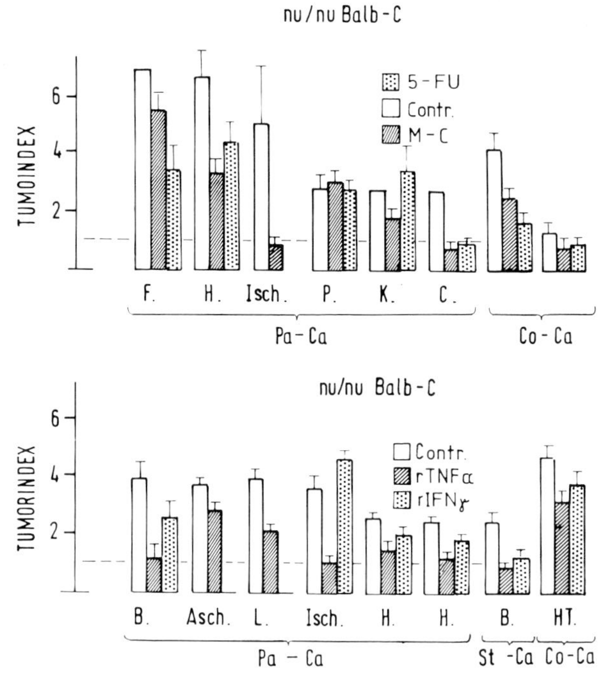

Fig. 3. Treatment of xenografts of human gastrointestinal-tract carcinomas established in nude mice (nu/nu Balb-c) by means of *(upper)* cytostatics (5-fluorouracil, *5-FU;* mitomycin C, *M-C*) and *(lower)* cytokines *(rTNF-α, rIFN-γ)*. The results demonstrate that single drugs may be active in some tumors; however, the different tumors studied show very heterogeneous responses. Treatment duration, 3 weeks; treatment dose, 5-FU, 80 mg/kg/week; M-C, 2.4 mg/kg/week; rTNF-α and rIFN-γ, 0.8 mg/kg/day i.p. *Pa,* pancreas; *St,* stomach; *Co,* colorectal; *Ca,* carcinoma

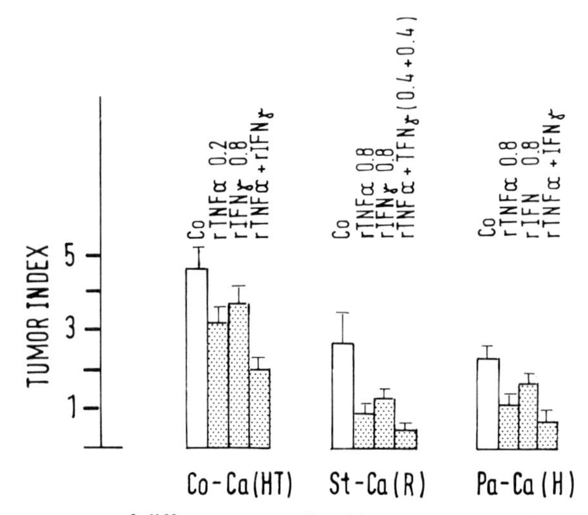

Fig. 4. Evidence for heterogeneous responses of different xenografts of human gastrointestinal-tract carcinomas to rTNF-α, rIFN-γ, or a combination of both drugs. Treatment duration, 21 days; *0.2 or 0.8,* 0.2 or 0.8 mg/kg/day respectively i.p. *Co-Ca,* colon carcinoma; *St-Ca,* stomach carcinoma; *Pa-Ca,* pancreas carcinoma

Table 1. Effects of "adjuvant" or palliative therapy with the Mab with ADCC BW 494/32 and 17-1A on various xenografts of human gastrointestinal and pancreatic carcinomas in nude mice. Administration route, i.p.; therapeutic efficacy varied in the adjuvant trials between complete inhibition of tumor growth (+ + +) and no effect, in the palliative trials between no effect and slight inhibition (as indicated by the mean values of tumor indices at the end of the treatment periods)

Xenograft	Dosage (μg/day)	Treatment Period (days)	Adjuvant Therapy	Palliative Therapy	Mean tumor indices after palliative treatment period[a]	
					controls	Mab-treated animals
Mab 494/32						
ASCH84 Pa	600	21	+ +			
EL84 Pa	600	21	no			
ISCH84 Pa	600	21	no	no	4.3	4.6
KF86 Pa	600	21		+	8.2	4.9
No86 Pa	600	21		+ ?	5.8	4.9
HT29 Co	600	21	+ + +	+	5.4	3.7
HSCH86 Co	600	21	no	+ + +	+	5.4
3.7						
Mab 17-1A						
ASCH84 Pa	600	21	+ + +			
ISCH84 Pa	400	14 (adjuvant) 21 palliative)	+ ?	?	4.3	3.8
HT29 Co	600	21	+ + +			
HSCH86 Co	600	21	+	no	2.6	2.3

Pa, pancreas; *Co,* colorectal.

[a] Ratio of tumor volume at end of therapy to tumor volume at beginning of therapy, calculated for controls and Mab-treated tumors.

by ^{131}I-labelled Mab after systemic or intratumoral administration in animal and clinical studies [5, 24, 44, 46].

3. Mab, cytokines, and cytostatics may be active in some tumors or xenografts. The various tumors, however, show a very heterogeneous response, varying between highly sensitive and insensitive (Figs. 3a, b, 4; Table 1).

4. Treatment trials with single Mab or cytokines may fail because of the complexity of the defense system of the host.

Theoretical Considerations Concerning Combinations of Mab, Cytokines and Cytostatics

Because of the complexity of the host defense system, the combination of different Mab or the combination of Mab with cytokines or other antitumoral drugs might produce more favorable results.

There is no doubt that experimental studies have shown a number of partly interacting effects of Mab, cytokines, or cytostatics that might result in additive or synergistic antitumoral effects when combined with single drugs (Table 2a, b; Fig. 5). However, combination therapy does not necessarily mean improvement in any

Table 2a. Effects of cytokines TNF, IFN, and IL2 that might improve the antitumoral activity of Mab with ADCC, as summarized in the literature

TNF	↑ Natural killer (NK) cells ↑ Neutrophils ↑ Effector arm of ADCC ↑ Expression of HLA class I antigens
IL2	↑ Cytotoxicity of NK cells ↑ B-cell mediated antibody response ↑ Antigen-specific T cells ↑ Expression of HLA class antigens
IFN	↑ Monocyte Fc receptor ↑ NK cells ↑ Expression of HLA class I/II antigens ↑ Expression of tumor-associated antigens ↑ B-cell mediated antibody response ↑ ADCC by low-dose IFN

Table 2b. Summary of results from the literature indicating that the combination of cytostatics with Mab or cytokines might also improve the antitumoral effects of immunotherapy

Cytostatics	
Cis-Platin	↑ NK activity
Cyclophosphamide	↑ Anti-idiotypic Ab response
Actinomycin D	↑ Cytotoxicity of TNF
Mitomycin C + IL2	↑ Antitumor activity
Adriamycin + IFN	↑ Antitumor activity
Bleomycin + IFN	↑ Antiproliferative activity (synergistic)
Mitomycin C + IFN	↑ Antiproliferative activity (additional)
Mafosfamide + immunotoxin (i.t.)	↑ Antitumor activity

[1, 2, 4, 6, 10, 14–18, 35, 41, 42, 48, 50, 53, 58–61] ↑, increases or stimulates.

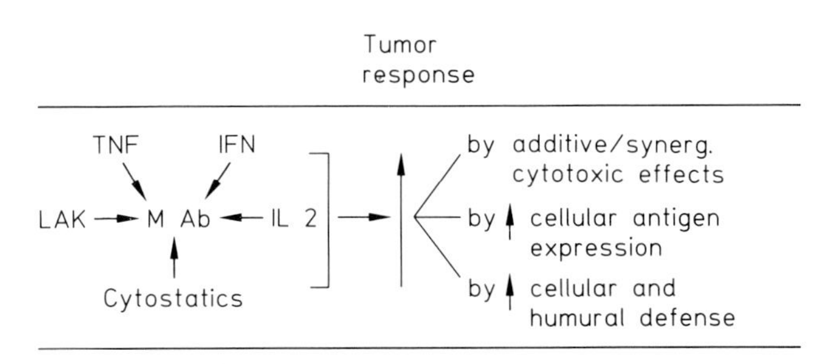

Fig. 5. Schema of potential interactions and additive/synergistic effects of combinations of Mab with cytokines and cytostatics. For definitions of abbreviations, see text

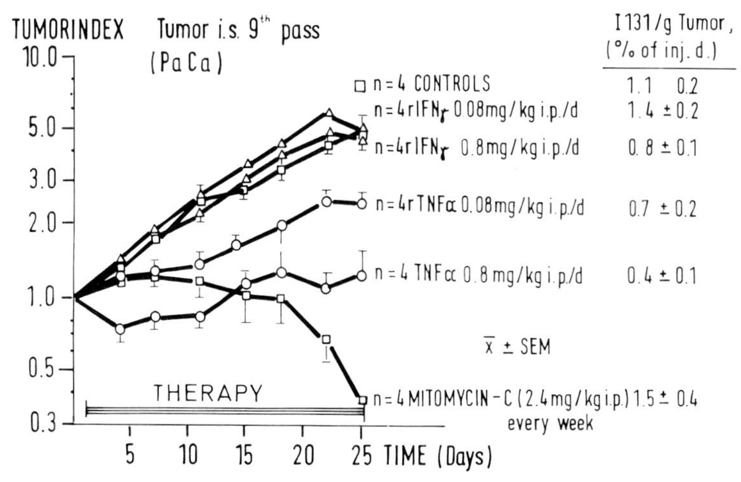

Fig. 6. Effects of treatment of xenografts of the pancreatic cancer ISCH 84 with low and high doses of rIFN-γ and rTNF-α, as well as mitomycin C, on tumor growth and tumor uptake of ^{131}I-labelled anti-CA 19-9. The radiolabelled Mab was injected i.v. 2 days before the animals were killed. Treatment duration, 21 days

case. Our studies of nude mice with human pancreatic carcinomas demonstrate that cytotoxic doses of rIFN-γ or rTNF-α may significantly inhibit tumor uptake of Mab, in this case ^{131}I-labelled anti-CA 19-9. A typical experiment is shown in Fig. 6. In this study, we treated pancreatic xenografts with low and high doses of rTNF-α and rIFN-γ or cytostatics for 3 weeks. Two days before the animals were killed we injected ^{131}I-labelled anti-CA 19-9 in order to measure the uptake of the Mab per unit of tumor weight in relation to the antitumoral activity of the different treatment regimens. In contrast to rTNF-α, treatment with mitomycin C, the most effective drug in this study, did not inhibit Mab uptake. Similar studies were performed to assess the uptake of ^{131}I-labelled BW 494/32 in different treatment regimens. In general, these studies confirmed the data presented in Fig. 6 (Fig. 7). These experiments therefore exemplify the possibility that high doses of these cytokines might decrease or inhibit the antitumoral effects of Mab with ADCC or radiolabelled Mab in the treatment of human xenografts or human tumors. In addition, they demonstrate that the effects of cytostatic or antiproliferative drugs on Mab uptake do not necessarily correlate with drug-induced inhibition of tumor growth.

Combinations of Mab, Cytokines and Cytostatics in Studies on Nude Mice with Xenografts of Human Gastrointestinal-Tract and Pancreatic Carcinomas

Based on these considerations and results, we started experiments in nude mice in order to look for potentially increased antitumoral effects of combinations of Mab with cytokines such as rTNF-α, rIFN-γ or combinations, interleukin 2 (IL2), and granulocyte-macrophage colony-stimulating factor (GM-CSF).

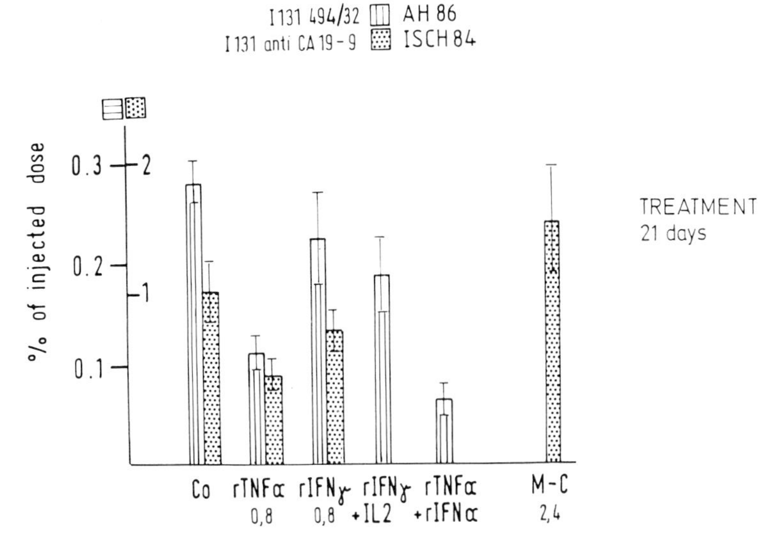

Fig. 7. Inhibition of tumor uptake of ^{131}I-labelled Mab BW 494/32 and anti-CA 19-9 by treatment of xenografts of human pancreatic carcinomas with rTNF-α or rIFN-γ, with combinations of cytokines, and with mitomycin-C. *Co,* controls; *0.8,* 0.8 mg/kg/day; *2.4,* 2.4 mg/kg/week; treatment duration, 21 days. The radiolabelled Mab were injected i.v. 2 days before the animals were killed

In spite of the problems known to hamper the extrapolation of experimental animal data to humans, the nude mouse represents an interesting model: About 90% of human gastrointestinal-tract of human tumors may be established in this animal, and xenografts show some important similarities to human tumors with respect to histology, grading, antigen expression, and tumor marker secretion [25, 27, 31]. Further, cytostatics, cytokines, and Mab may all be active in this model. Finally, similar to human tumors, the different xenografts show heterogeneous behavior after exposure to the various treatment modalities.

Mab and Cytokines

Some of our data are demonstrated in Fig. 8. In these studies, the combination of Mab with cytotoxic doses of rTNF-α or with rTNFα and rIFN-γ together did not enhance the antitumoral effect of the most effective single drug. Only the combination of Mab with rIFN-γ seems to result in a slightly increased effect. Preliminary studies with a combination of 17-1A and cytokines resulted in similar data.
These results might be explained by the experimental data shown in Figs. 6 and 7. In these studies, antiproliferative activity of rTNFα resulted in a significant decrease in Mab uptake into the tumor, which probably diminished the antitumoral activity of the Mab.

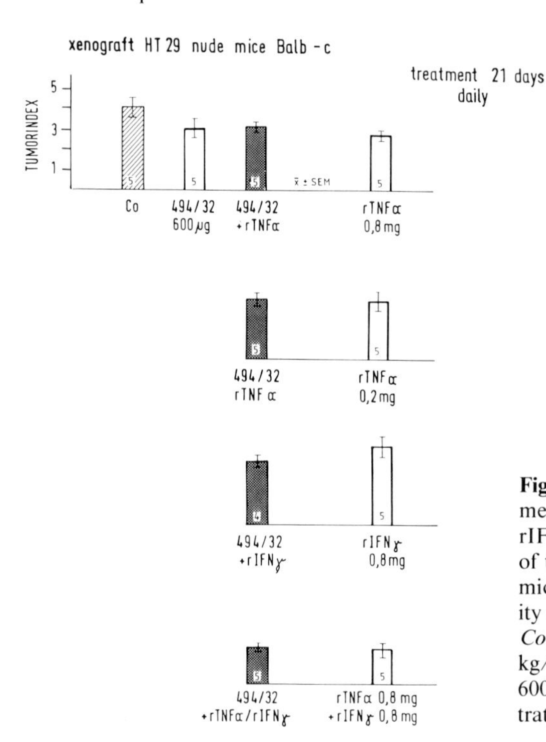

Fig. 8. Effects of combining Mab treatment with the cytokines rTNF-α and rIFN-γ on growth of established xenografts of the colorectal cell line HT 29 in nude mice, compared with the antitumoral activity of cytokines administered without Mab. *Co*, controls; *0.2 mg, 0.8 mg*, 0.2 or 0.8 mg/kg/day respectively for 21 days; *600* µg, 600 µg/day for 21 days; mode of administration, i.p.

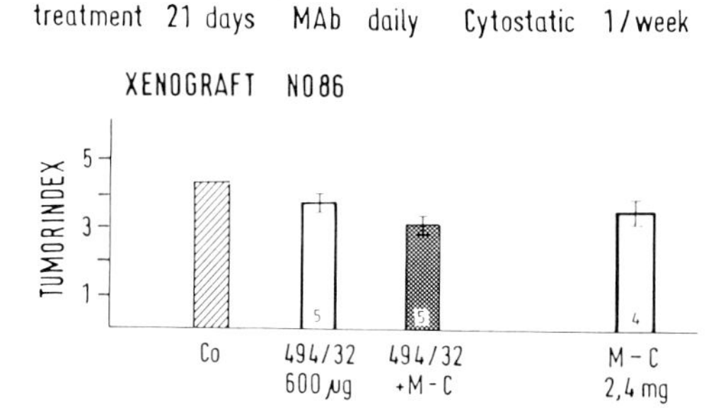

Fig. 9. Evidence for slightly enhanced antitumoral activity of BW 494/32 if combined with the cytostatic mitomycin C *(M-C)* in nude mice with established xenografts of the human colorectal carcinoma NO 86. *Co*, controls; *600* µg, 600 µg/day i.p.; *2.4 mg*, 2.4 mg/kg/week

Mab and Cytostatics

As shown in Fig. 9, the combination of Mab with mitomycin C showed a tendency toward increased antitumoral activity as compared with the drugs Mab BW 494/32 and mitomycin C when used singly. These results are in agreement with the results of the studies illustrated in Figs. 6 and 7, where mitomycin C did not induce a decrease in Mab uptake in spite of significant antitumoral activity.

Figure 10 shows the results of studies in which we investigated the potential value of combining the intratumoral administration of ^{131}I-labelled Mab for local antibody-mediated irradiation and systemic cytostatic treatment. These studies were based on (a) previous experiments demonstrating significant antitumoral effects of

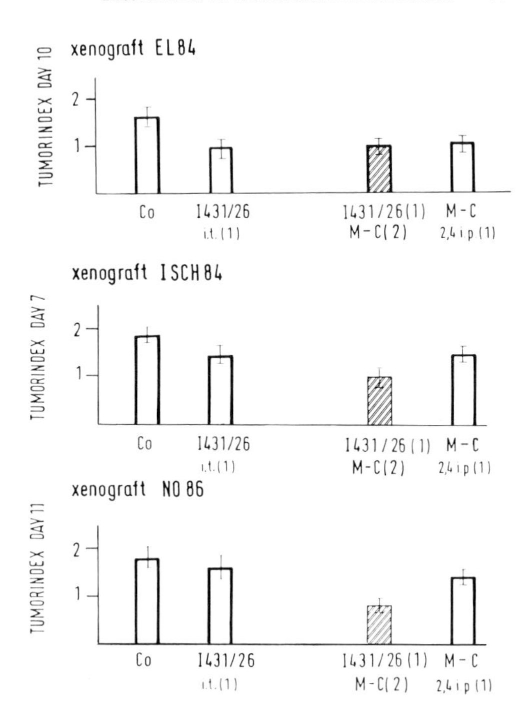

Fig. 10. Evidence in one (NO 86) of three tumors tested of synergistic effects resulting from a combination of intratumorally administered ^{131}I-labelled Mab BW 431/26 and mitomycin C. Dosages: 100 μCi ^{131}I-labelled Mab per 100 mm^3 tumor volume on day 1 *(1)*; 2.4 mg/kg mitomycin C i.p. on day 1 *(1)* or - in combination studies - on day 2 *(2)*

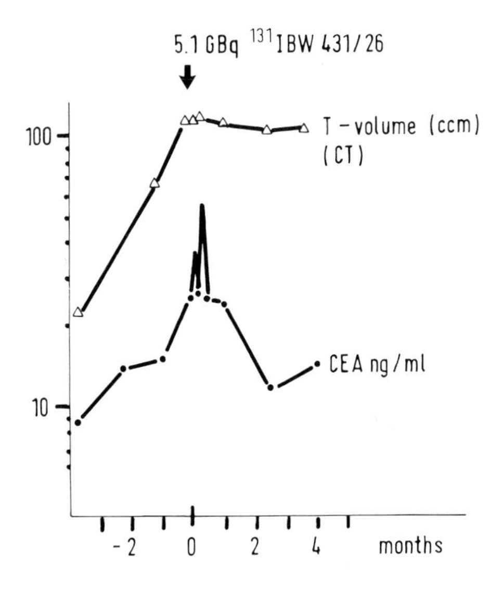

Fig. 11. Evidence for significant inhibition of tumor growth as determined by computerized tomography *(CT)* lasting 3-4 months of a metastasis of a colorectal carcinoma after intratumoral administration of 5.1 GBq ^{131}I-labelled Mab BW 431/26 (performed by fine-needle puncture guided by ultrasound). *CEA*, carcinoembryonic antigen

intratumorally administered radiolabelled Mab by direct irradiation [24] and (b) our first clinical investigations suggesting that intratumoral administration of radiolabelled Mab may also be active in humans (patients suffering from liver metastases due to gastrointestinal-tract cancer, Fig. 11) [46]. As shown in Fig. 10, intratumoral administration of ^{131}I-labelled Mab in combination with systemic

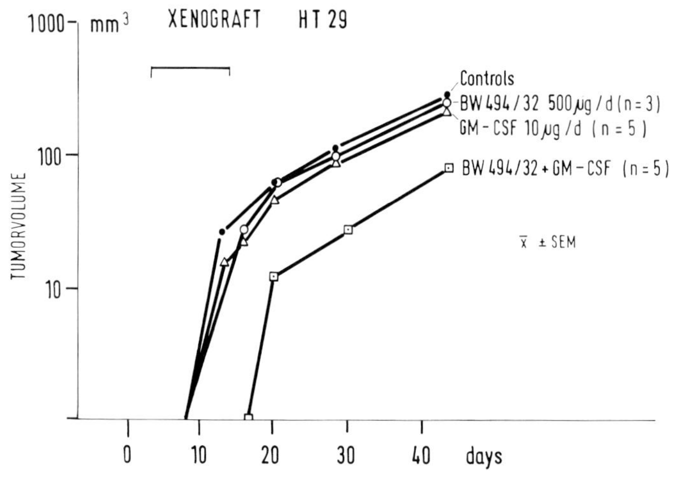

Fig. 12. Evidence for a slight increase in antitumoral activity of Mab BW 494/32 in combination with GM-CSF if applied in an "adjuvant" manner, i.e., when treatment is started immediately after transplantation of the xenografts of the cell line HT 29

mitomycin C treatment did not lead to a decrease in antitumoral activity. On the contrary, in two xenografts we found a significantly additive or synergistic effect. These data may be of clinical relevance, as they support the hypothesis that systemic Mab administration or local treatment of, for example, liver metastases may be initiated or performed simultaneously with systemic mitomycin C chemotherapy.

Mab and GM-CSF

Preliminary results of another experiment we have performed might also suggest that the combination of a Mab with ADCC and GM-CSF [43] might be of value (Fig. 12). The data presented in the figure reveal a more pronounced inhibition of the growth of freshly transplanted xenografts of the HT 29 cell line when BW 494/32 Mab was combined with 10 µg GM-CSF given i.p. over a period of 12 days. Studies with different GM-CSF doses, however, suggest dose-dependent effects. These preliminary data do not allow definitive conclusions at present, although they encourage further investigation of this combination.

Cytokines and Cytostatics

Combinations of cytokines and cytostatics seem to produce interesting results, as shown in Fig. 13, which summarizes data from studies in xenografts of human gastrointestinal-tract carcinomas. These data demonstrate additive and synergistic antitumoral effects of the combination of rTNF-α and mitomycin C, some of which were significant, as with tumors NO 86, ASCH 85, and CK 87.

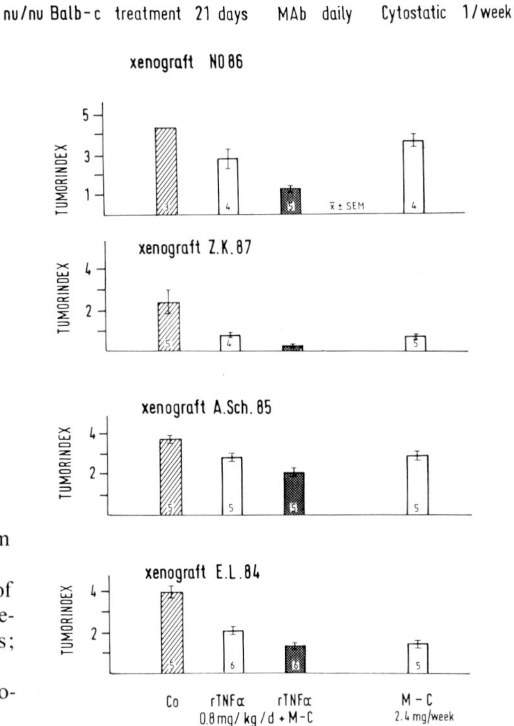

Fig. 13. Evidence for significantly increased antitumoral activity resulting from the combination of rTNF-α with mitomycin C administered i.p. to xenografts of various human gastrointestinal and pancreatic carcinomas in nude mice. *Co*, controls; *NO 86*, colorectal carcinoma; *Z.K.87*, *A.Sch. 85*, and *E.L.84*, pancreatic carcinoma

Summary

The concept of combining Mab with biological response modifiers or cytostatics represents an interesting approach to developing methods of improving the poor prognosis of gastrointestinal-tract cancers, to enhancing overall responsiveness of tumors to therapeutic agents, and to overcoming the important problem of the heterogeneous response of different tumors to a single drug. However, at present general recommendations cannot be given. Because of the complexity of the antitumoral defense system of the host, we are only beginning to elaborate this new concept. Much experimental and clinical work still remains to be done. At present, we can only hope that we will be able to improve the fate of these patients in the future by combining these different drug families.

References

1. Balkwill FR, Mowshowitz S, Seilman SS, Moodie EM (1984) Positive interactions between interferon and chemotherapy due to direct tumor action rather than effects on host drug-metabolizing enzymas. Cancer Res 44: 5249-5255
2. Balkwill FR, Proietti E, Stevonson MH, Bodmer J (1985) Use of an animal model to study the antitumor activity of human interferons. In: Stewart WE, Schellekens H (eds) The biology of the interferon system. Elsevier, Amsterdam, pp 379-382

3. Bartsch HH, Pfizemaier K, Rauschning W, Nagel G (1988) Tumor necrosis factor alpha administered i.m. or intratumoral in patients with advanced cancer. J Cancer Res Clin Oncol 114 [Suppl]: 44
4. Basham TY, Kaminski MS, Levy R, Merigan TC (1986) In vivo therapy of IFN and Mab for murine lymphoma. In: Stewart WE, Schellekens H (eds) The biology of the interferon system. Elsevier, Amsterdam, pp 389-395
5. Baum RP, Lorenz M, Senekowitsch R, Albrecht M, Hör G (1987) Klinische Ergebnisse der Immunszintigraphie und Radioimmuntherapie. Nuklearmedizin 26: 68-78
6. Berens ME, Saito T, Welander CE, Modest EJ (1987) Antitumor activity of new anthracycline analogues in combination with interferon alfa. Cancer Chemother Pharmacol 19: 301-306
7. Bosslet K, Kern HF, Kanzy EJ (1986) A monoclonal antibody with binding and inhibiting activity towards human pancreatic carcinoma cells. I. Immunohistological and immunochemical characterization of a murine monoclonal antibody selecting for well-differentiated adenocarcinomas of the pancreas. Cancer Immunol Immunother 23: 185-192
8. Büchler M, Kübel R, Malfertheiner P, Frieß H, Schulz G, Bosslet K, Beger HG (1988) Immuntherapie des fortgeschrittenen Pankreaskarzinoms mit dem monoklonalen Antikörper BW 494. Dtsch Med Wochenschr 113: 374-380
9. Chang BK (1983) Differential sensitivity of pancreatic adenocarcinoma cell lines to chemotherapeutic agents in culture. Cancer Treat Rep 67: 355-361
10. Dealtry GB, Naylo MS, Rubens RD, Padmanabhan N (1987) Effects of recombinant human interferon gamma on peripheral blood monocyte function. J Interferon Res 6 [Suppl 1]: 95
11. Dietel M, Arps H, Albrecht M, Simon WE, Klapdor R, Gerding D, Trapp M, Hölzel F (1986) Predictive determination of the sensitivity of gastrointestinal carcinomas to cytostatic drugs using the in vitro monolayer proliferation assay. In: Greten H, Klapdor R (eds) Clinical relevance of new monoclonal antibodies (3rd symposium on tumour markers, Hamburg). Thieme, Stuttgart, pp 447-455
12. Douillard JY, Lehur PA, Vignoud J, Blottière H, Maurel C, Thedrez P, Kremer M, LeMevel B (1986) Monoclonal antibody specific immunotherapy of gastrointestinal tumors. Hybridoma 5 [Suppl 1]: 139-149
13. Eggermont AM, Weimar W, Marquet RL, Lameris JD, Jeekel J (1985) Phase II trial of high-dose recombinant leukocyte alpha-2 interferon for metastatic colorectal cancer without previous treatment. Cancer Treat Rep 69: 185-187
14. Feinmann R, Henriksen-DeStefano D, Tsujimoto M, Vilcek J (1987) Tumor necrosis factor is an important mediator of tumor cell killing by human monocytes. J Immunol 138: 635-640
15. Fiers W, Brouckaert P, Guisez Y, Remaut E, van Roy F (1986) Recombinant interferon gamma and its synergism with tumor necrosis factor in the human and mouse systems. In: Stewart WE, Schellekens H (eds) The biology of the interferon system. Elsevier, Amsterdam, pp 241-248
16. Fransen L, v.d. Heyden J, Ruysschaert R, Fiers W (1986) Recombinant tumor necrosis factor: its effect and its synergism with IFN-g on a variety of normal and transformed human cell lines. Eur J Cancer Clin Oncol 22: 419-426
17. Giacomini P, Aguzzi A, Pestka S (1984) Modulation by recombinant DNA leukocyte (a) and fibroblast (b) interferons of the expression and shedding of HLA- and tumor associated antigens by human melanoma cells. J Immunol 133: 1649-1655
18. Greiner JW, Horan Hand P, Noguchi P, Fischer P, Pestka S, Schlom J (1984) Enhanced expression of surface tumor associated antigens on human breast and colon tumor cells after rIFN-αA treatment. Cancer Res 44: 3208-3214
19. Cudjonsson B (1987) Cancer of the pancreas - 50 years of surgery. Cancer 60: 2284-2303
20. Herlyn DM, Steplewski Z, Herlyn MF, Koprowski H (1980) Inhibition of growth of colorectal carcinoma in nude mice by monoclonal antibody. Cancer Res 40: 717-721
21. Ihse I, Isaksson G (1984) Pancreatic carcinoma: diagnosis and treatment. Clin Gastroenterol 13: 961-984
22. Klapdor R (1985) Clinical course and follow-up of patients suffering from pancreatic carcinoma. In: Greten H, Klapdor R (eds) New tumor-associated antigens (2nd symposium on tumour markers, Hamburg). Thieme, Stuttgart, pp 2-10
23. Klapdor R, Klapdor U, Bahlo M, Ufer Ch, Greten H (1986) Mitomycin and 5-fluorouracil in the treatment of xenografts of human pancreatic carcinomas. Dig Dis Sci 31: 1136

24. Klapdor R, Lander S, Bahlo M, Montz R (1986) Radioimmunotherapy of xenografts of human pancreatic carcinomas – intravenous and intratumoral application of ^{131}I-labelled monoclonal antibodies. Nuclearmedizin 25: 235–238
25. Klöppel G, Lingenthal G, Klapdor R, Klapdor U, von Bülow M, Rückert K, Kern HF (1986) Tumorgrading des menschlichen Pankreaskarzinoms im Nacktmausmodell und Resektionspräparat. In: Beger HG, Bittner R (eds) Das Pankreaskarzinom. Springer-Verlag, Berlin Heidelberg New York Tokyo, pp 97–106
26. Klapdor R, Lehmann U, van Ackeren H, Schreiber HW, Klöppel G, Greten H (1986) Chemotherapy des inoperablen Pankreaskarzinoms. In: Beger HG, Bittner R (eds) Das Pankreaskarzinom. Springer-Verlag, Heidelberg Berlin New York Tokyo, pp 401–419
27. Klapdor R, Bahlo M, Kühl JS, Lander S, Greten H, Ufer Chr, Dietel M, Montz R, Schreiber HW (1986) Xenografts of human pancreatic carcinomas in the nude mouse – a model for in vivo sensitivity tests against cytostatics, interferon, interleukin 2, TNF, monoclonal antibodies. In: Greten H, Klapdor R (eds) Clinical relevance of new monoclonal antibodies (3rd symposium on tumour markers, Hamburg). Thieme, Stuttgart, pp 435–446
28. Klapdor R, Kühl JS, Kunde C, Klapdor U, Arps H, Dietel M (1986) Therapy of pancreatic carcinomas with TNF and g-Interferon: studies on xenotransplants and tissue cultures. Dig Dis Sci 31: 1137
29. Klapdor R (1986) Neue Aspekte zur Chemotherapie des Pankreaskarzinoms. In: Nagel GA, Bach F, Bartsch HH (eds) Mitomycin-C 85: Klinik, Pharmakologie, Perspektive. Zuckschwerdt, Munich, pp 65–79
30. Klapdor R, Bahlo M, Schwarzenberg O, Riethmüller G (1987) Immunotherapy of exocrine pancreatic carcinoma xenografts in nude mice by the monoclonal antibody 17-1A. Dig Dis Sci 32: 1171
31. Klapdor R, Bahlo M, Dietel M, Montz R, Dimigen J (1987) Transplantation of exocrine pancreatic carcinomas to nude mice – a model to investigate immunoscintigraphy (^{131}I-anti-CA 19-9, anti-CEA, anti-CA 125), radioimmunotherapy and drug sensitivity. In: Rygaard J, Brünner N, Graem N, Spang-Thomson M (eds) Immune-deficient animals in biomedical research (5th international workshop on immune-deficient animals. Copenhagen). Karger, Basel, pp 390–395
32. Klapdor R, Guthoff A, Bahlo M, Schwarzenberg O, Hirschmann M (1987) Experimental and clinical aspects of immunotherapy of exocrine pancreatic cancer with BW 494/32. Dig Dis Sci 32: 1171
33. Klapdor R, Klapdor U, Montz R, Dietel M, Arps H, Schreiber HW, Greten H (1987) New tumor associated antigens and their monoclonal antibodies in the follow-up of exocrine pancreatic carcinoma. In: Greten H, Klapdor R (eds) New tumor-associated antigens and their monoclonal antibodies – actual relevance for diagnosis and therapy of solid tumors (4th symposium on tumor markers, Hamburg). Thieme, Stuttgart, pp 154–166
34. Klapdor R (1987) Treatment of pancreatic cancer with monoclonal antibodies with and without immunostimulation. In: Sugahara H (ed) New trends in gastroenterology: textbook of the second international symposium of the japanese society of gastroenterology, Kofu, Japan). pp 167–185
35. Klapdor R, Franke N, Bahlo M (1988) Combined therapy of xenografts of human colorectal and pancreatic carcinoma within mitomycin-C and rTNF-α. J Cancer Res Clin Oncol 114 [Suppl]: 45
36. Klapdor R, Montz R (1988) Clinical and immunological response to the therapy of pancreatic cancer with murine monoclonal antibodies. In: Epenetos AA, Oberhausen E, Reisfeld RA (eds) Immunotherapy and -scintigraphy of tumors with monoclonal antibodies. (Aktuelle Onkologie, vol 41). Zuckschwerdt, Munich, pp 87–100
37. Kühl JS, Klapdor R, Bahlo M, Arps H, Dietel M, Mohr H (1987) Effekte von Interleukin 2 und Lymphokin-aktivierten Killerzellen auf Zellkulturen sowie Transplantattumoren (Nacktmaus) humaner Pankreaskarzinome. Beitr Infusionsther Klinis Ernahr 18: 261–265
38. Kühl JS, Klapdor R, Bahlo M, Arps H, Dietel M (1987) Effects of gamma interferon and tumor necrosis factor on gastroinestinal and pancreatic tumors in vivo and in vitro under consideration of morphological and functional criteria. In: Greten H, Klapdor R (eds) New tumor-associated antigens and their monoclonal antibodies – actual relevance for diagnosis and therapy of solid tumors (4th symposium on tumor markers, Hamburg). Thieme, Stuttgart, pp 585–592

39. Kühl JS, Klapdor R, Arps H, Dietel M, Mohr H (1988) Cytokines and pancreatic cancer: I. The effect of rIFN-γ, HuLeIFN, rTNF-α and LAK cells on pancreatic and other gastrointestinal tumors in vitro. Int J Pancreatol (in press)
40. Kühl JS, Klapdor R, Bahlo M, Franke N, Kunde C, Arps H, Dietel M (1988) Cytokines and pancreatic cancer: II. Sensitivity of xenotransplants of predominantly pancreatic carcinomas to rIFN-γ and rTNF-α in nude mice. Int J Pancreatol (in press)
41. Lichtenstein AK, Pende D (1986) Enhancement of natural killer cytotoxicity by cis-diaminedichloroplatinum (II) in vivo and in vitro. Cancer Res 46: 639-644
42. Ligo M, Sakurai M, Saiji N, Hoshi A (1987) Synergistic effect of recombinant IL 2 on the inhibition of growth of adenocarcinoma 755 by mitomycin. Cancer Treat Rep 71: 567-570
43. Metcalf D (1985) The granulocyte-macrophage colony-stimulating factors. Science 229: 16-22
44. Montz R, Klapdor R, Rothe B, Heller M (1986) Immunoscintigraphy and radioimmunotherapy in patients with pancreatic carcinoma. Nuclearmedizin 25: 239-244
45. Moritz T, Niederle N, Kurschel E, May D, Osieka R, Schlick E, Schmidt CG (1988) Recombinant human tumor necrosis factor (rhuTNF) in the treatment of patients with advanced malignancies. J Cancer Res Clin Oncol 114 [Suppl]: 43
46. Müller-Gärtner HW, Montz R, Klapdor R, Spielmann R (1988) Radioimmunotherapie einer solitären Lebermetastase mittels intratumoraler Instillation des CEA-Antikörpers 131-J-BW 431/26. Nuklearmedizin 27: 35
47. Oettgen HF (1987) Interferone, Interleukin-2 and Tumor Nekrose Faktor. Neue Ansätze in der Krebsbehandlung. Drug Res 37: 251-255
48. Palladino M, Finkle B (1986) Immunopharmacology of tumor necrosis factor alpha and beta. TIPS 7: 388-389
49. Paul AR, Engström PF, Weiner LM, Steplweski Z, Koprowski H (1986) Treatment of advanced measurable or evaluable pancreatic carcinoma with 17-1A murine monoclonal antibody alone and in combination with 5-fluorouracil, adriamycin and mitomycin (FAM). Hybridoma 5 [Suppl 1]: 171-174
50. Pfizenmaier K, Bartschm H, Scheurich P, Seliger B, Ücer U, Vehmeyer K, Nagel G (1985) Inhibition of proliferation and modulation of immunogenicity as independent effects of g-interferon on tumor cell growth. Cancer Res 45: 3503-3509
51. Rayner AA, Grimm EA, Lotze MT, Chu EW, Rosenberg S (1985) Lymphokine-activated killer (LAK) cells. Analysis of factors relevant to the immunotherapy of human cancer. Cancer 55: 1327-1333
52. Sears HF, Herlyn D, Steplewski Z, Koprowski H (1985) Phase II clinical trial of a murine monoclonal antibody cytotoxic for gastrointestinal adenocarcinoma. Cancer Res 45: 5910-5915
53. Shaw ARE, Bleakley RC, Merryweather JP, Barr PJ (1985) Modulation of human natural killer cell activity by rIL 2. Cell Immunol 91: 193-200
54. Sherwin StA, Foon KA, Abrams PG, Heyman MR, Ochs JJ, Watson Th, Maluish A, Oldham RK (1984) A preliminary phase I trial of partially purified interferon-g in patients with cancer. J Biol Resp Mod 3: 599-607
55. Sindelar WF, Maher MM, Herlyn D, Sears HF, Steplewski Z, Koprowski H (1986) Trial of therapy with monoclonal antibody 17-1A in pancreatic carcinoma: preliminary results. Hybridoma 5 [Suppl 1]: 125-132
56. Sirinek KR, Aust JB (1986) Pancreatic cancer: Continuing diagnostic and therapeutic dilemma. Surg Clin North Am 66: 757-777
57. Tempero MA, Pour PM, Uchida E, Herlyn D, Zeplewski Z (1986) Monoclonal antibody CO 17-1A and leukopheresis in immunotherapy of pancreatic cancer. Hybridoma 5: 133-138
58. Trinchieri G, Kobayashi M, Rosen M, Loudon R, Murphy M, Perussia B (1986) Tumor necrosis factor and lymphotoxin induce differentiation of human myeloid cell lines in synergy with immune interferon. J Exp Med 164: 1206-1225
59. Uchida A, Vanky F, Klein E (1985) Natural cytotoxicity of human blood lymphocytes and monocytes and their cytotoxic factors: effect of interferon on target cell susceptibility. INCI 75: 849-857
60. Weil-Hillman G, Uckun FM, Manske JM, Vallera DA (1987) Combined immunochemotherapy of human solid tumors in nude mice. Cancer Res 47: 579-585
61. Weiner LM, Steplewski Z, Koprowski H, Sears HF (1986) Biologic effects of gamma interferon pre-treatment followed by monoclonal antibody 17-1A administration in patients with gastrointestinal carcinoma. Hybridoma 5 [Suppl 1]: 65-70

LYMPHOKINES

Cancer Treatment with Cytokines: Concepts and First Clinical Experience

A. LINDEMANN,[1] F. HERRMANN,[1] H. GAMM,[1] W. OSTER,[1] and R. MERTELSMANN[1]

Introduction

At present, the treatment of neoplastic disorders is based mainly on local surgical and radiotherapeutic means and the systemic use of cytotoxic drugs. The molecular basis of the differential sensitivity of cancer tissues for these drugs as compared with normal tissues remains, however, largely undefined. It has been postulated that differences in the kinetics of cell proliferation are the basis of this differential sensitivity. This has been demonstrated convincingly, however, for very few neoplastic diseases. Alternative explanations of chemotherapeutic efficacy include a relative decrease in efficient repair mechanisms in cancer cells, as well as chemotherapy-induced reduction of growth factor release, which is required for the proliferation of tumor cells. So far, chemotherapy remains the mainstay for the treatment of disseminated cancer. However, results of chemotherapy have remained largely disappointing, and cure rates been stagnating, especially for the more frequent cancers, such as lung, breast, and colon cancer [1]. Therefore, current researchers are looking for new concepts of cancer treatment based on a more profound understanding of tumor biology.

The oncogenetic defect in neoplastic disease appears to be a genetic alteration in the primordial cancer cell, which subsequently leads to clonal expansion and, in many instances, to clonal evolution with additional genetic alterations, leading to a proliferative advantage of cancer cells. Oncogenetic changes can be induced by different agents, such as viruses, ionizing radiation, or other substances altering the gene structure and expression. In addition, spontaneous genetic rearrangements leading to oncogenic growth seem probable, particularly in situations of proliferative stress. This oncogenetic change leads to a quantitatively or qualitatively abnormal production of proteins, which play a central role in the regulation of cell growth and differentiation. Molecules likely to be involved in this scenario include growth factors, their receptors, cytoplasmic transmitter molecules, or DNA-binding proteins regulating gene expression. Many of these key proteins have been identified, and aberrant expression in various experimental tumor systems has generated the term "proto-oncogenes" [2]. Once the oncogenic alteration has led to neoplastic transformation, the balance of gene expression is altered [3]. The transformed cell, however, does not appear truly autonomous in its growth, but remains, like its normal counterpart, dependent on interaction with physiolog-

[1] Department of Hematology, University Clinic Mainz, Langenbeckstraße 1, 6500 Mainz, FRG.

H. G. Beger et al. (Eds.), Cancer Therapy

ical systems of the host organism, as with for example the dependence on growth factors and/or hormones reminiscent of parasitic infections [4]. Thus, the alterations rendering a cell malignant seem to be very subtle and are often even imperceptible to the immune system. Only a small percentage of human cancers have been shown to be immunogenic. Immunogenicity of malignant cells occurs when the mutation-inducing malignancy involves a membrane protein or when the alteration of gene expression leads to cellular expression of previously hidden cryptic antigens.

This background information makes some basic approaches to cancer treatment possible. One promising, although complex strategy is the manipulation of the disturbed regulation of cancer cell growth and differentiation to restore growth and differentiation to a normal or nearly normal state by substituting regulatory factors that may be missing. Different efforts aimed at stimulating host defense mechanisms against cancer are already under intensive investigation, while the amelioration of the bone marrow toxicity of chemotherapy by means of factors that stimulate hematopoietic growth - probably the most feasible approach - has just begun to be studied.

A possible tool useful in all the approaches just described may be the therapeutic use fo cytokines. These are hormone-like polypeptides involved in intercellular communication of virtually all cell types capaple of regulating proliferation, differentiation, and functional activity. Thus, basic cellular functions related to both normal and neoplastic traits are under the control of these molecules. Some of the mediators identified so far are primarily involved in the regulation of immune responses, inflammatory reactions, and the control of hematopoiesis. Conceptually, therapeutic approaches with cytokines can be instrumental in cancer therapy in three ways:

1. Stimulation of the immune system in order to increase host immunity to cancer (e.g. interleukin 2)
2. Modulation of tumor cell growth and differentiation via cytotoxic, cytostatic or regulatory mechanisms (e.g., tumor necrosis factor and interferon)
3. Stimulation of nonspecific host restistance and amelioration of the side effects of the intensive cancer treatment as practiced today (e.g., colony stimulating factors and erythropoietin)

Such a classification remains artificial, especially with regard to the pleiotropic and contingent effects of cytokines. All these factors can have both growth-stimulating and -inhibitory properties, depending on the functional state of the respective target cell, receptor affinity, receptor density, and concentration of the ligand. In addition, it has become increasingly clear that the original hypothesis "one producer cell - one target cell" no longer reflects biological reality. Recent research has shown that a given cytokine can be produced by multiple cell types and that its effects can be exerted on multiple target cell types. Therefore, clinical studies of cytokines are very complex when compared with the clinical evaluation of cytotoxic drugs. Furthermore, cytotoxic drugs are generally used at their maximal tolerated dose, while the maximal tolerated dose of cytokines is not the optimal biological response-modifying dose, in many instances. Thus, it is necessary to take into account that the tumor-host interaction is an integral part of a coordi-

nated regulatory network of normal cells and cytokines similar to the endocrine system. Moreover, modulation of one parameter will frequently generate a broad spectrum of indirect effects via activation of target cells and the secondary release of other cytokines.
Among the cytokines studied in vivo so far, interferon-alpha has already demonstrated clinical activity, particularly in the treatment of hairy cell leukemia [5], chronic myelogenous leukemia [6], and, to a lesser extent, in certain solid tumors that are largely refractory to conventional chemotherapy, such as malignant melanoma, renal cell cancer, superficial bladder cancer, and cancer of the ovary [7-11]. Most other cytokines are still in the early stages of clinical evaluation. Interleukin 2 (IL-2) and tumor necrosis factor-alpha (TNF-alpha) have been evaluated most extensivly in patients with cancer, while granulocyte-macrophage colony-stimulating factor (GM-CSF) and granulocyte colony-stimulating factor (G-CSF) have so far been evaluated primarily in chemotherapy-induced pancytopenias. The following review will focus on IL-2, TNF-alpha, GM-CSF and G-CSF, which are the agents currently under extensive investigation in our department and other institutions in the United states and Europe.

Interleukin 2

IL-2 is probably the most important example of an agent that works primarily through the stimulation of immunity against tumor cells. It appears to have clinical activity with or without in vitro lymphokine-activated killer (LAK) cells or low doses of cyclophosphamide (LD-CP) in malignant melanoma and, possibly, in malignant lymphoma, while the combination of IL-2 with LAK cells appears to be necessary for therapeutic responses in renal cell cancer. Our own multicenter study has confirmed that partial responses can be obtained with tolerable doses of IL-2 in combination with LD-CP in malignant melanoma, while only mixed responses were seen in renal cell cancer [12].
The T-cell product IL-2 ist involved in the proliferation and the functional activation of immune competent cells, which also appear to play a central role in the surveillance and elimination of tumor cells. In an autocrine pathway, IL-2 is active as a growth factor and functional activator for T-helper cells. In a paracrine pathway, IL-2 stimulates natural killer (NK) cells, preactivated cytotoxic T cells, B cells, and macrophages [13]. To exert its function, IL-2 has to bind to a specific target structure, the IL-2 receptor. The IL-2 receptor is a bimolecular structure consisting of an alpha-chain of 55 kD and a beta-chain of 75 kD [14]. Both chains form a dimer with a 100-fold higher affinity for IL-2 than the single chains. Resting T cells or NK cells do not express high-affinity IL-2 receptors and therefore do not respond to physiological serum concentrations of IL-2 unless activated. Higher concentrations of IL-2 (100 units/ml), however, are capable of activating NK cells and, to a certain extent, also T cells to synthesize alpha-chains, which then form dimers with preexisting beta-chains and lead to subsequent proliferation and activation of cytotoxic functions [15]. IL-2-activated, cytotoxic T cells (like NK cells) are capable of binding to tumor target cells via nonspecific adhesion structures, such as leukocyte function-associated antigen LFA-1 or LFA-2

(equivalent to the cluster designated CD-2) or CD-16, in addition to the interaction via the antigen-specific T-cell receptor with its target antigens.
The phenomenon of IL-2-induced, lymphocyte-mediated tumor lysis in vitro and in vivo has been extensivly studied by Grimm and Rosenberg, who coined the term "lymphokine-activated killer cell phenomenon" (LAK), [16]. Investigations in various murine models have demonstrated that, by administration of ex vivo activated cytotoxic cells (LAK cells), tumor regressions can be achieved in a variety of tumor models, in particular when combined with the systemic application of IL-2 [17]. When administered at very high doses as a single agent, IL-2, was also capable of inducing LAK activity leading to tumor regressions in certain model systems in vivo [18].
The promising results that have been obtained in the murine tumor models have led to the development of similar strategies in man. First clinical studies with purified IL-2 at the National Cancer Institute of the United States in Bethesda, Maryland [19], as well as at Memorial Sloan-Kettering Cancer Center in New York [20], failed to exhibit significant tumor regressions, although immunomodulatory effects were clearly demonstrated. These observations included the activation of T and NK cells, as well as the polyclonal expansion of IL-2 receptor-positive T lymphocytes in vivo. Subsequent studies using recombinant IL-2 with or without the simultaneous administration of ex vivo IL-2-activated killer cells have been pursued at the National Cancer Institute as well as at other institutions [21]. A different strategy has focused on combination therapy with low-dose cyclophosphamide and IL-2. These two agents have been shown in animal models to act synergistically to eliminate tumor metastasis [22]. This approach was explored in a study at Memorial Sloan-Kettering Cancer Center [23] and in a recently completed cooperative trial in the Federal Republik of Germany [12]. While the original study [23] had shown reproducible immune stimulation in the majority of patients, no remissions were observed. The German study, using a threefold higher dose of IL-2, is currently undergoing evaluation. Preliminary analysis has demonstrated a partial remission rate of approximately 20% in malignant melanoma, with no partial remissions observed in renal cell carcinoma. However, mixed responses (the disappearance of some metastases with continued growth of other metastases) were also observed in patients with metastatic renal cell cancer.
The NCI protocol [21] uses a much higher IL-2 dose, administered as a 30-min infusion every 8 h for 5 days. After 2 days without therapy, during which a rebound lymphocytosis occurs lymphocytes are harvested by leukapheresis. These cells are subquently cultivated in vitro and stimulated by a high concentration of IL-2 to induce LAK activity. In the NCI study, partial remissions were seen in 30% of the patients with malignant melanoma with both approaches, high-dose IL-2 alone as well as with the combination of IL-2 and LAK cells. In renal cell cancer, high-dose IL-2 alone has not yielded significant antitumor responses, while the combination of IL-2 with LAK cells resulted in 20% partial remissions [21]. Using a modified protocol, West et al. [24], reported similar response rates using a continuous infusion schedule for IL-2 in combination with LAK cells, which appears to be much better tolerated than the NCI protocol. Interestingly, mixed responses have been seen in all studies, suggesting that the sensivity of metastases depends on their anatomic location. Whether this is due to differential gene expression or

clonal evolution in different metastatic sites or to the anatomic distribution itself, resulting in a differential accessibility to killer cells, remains to be determined.

Side effects of IL-2 treatment with or without LAK cells are dose-related and consist of fever and chills, presumably caused by endogenous induction of IL-1 [25]. The dose-limiting toxicity in all trials was a capillary leakage syndrome, resulting in interstitial pulmonary edema in some patients. The pathophysiological basis of this IL-2-associated syndrome is not completely understood at this time. Similar symptoms can also be seen at higher doses in patients receiving TNF, probably because both cytokines have the capacity to induce interferon-gamma [26]. Most IL-2-associated side effects are clearly dose dependent and are rapidly reversible upon discontinuation of IL-2 administration, as is also true for the limited but definite bone marrow toxicity. Both anemia and thrombocytopenia have been observed. Bone marrow toxicity, however, does not appear to be dose limiting. Biological effects include a polyclonal expansion of IL-2 receptor positive T lymphocytes and of natural killer activity, as well as a considerable bone marrow and blood eosinophilia, which is probably caused by endogenous induction of IL3, IL-5, and GM-CSF.

Pharmacokinetics of IL-2 have demonstrated a half-life of approximately 30 min. The inactivation appears to occur in the kidneys with a biologically inactive metabolite excreted in the urine. The i.v. infusion over 2 h of 3×10^6 units/m^2 IL-2 induces serum concentrations of more than 300 units/ml, which fall to 20 units/ml within 4 h. Long-term concentrations of 15 units/ml can be achieved by continuous infusion or subcutaneous administration [27].

Although the clinical responses have been dramatic at times, overall therapeutic results have not been satisfactory. It remains to be determined whether better tolerated and more effective schedules of IL-2 administration with or without the combination with in vitro activated killer cells can be developed. It also remains to be studied whether the activated killer cells, which presumably are responsible for killing cancer cells in vivo, also cause the major side effects of IL-2, which consist of damage to endothelial cells and the capillary leakage syndrome. Further studies are focusing on the characterization and cloning of specific killer cell populations and include patients with smaller tumor burdens. Other approaches currently under investigation deal with combinations of IL-2 with conventional chemotherapeutic agents, bifunctional monoclonal antibodies, and other cytokines, including interferon-alpha and -gamma, TNF, and IL-4.

Tumor Necrosis Factor

An example of a cytokine demonstrating direct antitumor effects in vitro and in vivo against a broad spectrum of tumor cell types is the tumor necrosis factor (TNF-alpha). This molecule, which was first characterized molecularly be Carswell et al. in 1975 [28], is a product of activated macrophages. It is functionally characterized by the induction of hemorrhagic necrosis in the meth-a-sarcoma of mice. T lymphocytes, B lymphocytes, and neutrophil granulocytes also can secrete this molecule under appropriate conditions of induction [29]. In view of its dramatic effect in the meth-a-sarcoma model, as well as its activity in various other in vitro models, TNF has been intensively evaluated with respect to antitumor activity in various tumor models and also, more recently, in humans. However, its primary physiological role appears to be the mediation of inflammatory and immune reactions. A variety of laboratory studies in recent years have shown that TNF stimulates both the antibody-dependent cytotoxicity of neutrophil granulocytes and their functional repertoire, including oxygen radical production. Furthermore, it induces cytotoxicity in monocytes and in NK cells and modulates IL-2 receptor expression and interferon-gamma production by T cells [30–33]. Other properties of TNF include induction of adhesion molecules, cell surface differentiation antigens, and major histocompatibility complex (MHC) molecules, as well as the induction of other cytokines, such as IL-1, IL-6, CSF, and of growth and activation inducing factors for platelets in receptive target cells [34, 35].

In vivo studies in murine model systems using recombinant TNF-alpha have produced nearly identical results to those previously obtained with natural TNF. In vitro, recombinant TNF exhibits both cytotoxic and cytostatic effects on a broad spectrum of tumor cell lines derived from different tissues. In contrast, normal diploid renal cells, melanocytes, colon epithelium, endothelial cells, and fibroblasts have been shown to be TNF restistant in vitro. Since TNF-alpha exerts direct antitumor effects and serves as a costimulant for activated immuno competent cells [33, 36], the clinical evaluation in cancer patients has seemed promising.

In phase I studies at the M. D. Anderson Hospital in Houston, Texas, [37] and in our own department [38], TNF-alpha was administered in different schedules with dose increases from 1 to 400 μg/m^2 per day. Peak serum concentrations of TNF during 30-min i. v. infusions reach 10 pg/ml, while by i. m. application of the same dose, up to 5 pg/ml were achieved. The half-life of intravenous TNF-alpha was 14–18 min with a dose-dependent increase up to 30 min at higher TNF doses. The clinical side effects of TNF-alpha appear somewhat similar to those previously described for IL-2. However, even at lower doses, fever and chills dominate the clinical picture; the dose-limiting toxicity is fluid retention, probably due to a capillary leakage syndrome, similar to that occurring in patients treated with IL-2. Intramuscular injection of TNF-alpha can cause local irritation at the injection site. While TNF is being infused, a rapid disappearence of neutrophils from the circulation can be observed, probably due to the induction of adhesion structures on endothelial cells and neutrophils, leading to a rapid redistribution of white blood cells. White blood cell counts quickly recover to normal within 30–60 min after discontinuation of TNF infusion. No significant hematological toxicity of TNF was observed.

In our own recently completed phase I clinical trial of recombinant human TNF-alpha in 65 patients with advanced cancer, the maximum tolerated dose of TNF was found to be 200 μg/b. i. d. Tumor responses were induced only sporadically. Partial remissions in one patient with colon cancer and one patient with pancreatic cancer were observed. Stable disease lasting for 10 months was seen in an additional patient with colon cancer. No significant tumor regressions were seen in a broad spectrum of other malignancies. The maximum tolerated dose for an injection of TNF was consistently shown to be 200 μg/m^2, while our own schedule of administration twice daily allowed a total daily dose of 400 μg/m^2 given by two injections 6 h apart. In spite of these high doses of TNF, the overall antitumor effects were unsatisfactory. When considering the data reported by other investigators, [37, 39], colorectal cancers and renal cell cancers might be targets for future phase II studies, although our own conclusion has been that TNF alone is unlikely to be of major benefit to patients with cancer. It has to be concluded that the great expectations with respect to TNF, which were awakened by its very designation, have not been fulfilled. It remains to be seen whether higher doses of TNF can be administered with better control of side effects or whether combinations of TNF with IL-2 or other biological response-modifying agents will lead to more frequent and more predictable antitumor effects.

Granulocyte-Macrophage Colony-Stimulating Factor

GM-CSF is a member of the family of hematopoietic growth factors that regulate proliferation, differentiation, and functional activation of hematopoietic progenitor cells [40]. The clinical use of growth factors in cancer therapy depends on objectives different from those of cytotoxic or immune stimulatory factors. Preclinical investigations of GM-CSF in a primate model [41] have demonstrated that GM-CSF promises to reduce the chemotherapy-associated morbidity, which is caused by neutropenia-associated infections. In clinical situations where bone marrow toxicity is the dose-limiting factor of a cytotoxic drug, GM-CSF treatment might lead to increased bone marrow capacity, allowing more frequent administration of chemotherapy or the administration of higher doses. In the setting of autologous bone marrow transplantation, the clinical evaluation of GM-CSF appears to be worthwhile. In addition, it has been shown that GM-CSF stimulates the activation of granulocytes and macrophages, which could induce indirect and direct antitumor effects. For example, GM-CSF induces the release of tumoricidal molecules, such as TNF-alpha, by monocytes [42] and stimulates antibody-dependent cytotoxicity of granulocytes as well as oxygen radical formation and cytotoxicity of monocytes [43, 44]. Groopman and colleagues [45] have demonstrated in vivo biological activity of GM-CSF in leukopenic patients with AIDS. In our own phase I clinical study [46], 20 cancer patients refractory to chemotherapy have received recombinant GM-CSF at six dose levels ranging 30 to 1000 $\mu g/m^2$ per day in 5-day and 14-day cycles given by i.v. bolus injection as well as by 24-h continuous infusion. A broad spectrum of reproducible and predictable hematological effects were observed. The continuous infusion of 1000 $\mu g/ml$ GM-CSF over 14 days resulted in a 17-fold increase in total white blood counts consisting predominantly of neutrophil granulocytes, with increased numbers of eosinophils and monocytes as well. Bone marrow cellularity was highly increased. In doses of 500 $\mu g/m^2$ and above, an increase of circulating myeloid progenitor cells could be demonstrated. No significant effect was observed on circulating lymphocytes, platelets, or reticulocytes. Within 1 week of discontinuing GM-CSF, leukocyte counts returned to baseline. Compared with other cytokines, GM-CSF treatment was associated with minor side effects. Toxicity was observed in four patients at higher doses, consisting of dyspnea during the 30 min infusion, possibly related to rapid redistribution of neutrophils into the pulmonary circulation, associated with a temporary decrease in circulating neutrophils. The enhancement of leukocyte-

endothelial cell interactions by GM-CSF could be the basis for this clinical effect [47]. All side effects were, however, rapidly reversible.
Although objective tumor responses were not seen in patients receiving GM-CSF, both our own early data with GM-CSF after chemotherapy and data obtained at Memorial Sloan-Kettering Cancer Center in a similar study with G-CSF [48] strongly support the hypothesis that the administration of one of the CSFs will significantly reduce chemotherapy-associated neutropenia.

Granulocyte Colony-Stimulating Factor

The second CSF, currently undergoing phase I and II clinical evaluation, is granulocyte CSF (G-CSF). This 175-amino-acid protein has a molecular weight of about 18800 kD. The recombinant human G-CSF produced by Amgen (Thousand Oaks, California) differs from the natural protein in one amino acid, and it is not glycosylated. G-CSF is a hematopoietic regulator, which has the ability to promote the growth and maturation of myeloid cells and, in particular, the proliferation and differentiation of granulocytes both in vitro as well as in vivo. Human G-CSF has recently been purified [49], molecularly cloned, and successfully expressed in a cell line [50], allowing production of large quantities of purified, recombinant human (rhG-CSF). Highly purified human G-CSF and rhG-CSF have identical biological activity in vitro [50] and have effects on immature bone marrow progenitors, terminally differentiated myeloid cells, and leukemic myeloid cells in vitro. In preclinical studies, rhG-CSF has been shown to induce significant rises in neutrophil counts, which are dose-dependent, reproducible, and predictable both in a normal hamster model and in a primate model [51, 52]. It has also been shown that drug- or irradiation-induced cytopenia in the primate model can be significantly reduced by the simultaneous or subsequent administration of G-CSF. Interestingly, G-CSF has differentiation-inducing activity on malignant myeloid progenitor cells, which has also recently been demonstrated in the murine WEHI-3b (D^+) myelomonocytic tumor cell line. In this model, the survival of mice with this type of leukemia was significantly prolonged when G-CSF was administered [50]. In our own phase I study of recombinant G-CSF, very few side effects were observed, achieving neutrophil counts of up to $50000/m^3$ at doses of 30 μg/kg, while at higher doses, thrombocytopenia might be dose limiting. In a phase I/II study of the combination of G-CSF with chemotherapy in bladder cancer using the M-VAC protocol, prevention of neutropenia has also been demonstrated [48].

Cytokines in Cancer Therapy

While interferon alpha is established in the management of a selected, small group of patients with cancer, CSFs may well play a role in supportive care. The use of GM-CSF and G-CSF in cancer patients is at present the main focus of our clinical efforts. Evaluation of the stimulatory effects of cytokines on normal hematopoiesis in vivo has shown dose/response curves for both GM-CSF and G-CSF in vivo. White blood cell counts of up to $50000/mm^3$ can be obtained with either agent with minimal side effects. Thus, reduction of chemotherapy-associated neutropenia seems probable according to preliminary clinical data. Further studies will have to analyze whether the additional application of CSFs to reduce therapy-related morbidity and to allow more aggressive treatment protocols will make possible higher cure rates in patients treated by chemo- or radiotherapy. Whether erythropoietin will also reduce transfusion requirements in anemic cancer patients remains to be determined.

The clinical results with those cytokines thought to demonstrate direct tumoristatic or tumoricidal effects have so far been largely disappointing. The intercellular network of amplifying mechanisms in vivo is insufficiently understood, resulting in unpredictable side effects and a lack of predictable antitumor effects, except with the administration of interferon-alpha in hairy cell leukemia and chronic myeloid leukemia. The heterogeneity of tumors and their respective hosts is of major relevance, since all murine in vivo results have only been reproducible in specific strains of mice and in cloned tumor cell lines that do not reflect the complexity of the human organism. A definite place for IL-2 and TNF as single agents appears somewhat unlikely at this point, although remissions have been seen in a number of patients. The future for those agents, which predominantly suppress or kill tumor cells, will probably be in combination therapy, which has proven advantageous in the case of chemotherapy in the majority of sensitive tumors.

Further research is needed on the cytokine cascade to allow better control of side effects accompanying directly cytotoxic factors. This could enable higher doses to be applied, leading to higher efficacy. In addition, better parameters for measuring biological responses associated with tumor regression appear to be crucial before the development of these agents can proceed more successfully. At present, the factors stimulating hematopoiesis, which, in addition to GM-CSF and G-CSF, include erythropoietin and other factors, promise at least a palliative benefit for many cancer patients in the near future.

References

1. Bailar JC, Smith EM (1986) Progress against cancer? N Engl Med J 314: 1226
2. Vogt PK (1987) Oncogenes and signals of cell growth. Drug Res 37: 243
3. Goyette M, Petrapoulos CJ, Shank PR, Fausto N (1983) Expression of a cellular oncogene during liver regeneration Science 219: 510
4. Dvorak HF (1986) Tumors: wounds that do not heal. Similarities between tumor stroma generation and wound healing. N Engl J Med 315: 1651
5. Goulomb H, Jacobs A, Fefer A, Ozer H, Thompson J, Portlock C, Ratain M, Golde D, Vardiman J, Burke JS, Brady J, Bonnem E, Spiegel R (1986) Alpha-2 interferon therapy of hairy cell leukemia: a multicenter study of 64 patients. J Clin Oncol 4: 900
6. Talpaz M, Kantarjian HM, Mc Credie K, Trujillo JM, Keating MJ, Gutterman JU (1986) Hematologic remission and cytogenetic improvement induced by recombinant human interferon alpha in chronic myelogenous leukemia. N Engl J Med 314: 1065
7. Ozer H, Anderson JR, Peterson BA, Budman DR, Henderson ES, Bloomfield CD, Gottlieb A (1987) Combination trial of subcutaneous interferon alpha-2b and oral cyclophosphamide in favorable histology, non-Hodgkin's lymphoma. Invest New Drugs 5: 27
8. Robinson WA, Mughal TI, Thomas MR, Johnson M, Spiegel RJ (1986) Treatment of metastatic malignant melanoma with recombinant interferon alpha 2. Immunobiol 172: 275

9. Muss HB, Constanzi JJ, Leavitt R, Williams RD, Kempf RA, Pollard R, Ozer H, Zekan PJ, Grunberg SU, Metchell US, Caponera M, Gavigan M, Ernest ML, Venturi C, Greiner J, Spiegel RJ (1987) Recombinant alpha interferon in renal cell carcinoma: a randomized trial of two routes of administration. J Clin Oncol 5: 286
10. Torti FM, Lum BL, Aston D, MacKenzie N, Faysel M, Shortliffe LD, Freiha F (1986) Superficial bladder cancer: the primacy of grade in the development of invasive disease. Sem Oncol 8 [Suppl 2]: 57
11. Berek JS, Hacker NF, Lichtenstein A, Jung T, Spina C, Knox RM, Brady J, Greene T, Ettinger LM, Lagasse LD, Bonnem EM, Spiegel RJ, Zighelboim J (1985) Intraperitoneal recombinant alpha-interon for "salvage" immunotherapy in stage III epithelial overarin cancer: a gynecologic oncology group study. Cancer Res 45: 4447
12. Lindemann A, Oster W, Schmidt RE, Höffken K, Herrmann F, Mertelsmann R (1988) Phase-II-Studie mit rekombinantem humanen Interleukin 2 bei Patienten mit malignem Melanom und Hypernephrom. Klin Wochenschr [Suppl] 66: 252 (abstract 551)
13. Waldmann TA (1986) The structure, function, and expression of interleukin-2 receptors on normal and malignant lymphocytes. Science 232: 727
14. Wang HM, Smith (1987) The interleukin-2 receptor. J Exp Med 166: 1055
15. Siegel JP, Sharon M, Smith KL, Leonard WJ (1987) The IL-2 receptor beta chain (p70): role in mediating signals for LAK, NK and proliferative activities. Sciene 238: 75
16. Grimm EA, Mazumder A, Zhang HZ, Rosenberg S (1981) Lymphokine activated killer cell phenomenon. Lysis of natural killer-resistant fresh solid tumor cells by interleukin-2 activated autologous human peripheral blood lymphocytes. J Exp Med 155: 1823
17. Mule JJ, Shu S, Schwarz L, Rosenberg SA (1984) Adoptive immunotherapy of established pulmonary metastases with LAK cells and recombinant interleukin-2. Science 255: 1487
18. Rosenberg SA, Mule JJ, Spiess PJ, Reichert CM, Schwarz SL (1985) Regression of established pulmonary metastases and subcutaneous tumor mediated by the systemic administration of high-dose recombinant interleukin-2. J Exp Med 161: 1169
19. Lotze UT, Frana LW, Sharrow SO, Robb RJ, Rosenberg SA (1985) In vivo administration of purified human interleukin-2. I. Half life and immunologic effects of the Jurkat cell line-derived interleukin-2. J Immunol 134: 157
20. Kolitz JE, Welte K, Wong GY, Holloway K, Merluzzi VJ, Enger A, Bradley EC, Konrad M, Polivka A, Gabrilove JL, Sykora FW, Miller GA, Fiedler W, Krown S, Oettgen HF, Mertelsmann R (1987) Polyclonal expansion of activated T-lymphocytes in patients treated with recombinant interleukin-2. J Biol Response Mod 6: 412
21. Rosenberg SA, Lotze MT, Muul LM, Chang AE, Avis FP, Leitman S, Lineken WM, Robertson GN, Lee RE, Rubin JT, Seipp CA, Simpson CG, White DE (1987) A progress report on the treatment of 157 patients with advanced cancer using lymphokine-activated killer cells and interleukin-2 or high dose interleukin-2 alone. N Engl J Med 55: 1063
22. North RJ (1982) Cyclophosphamide-facilitated adoptive immunotherapy of an established tumor depends on elimination of tumor-induced suppressor T cells. J Exp Med 55: 1063
23. Kolitz JE, Wong GY, Welte K, Merluzzi VJ, Engert A, Bialas T, Polivka A, Bradley EC, Konrad M, Gnecco C, Oettgen HF, Mertelsmann R (1988) Phase I trial of recombinant interleukin-2 and cyclophosphamide: augmentation of cellular immunity and T-cell mitogenic response with long-term administration of rIL-2. J Biol Response Mod (to be published)
24. West WW, Tauer KW, Yanelli JR, Marshall GD, Orr DW, Thurman GB, Oldham RK (1987) Constant-infusion recombinant interleukin-2 in adoptive immunotherapy of advanced cancer. N Engl J Med 316: 898
25. Herrmann F, Cannistra SA, Lindemann A, Mertelsmann RH, Rambaldi A, Griffin JD (1988) Functional consequences of monocyte interleukin-2 receptor expression: induction of monokines by interferon-gamma and interleukin-2. J Immunol in press
26. Lotze MT, Matory YL, Ettinghausen SE, Rayner AA, Sharrow SO, Seipp CAY, Custer MC, Rosenberg SA (1985) In vivo administration of human interleukin-2. II. Half life, immunologic effects, and expansion of peripheral lymphoid cells in vivo with recombinant IL-2. J Immunol 135: 2865
27. Thompson JA, Lee DJ, Welby-Cox W, Lindgren CG, Collins C, Neraas KA, Dennin RA, Fefer A (1987) Recombinant interleukin-2 toxicity, pharmacokinetics, and immunomodulatory effects in a phase I trial. Cancer Res 47: 4202

28. Carswell EA, Old LJ, Kassel RL, Greens S, Fiore N, Williamson B (1975) An endotoxin-induced serum factor that causes necrosis of tumors. Proc Natl Acad Sci USA 72: 3666
29. Herrmann F (1988) Tumornekrosefaktor. Molekularbiologische und biochemische Grundlagen, biologische Aktivität, klinische Anwendungsmöglichkeiten. MMW 128: 630
30. Klebanoff SJ, Vadas MA, Harlan JM, Sparks LH, Gamble JR, Agosti JM, Waltersdorph AM (1986) Stimulation of neutrophils by tumor necrosis factor. J Immunol 136: 4220
31. Philip R, Epstein LM (1986) Tumor necrosis factor as immunomodulator and mediator of monocyte cytotoxicity induced by itself, gamma-interferon and interleukin-1. Nature 323: 80
32. Ortaldo JR, Ransom JR, Sayers TJ, Herbermann RB (1986) Analysis of cytostatic/cytotoxic lymphokines: relationship of natural killer cytotoxic factor to recombinant lymphotoxin, recombinant tumor necrosis factor, and leukoregulin. J Immunol 137: 2587
33. Scheurich P, Thoma B, Ücer U, Pfizenmaier K (1987) Immunoregulatory activity of recombinant human tumor necrosis factor (TNF)-alpha: Induction of TNF receptors on human T cells and TNF-alpha-mediated enhancement of T cell responses. J Immunol 138: 1786
34. Old LJ (1985) Tumor necrosis factor (TNF). Science 230: 630
35. Beutler B, Cerami A (1987) Cachectin: more than a tumor necrosis factor. Nature 316: 379
36. Kehl JH, Miller A, Bauci AS (1987) Effect of tumor necrosis factor alpha on mitogen-activated human B cells. J Exp Med 166: 786
37. Blick M, Sherwin SA, Rosenblum M, Guttermann J (1987) Phase I study of recombinant tumor necrosis factor in cancer patients. Cancer Res 47: 2986
38. Mertelsmann R, Gamm H, Flener R, Herrmann F (1987) Recombinant human tumor necrosis factor alpha in advanced cancer. A phase I clinical trial. Proc Am Ass Cancer Res 28: 399 (abstract 1583)
39. Chapman PB, Lester TL, Casper ES, Gabrilove JL, Wong GY, Kempin SJ, Gold PJ, Welt S, Warren RS, Starnes HF, Sherwin SA, Old LJ, Oettgen HF (1987) Clinical pharmacology of recombinant human tumor necrosis factor in patients with advanced cancer. J Clin Oncol 5: 1942
40. Herrmann F (1988) Polypeptides controlling hemopoietic growth and function. Blut (to be published)
41. Donahue RE, Wang EA, Stone D, Kamen R, Wong GG, Seghal PK, Nathan DG, Clark SC (1986) Stimulation of hematopoiesis in primates by continuous infusion of recombinant human GM-CSF. Nature 321: 872
42. Lindemann A, Oster W, Ziegler-Heitbrock HWL, Mertelsmann R, Herrmann F (1988) Granulocyte-macrophage colony-stimulating factor induces cytokines secretion by polymorphonuclear neutrophils. J Clin Invest (to be published)
43. Lopez AF, Williamson DJ, Gamble JR, Begley CG, Harlan JU, Klebanoff SJ, Waltersdorph A, Wong G, Clark SC, Vadas MA (1986) Recombinant human granulocyte-macrophage colony-stimulating factor stimulates in vitro human neutrophil and eosinophil function, surface receptor expression, and survival. J Clin Invest 78: 1220
44. Grabstein KH, Urdal DL, Tuschinski J, Mochizuki DY, Price VL, Cantrell MA, Gillis S, Conoln PJ (1986) Induction of macrophage tumoricidal activity by granulocyte-macrophage colony-stimulating factor. Science 232: 506
45. Groopman JE, Mitsuyasu RT, DeLeo MJ, Oette DH, Golde DW (1987) Effect of recombinant human granulocyte-macrophage colony-stimulating factor on myelopoiesis in the acquired immunodeficiency syndrome. N Engl J Med 317: 593
46. Herrmann F, Schulz G, Lindemann A, Meyenburg W, Oster W, Krumwieh D, Mertelsmann R (1988) Hematopoietic responses in patients with advanced malignancy treated with recombinant human granulocyte-macrophage colony-stimulating factor. J Clin Oncol (to be published)
47. Arnaout MA, Wang EA, Clark SC, Sieff CA (1986) Human recombinant granulocyte-macrophage colony-stimulating factor increases cell-to-cell adhesion and surface expression of adhesion promoting surface glycoproteins on mature granulocytes. J Clin Invest 78: 597
48. Gabrilove J, Jacubowski A, Fain K, Scher H, Grous J, Sternberg C, Yogoda A, Clarkson B, Moore MAS, Bonilla MA, Oettgen HF, Alton K, Downing M, Welte K, Souza LM (1987) A phase I/II study of rhG-CSF in cancer patients at risk for chemotherapy-induced neuropenia. Blood [Suppl 1] 70: 135a (abstract 394)

49. Welte K, Platzer E, Lu L, Gabrilove J, Mertelsmann R, Moore MAS (1985) Purification and biochemical characterization of human pluripotent hematopoietic colony-stimulating factor. Proc Natl Acad Sci USA 82: 1526
50. Souza LM, Boone TC, Gabrilove J, Lai PH, Zsebo KM, Murdock DC, Chazin VR, Bruszewski J, Lu H, Chenk K, Barendt J, Platzer E, Moore MAS, Mertelsmann R, Welte K (1986) Recombinant human granulocyte colony-stimulating factor: effects on normal and leukemic myeloid cells. Science 232: 261
51. Cohen AM, Zsebo KM, Inoue H, Hines D, Boone TC, Chazin VR, Tsai L, Ritch T, Souza LM (1986) In vivo stimulation of granulopoiesis by recombinant human granulocyte colony-stimualting factor. Proc Natl Acad Sci USA 84: 2484
52. Welte K, Bonilla MA, Gillio AP, Potter GK, Boone TC, Potter GK, Gabrilove JC, Moore MAS, O'Reilly R, Souza LM (1987) Recombinant human granulocyte colony-stimulating factor. Effects on hematopoiesis in normal and cyclophosphamide-treated primates. J Exp Med 165: 941

Low-dose Cyclophosphamide and IL-2 in the Treatment of Advanced Melanoma*

M.S. MITCHELL[1]

We have recently described a new combinantion of biomodulators, low-dose cyclophosphamide (CY) and interleukin-2 (IL-2), which has been successful in the treatment of advanced melanoma in 24 patients [1]. In this report, we present results on the first 30 patients treated with this regimen. Our rationale for giving low-dose CY was to inhibit suppressor T cells, the number and activity of which might be increased by IL-2, thereby possibly preventing an increase in the number of helper and cytolytic T cells and in lymphokine-activated killer (LAK) cells as well. The dose of IL-2 was chosen to be at or near the projected maximum tolerated single dose level, as estimated from Phase I data.

A dose of 350 mg/m^2 CY was administered by a rapid intravenous infusion on a Friday, 3 days before beginning treatment with IL-2 at a dose of 3.6 million Cetus units per m^2 per day by a 15-min i.v. infusion, 5 days a week, 2 weeks in a row. After an interval of 6 days, the CY administration was repeated on the following Friday to begin the second cycle of therapy. After a third cycle, the patient's lesions were formally re-evaluated. Originally, attempts were made to increase the dose of IL-2 during the second cycle to 5.4 million units per m^2, and on the third cycle to 7.2 million units per m^2. However, when patients responded well to repeated courses of 3.6 million units per m^2, which were generally well tolerated, that dose was consistently given throughout the patient's treatment. Patients who had at least a 25%-50% shrinkage of all measured lesions were given another 3 cycles of CY + IL-2, with a least a 2-3 week interval between the first set of 3 cycles and the next. Therapy was continued as long as there was progressive tumor shrinkage. If there was no further shrinkage on continued treatment, we put the patient on a maintenance regimen. Maintenance therapy consisted of 1 cycle of CY and IL-2 administered every 6 weeks. Patients achieving a complete remission were given at least 2 further cycles and then observed without further treatment. The results of treatment in the first 33 patients, 30 of whom were evaluable for response, are shown in Tables 1 and 2. These patients ranged in age from 18 to 75. Twenty-seven percent of the melanoma patients achieved a complete or partial response, with two complete remissions and six partial remissions, and 5 others had a minor response. The remaining 17 of the 30 patients failed to respond.

---

* Supported by a contract with the Cetus Corporation, a grant from the Concern Foundation, and gifts from Mr. Alan Gleitsman, the Morey and Claudia Mirkin Foundation, the Lenihan Trust, and Mrs. Virginia L. Andleman.

[1] Division of Medical Oncology, Compr. Cancer Center, University of Southern California, Los Angeles, CA 90033, USA.

H. G. Beger et al. (Eds.), Cancer Therapy

Table 1. Results of treatment

Type of response	Patients[a] (n) (%)
Complete remission	2 (6.7)
Partial remission	6 (20)
Minor response	5 (16.7)
None	17 (56.7)
Total	30 (100)

[a] Three patients who received only one 2-week cycle of therapy were not included in this analysis.

Table 2. Results of treatment by site

Site of disease	Number of patients	Responses	Duration[a] in months	Status of responders
Liver	7	1 CR	17 +	Living, off study
		2 PR	13	Dead
			10	Living, off study
Lung	11	1 CR	6 +	Living, on study
		2 PR	21	Living, off study
			3	Living, on study
		1 MR	2	Living, off study
Subcutaneous	16	2 CR	17 +	Living, on study
			1.5	Dead
		4 PR	16	Living, off study
			1	Dead
			1	Dead
			2	Dead
		6 MR	14 +	1 Living, on study
			< 2	5 dead
Lymph node	9	2 PR	15	Living, on study
			14 +	Living, on study
		4 MR	< 2	2 dead 2 living, one on study
Bone	5	0		
Adrenal	3	0		
Pelvis, kidney	5	0		

CR, complete remission, *PR*, partial remission; *MR*, minor response.
[a] Durations of response are given from the date a CR was achieved or the date therapy was begun for a PR, as per convention.

We were pleased to observe that responsive sites of disease included the liver, with remissions noted in 3 of 7 patients with metastatic lesions of that organ. Subcutaneous nodules (in 7 of 16 patients), lymph node metastases (2 of 9 patients), and pulmonary metastases (3 of 11 patients) also responded, but adrenal and bone metastases did not. Brain lesions on computed tomographic scans or magnetic resonance imaging precluded admission onto the protocol. Durations of response were as brief as 1–2 months in some patients, but the mean was > 6 months, with two remissions continuing for more than 1 year.

A 59-year-old woman with subcutaneous nodules had a complete remission lasting 6 weeks. A second complete remission was achieved after only three cycles of CY + IL-2 in a 34-year-old man with three pulmonary nodules and an enlarged hilar lymph node. After two further cycles, therapy was discontinued, per protocol, and he has remained in unmaintained, complete remission for over 6 months (since July 1987). A 42-year-old woman had a remarkable complete disappearance of eight large lesions in the liver of up to 5 cm in diameter, together with three small subcutaneous nodules and two out of three pulmonary nodules. Because of one residual 1-cm pulmonary nodule, her response was termed a partial remission, but we elected to treat her as though she had a complete remission, stopping all treatment after 15 cycles. She remained in unmaintained partial remission for more than 6 months, or a total of 21 months from the onset of therapy (April 1986–December 1987). In fact, her disease did not relapse in the sites that had responded but rather in the central nervous system. Two other patients with liver disease had partial remissions lasting 6 months. They, too, relapsed with brain lesions.

A patient with a partial remission in skin and lymph nodes was kept on maintenance therapy for over 1 year, relapsing first in the central nervous system and only later, after a lapse in therapy, in the original sites of disease. It is of interest that a man whose overall response has been designated as minor, with a flattening but not a complete disappearance of intradermal nodules, nevertheless has had > 50% shrinkage of a 3.0 × 3.0-cm inguinal lymph node. His disease has remained completely stable for nearly 1 year (over 14 months since the start of therapy) on maintenance treatment. Both of these individuals were well enough to resume strenuous work.

The regimen was well tolerated, with fewer than 20% of patients showing severe toxicity (Table 3). (Note that the table also includes data from two patients with renal cell carcinoma, with a total of 35 subjects evaluated.) All treatment was administered in a day-hospital, i.e., outpatient setting, and only two patients were admitted briefly (because of postural hypotension requiring an infusion of saline). The same spectrum of effects was seen as in other studies with high doses of IL-2, but most patients, including elderly individuals, found it tolerable.

Immunological correlates included the development of LAK cells in 21 patients, 8 of whom had a clinical remission (Table 4). In contrast, none of the 9 patients who failed to show an increase in the number of LAK cells achieved a complete or partial remission. This was highly significant by Fisher's exact test, at $P = 0.003$. The level of significance was, in fact, considerably higher than in our evaluation of the first 24 patients. Incremental increases in LAK cells, calculated in lytic units, were generally achieved with each succeeding course of immunotherapy, at least until the third or fourth cycle in succession. After that, repeated courses did not seem to achieve an increase. However, the respite of 2–3 weeks between one set of 3 cycles and the next may have been beneficial to the immune response because the woman who received 15 cycles, with many such intervals, developed nearly 5,000 lytic units of LAK cells. A significant proportion of those killer cells were found to be cytolytic T lymphocytes, judging from cold target competition assays, which indi-

Table 3. Toxicity of CY + IL-2

Toxic Effect[a]	Patients experiencing effect (*n*)	WHO Grade III (*n*)
Fatigue	35	6
Fever	34	4
Nausea, vomiting	33	5
Chills, Rigors	28	3
Diarrhea	24	2
Hypotension	23	5
Arthritis	22	2
Fluid retention	21	2
Dry cough, dyspnea	19	2
Myalgia	18	1
Allergies, rash	16	1
Anemia	11	0
Catarrhal symptoms	8	0

[a] World Health Organization criteria were used except for hypotension, which was modified as described in the text, and fluid retention (weight gain), which was a category specifically added for IL-2 protocols by Cetus.
CY, cyclophosphamide; *IL-2*, interleukin-2.

Table 4. Immunological correlates of clinical response

Induction of LAK Cell Activity versus Response	Response[a]	No Response	Total
LAK increased[b]	8	13	21
LAK not increased	0	9	9

[a] Comprises complete and partial remissions.
[b] Maximal increase of > 10 lytic units during treatment.
$P = 0.003$ by Fisher's exact test.

cated their specificity for melanoma cells. There was no correlation of either natural killer (NK) cell activation or eosinophilia with clinical remission.
A major problem that we have encountered, ironically in those patients who have had the best systemic control of their disease, has been the development of a large solitary brain metastasis. Three patients whose liver disease remained under control for 6–21 months and another, whose partial remission of skin and lymph node metastases lasted 15 months, relapsed in the central nervous system while on maintenance treatment with CY and IL-2. It is obvious that an additional strategy will have to be developed to combat this late complication of otherwise successful therapy.
In summary, the regimen we have devised, consisting of low-dose CY and low-dose IL-2, was well tolerated and had an efficacy comparable or superior to that of higher dose regimens of IL-2, which also require the reinfusion of LAK cells activated ex vivo [2]. The ability to induce LAK activity in vivo may, in fact, obviate the need for ex vivo activation, although it remains to be seen whether suffi-

cient numbers can routinely be generated by in vivo activation alone. The relative tolerability of the regimen suggests that it may be applicable to the adjunctive setting after resection of the primary tumor and involved lymph nodes. It will be interesting to see whether CY + IL-2 or a similar regimen will prove effective in other types of tumor, particularly renal cell, colon, and breast carcinomas, all of which have shown some response to IL-2 and LAK cells.

References

1. Mitchell MS, Kempf RA, Harel W, Shau H, Boswell WD, Lind S, Bradley EC (1988) Effectiveness and tolerability of low-dose cyclophosphamide and low-dose intravenous interleukin-2 in the treatment of disseminated melanoma. J Clin Oncol 6 (3): 409-424
2. Rosenberg SA, Lotze MT, Muul LM, Chang AE, Avis FP, Leitman S, Linehau WM, Robertson CN, Lee RE, Rubin JT, Seipp CA, Simpson CG, White DE (1987) A progress report on the treatment of 157 patients with advanced cancer using lymphokine-activated killer cells and interleukin-2 or high-dose interleukin-2 alone. New Engl J Med 316: 889-897

Application of Granulocyte-Macrophage Colony-Stimulating Factor in Patients with Malignant Hematological Diseases

A. GANSER,[1] B. VÖLKERS,[1] J. GREHER,[1] F. WALTHER,[2] and D. HOELZER[1]

Introduction

Colony-stimulating factors (CSF) are a group of glycoproteins produced by a variety of human and murine cell types [1]. These factors primarily regulate hemopoiesis by promoting the proliferation and differentiation of hemopoietic progenitor cells [1-3]. Recently, a cDNA for human GM-CSF has been cloned from the HUT 102 cell line, and using a yeast expression system, recombinant human GM-CSF (rhGM-CSF) has been produced and purified to homogeneity [4]. It has also been possible to clone rhGM-CSF from the human Mo-cell line [5].

In vitro studies have shown that rhGM-CSF has effects on both normal precursor cells and mature granulocytes [6, 7]. It stimulates the formation of human granulocyte, macrophage, and eosinophil colonies [7-9]. In the presence of erythropoietin, GM-CSF also induces the proliferation and differentiation of early erythroid (burst-forming units-erythoid, BFU-E) and multipotent progenitors (colony-forming unit-granulocyte, erythrocyte, macrophage, megakaryocyte, CFU-GEMM). Activation of granulocytes and macrophages both to antibody-dependent cellular cytotoxicity against human tumor and leukemic cell lines and to phagocytosis of yeast organisms and extracellular kill of tumor targets has also been demonstrated [7-10]. In addition, GM-CSF increases cell-to-cell adhesion of mature granulocytes.

In preclinical studies [11] and in patients with the acquired immunodeficiency syndrome [12], rhGM-CSF has been shown to increase peripheral blood neutrophil counts in a dose-dependent manner. Therefore, a rhGM-CSF trial was undertaken in patients with myelodysplastic syndromes (MDS). Leukopenia, especially neutropenia, is found in half of the patients with myelodysplastic syndromes at the time of diagnosis, leading to serious infection as a cause of death in 20%-40% of the patients [13]. Hence, it was the aim of a phase I/II trial to study the toxicity and the therapeutic effects of rhGM-CSF on hematopoiesis in patients with MDS.

[1] Department of Hematology, Center for Internal Medicine, Johann Wolfgang Goethe University, Theodor-Stern-Kai 7, 6000 Frankfurt/Main 70, FRG.
[2] Department of Internal Medicine, Bethanien Hospital, 6000 Frankfurt/Main, FRG.

H. G. Beger et al. (Eds.), Cancer Therapy

Materials and Methods

Preparation of rhGM-CSF

The molecular cloning and purification of rhGM-CSF were done by Immunex, Inc. (Seattle, WA, USA) and Behringwerke (Marburg, Federal Republic of Germany) as has been described [4]. The rhGM-CSF produced in a yeast expression system is glycosylated and has a molecular weight of between 14 and 22 kD, depending on the pattern of glycosylation. The rhGM-CSF used had a specific activity of about 5×10^7 colony-forming units per mg protein. The endotoxin concentration was <1 ng/mg protein. Sterility, general safety, and purity studies met the Food and Drug Administration (FDA) standards.

Patient Selection and Study Design

Only patients with clinical and hematological confirmation of MDS, i.e. refractory anemia (RA), refractory anemia with an excess of blast cells (RAEB), RAEB-T (T = in transformation to acute leukemia), and chronic myelomonocytic leukemia (CMML), who had not been treated with antileukemic drugs for at least 4 weeks were included. Eligibility criteria included a performance status of >50% (Karnofsky scale), a life expectancy of more than 3 months, an age below 75 years, and preserved hepatic, renal, and hemostatic function. Patients eligible for bone marrow transplantation or conventional high-dose chemotherapy were excluded. The study was approved by the FDA as well as by the local Ethics Committee. Informed consent was obtained from the patients prior to rhGM-CSF therapy.
The treatment schedule consisted of four dose levels of rhGM-CSF: 15 $\mu g/m^2$, 30 μ/m^2, 60 $\mu g/m^2$, and 150 $\mu g/m^2$. The first two patients received 15 $\mu g/m^2$ i.v. (level 1), the next two patients received 30 $\mu g/m^2$ i.v. (level 2), etc. Two patients were entered sequentially at dose levels 1-4 and received treatment on days 1-7 and 22-28. On day 1, the daily dose was given within 5 min, while on the other days the intravenous infusions were given over an 8-h period. From dose level 4, the initial bolus injection was omitted, and the first course of rhGM-CSF was extended to 14 days since, based on the initial results, an effect on hematopoiesis was expected to occur not before day 7 or 8 of therapy.
Patients were monitored daily, and all constitutional symptoms were recorded. Vital signs were checked before injections and at 1, 2, 4, and 6 h after the start of infusion on days 1, 2, 5, 8, 22, and 29. A history was taken, and physical examination performed before the initial dose and weekly thereafter. Patients were weighed weekly. An electrocardiogram was recorded and chest X-ray films were taken before the study and after the final administration of therapy. A serum chemistry profile, coagulation profile, and urinalysis were obtained before therapy was begun and on days 1, 2, 5, 8, 15, 22, 26, 29, and 32. A complete blood count, including differential and reticulocyte counts, was taken prior to and on days 1-8, 15, 22, 24, 26, 29, and 32.
Lymphocyte subpopulations (CD4 and CD8) and the presence of the interleukin 2 receptor on the lymphocytes were estimated in the peripheral blood on days 1, 8,

15, 22, and 29 using a commercial kit from Becton-Dickinson (Heidelberg, Federal Republic of Germany) and the FACStar flow cytometer. Bone marrow aspirations were performed before and after the end of the study for cytological examination and cultures of the hemopoietic progenitor cells.
Toxicity was graded according to the World Health Organization (WHO) criteria. Dose-limiting toxicity was generally defined as toxicity of grade 3 or higher by WHO criteria. The maximally tolerated dose was defined as the dosage at which approximately 75% of the patients achieved a reversible grade 3 toxicity. The preliminary data on the toxicity of rhGM-CSF have been reported [14].

Results

Eleven patients with various forms of MDS and ranging in age from 46 to 75 years, with a median age of 62 years, were entered into the study. Three patients had RA, four patients had RAEB, two patients had RAEB-T, and two patients had CMML [14]. All patients were severely cytopenic: 5 out of 11 patients were neutropenic (<1500/μl), 10 out of 11 were thrombocytopenic (<40000/μl), and all were anemic, with hemoglobin <12 g/dl. No chemotherapy had been given prior to rhGM-CSF, with the exception of one patient, who had received two courses of low-dose cytarabine. All patients frequently required substitution with erythrocytes and/or platelets. Because of their advanced ages (median 62 years), none of the patients was a candidate for bone marrow transplantation.

Hematological Effects

When the initial leukocyte count is compared with the maximal increase during rhGM-CSF therapy, 10 out of 10 patients responded with an increase (Table 1). This increase was apparently related to the dosage of rhGM-CSF (Table 2). This

Table 1. Change in leukocyte count after administration of rhGM-CSF in patients with myelodysplastic syndromes

Patient	Dose (μg/m²)	Maximal increase (%)
1	15	130
2	15	
3	30	160
4	30	180
5	60	180
6	75	720
7	150	290
8	150	200
9	150	1800
10	150	680
11	150	200

dose-related increase was seen for granulocytes, monocytes, eosinophils, and lymphocytes. One patient at dose level 1 responded with a transient platelet increase from 20000/μl to 90000/μl, while two patients receiving 150 μg rhGM-CSF/m^2 showed a transient rise in reticulocytes.

The increase in the number of circulating lymphocytes, which directly correlated to the dosage of rhGM-CSF administered, affected both CD4- and CD8-positive T-lymphocyte populations without changing the CD4/CD8 ratio. No activation of the lymphocytes as determined by the expression of the interleukin 2 receptor occurred. In vitro studies performed prior to and during GM-CSF therapy showed a nearly unchanged incidence of granulocyte/macrophage progenitor cells CFU-GM in the bone marrow of the patients.

As an adverse effect, an increase in the percentage of leukemic blast cells occurred in the bone marrow of 4 out of the 11 patients. This increase in blast cells was, however, only observed in patients with an initial blast cell content in the bone marrow of over 14% (Table 3).

For the patients with an increase of blast cells in the bone marrow and/or blood, a cytotoxic therapy with low-dose cytarabine was considered. These patients received one or more 14-day courses of low-dose cytarabine (Table 4). One patient responded with a blast cell decrease and transient platelet increase after two courses of low-dose cytarabine, which, however, had to be stopped after the fifth cycle because of refractory disease. The second patient responded initially with a blast cell decrease and platelet increase, but the disease progressed after two courses of low-dose cytarabine, so the patient has now undergone combination chemotherapy. In the other two patients, the percentage of blast cells did not change after a single course of low-dose cytarabine, and the disease either progressed , necessitating conventional chemotherapy, or the patient died following pulmonary hemorrhage due to the pre-existing thrombocytopenia.

Table 2. Effect of rhGM-CSF on blood counts[a]

	Present study	Vadhan-Raj et al. [15]
Increase in:		
White blood count	10/11	8/8
Monocytes	7/11	8/8
Eosinophils	6/11	7/8
Lymphocytes	11/11	8/8
Blast cells	5/11	0/8

[a] The number of patients with a rise of the indicated cell type is given.

Table 3. Effect of rhGM-CSF on leukemic cells

Patients *(n)*	Present study	Vadhan-Raj et al. [15]
>15% bone marrow blasts	4	2
Progression of disease	3	0
<15% bone marrow blasts	7	5
Progression of disease	1	0

Table 4. Sequential therapy with rhGM-CSF and low-dose cytarabine in patients with myelodysplastic syndromes

Patient	Diagnosis	GM-CSF dose (μg/m²)	Low-dose cytarabine) (days)	Treatment outcome
3	CMML	30	1 × 14	Blast cells unaffected, progression
5	RAEB	60	5 × 14	Blast cell decrease, platelet increase
7	RAEB	150 75	2 × 14[a]	Blast cell decrease, platelet increase, progression after two courses of low-dose cytarabine courses
8	RAEB	150	1 × 14	Blast cells unaffected, persistent thrombocytopenia, death following pulmonary hemorrhage

[a] Refractory to low-dose cytarabine before rhGM-CSF.
CMML, chronic myeolomonocytic leukemia; *RAEB*, refractory anemia with an excess of blast cells.

Discussion

This phase I/II study demonstrates that rhGM-CSF is able to induce an increase in circulating leukocytes in the majority of patients with various forms of MDS and long-lasting cytopenia. Our results coincide with the results of a phase I/II trial performed in Houston [15]. Several factors may contribute to this increase in the white blood cell count. An initial factor could be the release of granulocytes from the bone marrow and/or vessel walls. A second factor could be increased proliferation of the morphologically recognizable granulocytic precursors, i.e., myelocytes and promyelocytes, as observed in two of our patients.

While an influence of rhGM-CSF on cell lineages other than granulopoiesis and monocytopoiesis, i.e., erythropoiesis and megakaryopoiesis, was seen in preclinical studies in vitro [3] and in animals [11], effects on platelets and erythrocytes was observed only in the minority of our patients. It should, therefore, be considered whether rhGM-CSF should be given in combination with other hemopoietic growth factors, such as erythropoietin and interleukin-3, to see whether synergistic multilineage effects on hematopoisis can be obtained.

A major point for the clinical application of rhGM-CSF in patients with MDS is related to the question of the growth stimulation of leukemic cell clones. The application of rhGM-CSF in four cases resulted in an increase in leukemic blast cells in the bone marrow, indicating that rhGM-CSF stimulates the proliferation of human leukemic blast cells as well as of normal hemopoietic cells. In contrast to another study [15], we achieved neither a decrease in the percentage of bone marrow blast cells nor an improvement in the ratio of differentiation. Since this increase in blast cell counts only occurred in patients with a blast cell percentage $>14\%$ in the bone marrow, rhGM-CSF should not be used as a single agent in such cases. Furthermore, both of our patients with CMML had progressive disease during treatment with rhGM-CSF and should, therefore, be excluded from further trials with this therapy.

The observed stimulation of blast cells is quite evidently harmful and limits the use of rhGM-CSF or other hemopoietic growth factors. However, GM-CSF treatment seems indicated in myelodysplastic patients with neutropenia without blast cells because of its marked effect on the stimulation and differentiation of normal granulopoietic cells.

References

1. Burgess AW, Metcalf D (1980) The nature and action of granulocyte-macrophage colony stimulator factors. Blood 56: 947-958
2. Metcalf D (1984) The hemopoietic colony stimulating factors. Elsevier, Amsterdam
3. Clark SC, Kamen R (1987) The human hematopoietic colony-stimulating factors. Science 236: 1229-1237
4. Cantrell MA, Anderson D, Ceretti D, Price V, McKeregham K, Tushinski RJ, Mochizuki DY, Larsen A, Grabstein KH, Gillis S, Cosam D (1985) Cloning, sequence, and expression of a human granulocyte/macrophage colony-stimulating factor. Proc Natl Acad Sci USA 82: 6250-6254
5. Wong GG, Witek JS, Temple PA, Wilkens KM, Leary AC, Luxenberg DP, Jones SS, Brown EL, Kay RM, Orr EC, Shoemaker C, Golde DW, Kaufmann RJ, Hewick RM, Wang EA, Clark SC (1985) Human GM-CSF. Molecular cloning of the cDNA and purification of the natural and recombinant proteins. Science 228: 810
6. Weisbart RH, Golde DW, Clark SC, Wong GG, Gasson JC (1985) Human granulocyte-macrophage colony-stimulating factor is a neutrophil activator. Nature 314: 361-366
7. Metcalf D, Begley CG, Johnson GR, Nicola NA, Vadas MA, Lopez AF, Williamson DJ, Wong GG, Clark SC, Wang EA (1986) Biologic properties in vitro of a recombinant human granulocyte-macrophage colony-stimulating factor. Blood 67: 37-45
8. Lopez AF, Nicola NA, Metcalf D, Burgess AW, Metcalf D, Battye FL, Sewell WA, Vadas M (1983) Activation of granulocyte cytotoxic function by purified mouse colony-stimulating factors. J Immunol 131: 2983
9. Gasson JC, Weisbart RH, Kaufman SE, Clark SC, Hewick RM, Wong GG, Golde DW (1984) Purified human granulocyte-macrophage colony-stimulating factor: direct action on neutrophils. Science 226: 1339
10. Grabstein KH, Urdal DL, Tushinski RJ, Mochizuki DY, Price VA, Cantrell MA, Gillis S, Conlon PJ (1986) Induction of macrophage tumoricidal activity by granulocyte-macrophage colony stimulating factor. Science 232: 506-508
11. Donahue RE, Wang EA, Stone DK, Kamen R, Wong GG, Seghal PK, Nathan DG, Clark SC (1986) Stimulation of haematopoiesis in primates by continuous infusion of recombinant human GM-CSF. Nature 321: 872-875
12. Groopman JE, Mitsuyasu RT, DeLeo MJ, Oette DH, Golde DW (1987) Effect of recombinant human granulocyte-macrophage colony-stimulating factor on myelopoisis in the acquired immunodeficiency syndrome. N Engl J Med 317: 593-598
13. Hoelzer D, Ganser A, Heimpel H (1984) "Atypical" leukemias: preleukemias, smoldering leukemia and hypoplastic leukemia. In: Thiel E, Thierfelder S (eds) Leukemia: recent developments and therapy. Springer, Berlin Heidelberg New York Tokyo, pp 69-101 (Recent results in cancer research, vol 93)
14. Ganser A, Völkers B, Greher J, Walther F, Hoelzer D (1988) Recombinant human granulocyte-macrophage colony-stimulating factor in patients with myelodysplastic syndromes - a phase I/II trial. Onkologie 11: 53-55
15. Vadhan-Raj S, Keating M, LeMaistre A, Hittelman WN, McCredie K, Trujillo JM, Broxmeyer HE, Henney C, Guttermann JU (1987) Effects of recombinant human granulocyte-macrophage colony-stimulating factor in patients with myelodysplastic syndromes. N Engl J Med 317: 1545-1552

Enhancement of Autologous Bone Marrow Transplantation with Recombinant Human Granulocyte-Macrophage Colony-Stimulating Factor (rhGM-CSF)

H. LINK,[1] M. FREUND,[1] H. KIRCHNER,[1] M. STOLL,[1] H. SCHMID,[1]
P. BUCSKY,[1] J. SEIDEL,[1] G. SCHULZ,[2] R. E. SCHMIDT,[1] H. RIEHM,[1]
H. POLIWODA,[1] and K. WELTE[1]

Introduction

Intensive combination chemotherapy makes long-term survival possible after several lymphoid malignancies. However, a substantial number of patients have poor prognostic factors for remaining in remission and should therefore be treated with additional aggressive chemotherapy during remission. Many studies have shown that high-dose chemotherapy alone or in combination with total-body irradiation followed by bone marrow transplantation (BMT) improves the chances of survival for poor-risk patients with acute lymphoblastic leukemia (ALL) [3, 8]. The prognosis for patients with relapsed intermediate or high-grade non-Hodgkin's lymphoma (NHL) can be improved by high-dose radiochemotherapy followed by BMT [2, 16]. Patients with Hodgkin's disease (HD) who do not enter a complete remission with conventional chemotherapy have an unfavorable prognosis [1, 6], as do relapse patients who require treatment with chemotherapy. These patients' chances of being cured are greater with high-dose chemoradiotherapy followed by bone marrow transplantation than with the usual salvage treatment. Neuroblastoma stage III/IV can only be cured by high-dose chemotherapy followed by BMT during remission as consolidation [15]. However, infectious complications due to bone marrow insufficiency during the immediate post-transplant phase after BMT contribute significantly to morbidity and mortality [12, 17]. These infections tend to be more severe than during the granulocytopenia following conventional cytotoxic therapy. The association of the degree and duration of granulocytopenia and an increased risk of infection has long been recognized [10]. In autologous BMT for ALL, the median time for recovery to 500 neutrophils per microliter is 22 days, with a range of 14–40 days [7, 11]. The risk of severe infections and of high morbidity could be reduced markedly if the duration of neutropenia could be shortened significantly.

Recombinant Human Granulocyte-Macrophage Colony Stimulating Factor (rhGM-CSF)

In normal hematopoiesis, cell proliferation and differentiation are controlled by a group of growth factors known as colony-stimulating factors (CSF) [13, 14]. These

[1] Bone Marrow Transplant Ward, University Hospital Hannover, Konstantin-Gutschow-Straße 8, 3000 Hannover 61, FRG.
[2] Clinical Research, Behringwerke AG Marburg, 3550 Marburg 1, FRG.

H. G. Beger et al. (Eds.), Cancer Therapy

factors support the proliferation and differentiation of hematopoietic progenitor cells in semisolid culture systems and activate the function of peripheral blood granulocytes and macrophages.

In man, GM-CSF is secreted by T-lymphocytes. Naturally occurring human GM-CSF has been only partially purified [9]. However, GM-CSF has been produced for clinical use with recombinant DNA technology using a yeast expression system [5]. In animal experiments, GM-CSF proved to be effective in accelerating bone marrow recovery after cytostatic therapy or total-body irradiation. In man, phase I trials showed only mild toxicity. Biologic activity was observed even with low doses of 30 $\mu g/m^2$ daily. Most effective was the application as a continuous infusion over 24 h.

In this study, rhGM-CSF from a yeast expression system was used with a specific activity of 5×10^5 colony-forming units-culture (CFU-C)/μg rhGM-CSF.

Aims of the Study

Our purpose was to:

1. Assess the effects of rhGM-CSF on the hematologic and immunologic reconstitution of autologous marrow graft recipients
2. Determine the therapeutic dosage of rhGM-CSF that can increase the peripheral blood neutrophil count in patients after autologous BMT
3. Assess the safety, tolerance, and toxicity of multiple intravenous infusions of rhGM-CSF when administered daily to recipients of bone marrow grafts

Patients and Methods

Patients included in the study have ALL in complete remission, intermediate- or high-grade NHL, HD, or neuroblastoma (NB) and are eligible for autologous BMT as specified in the corresponding treatment protocols. The patient characteristics are summarized in Table 1.

Table 1. Patient characteristics

Number	Unique patient number	Age (years)	Sex	Diagnosis	Mononuclear cells per kg $\times 10^8$
1	39	4	f	Neuroblastoma IV, CR	0.65
2	40	26	f	Hodgkin's disease IV, CR	1.26
3	44	15	f	ALL, 2nd CR	1.08
4	46	10	m	Neuroblastoma IV, PR	0.72
5	47	6	f	Neuroblastoma IV, CR	0.74
6	55	16	f	Alveolar rhabdomyosarcoma, CR	0.55

CR, complete remission; *PR*, partial remission; *ALL*, acute lymphoblastic leukemia.

Table 2. Conditioning regimens for BMT

Acute lymphoblastic leukemia and non-Hodgkin's lymphoma		
Fractionated total-body irradiation		total dose: 12 Gy
On days		-10,-9,-8,-7
Daily fractions		2
Lung dose		10 Gy
VP-16		15 mg/kg per day:
On days		-6,-5,-4,-3;
Hodgkin's disease		
Cyclophosphamide	1.5 g/m^2	days -6,-5,-4,-3
VP-16	250 mg/m^2	days -6,-5,-4,-3
BCNU	200 mg/m^2	days -6,-5,-4,-3
Neuroblastoma		
Cisplatin	120 mg/m^2	day -19
Irradiation	2100 cGy	days -18 to -10
to former sites of bulky disease (2 fractions per day)		
BCNU	200 mg/m^2	day -9
Melphalan	2 × 30 mg/m^2	days -8,-7,-6
VP-16	300 mg/m^2	days -5,-4,-3

VP-16, etoposide; *BCNU*, 1,3-bis(2-chloroethyl)-1-nitrosourea.

Conditioning Regimens for BMT

Table 2 summarizes the conditioning regimens administered to patients with ALL and NHL or with HD prior to undergoing BMT.

Autologous BMT

Autologous BMT was carried out after high-dose chemotherapy alone or in combination with total-body irradiation as preparative (conditioning) regimens for BMT. No bone marrow treatment was performed. Day 0 was the day of BMT.

Treatment Schedule with rhGM-CSF

Doses of 500 μg/m^2 rhGM-CSF a day were given by intravenous infusion over a period of 24 h in 0.9% normal saline with 1% albumin. The first dose was administered within 1 h of the completion of BMT. This dose was maintained until the absolute neutrophil count reached 1000/μl or more for 3 consecutive days. The rhGM-CSF dose was then reduced to 250 μg/m^2 a day. If the neutrophil count increased further or remained greater than 1000/μl for at least 3 consecutive days, the dose was further reduced to 125 μg/m^2. After 3 more days at this dose level and with neutrophils stable at more than 1000/μl, the dose was further reduced to 50 μg/m^2 for 3 days. Then, rhGM-CSF treatment was discontinued. Therapy should not extend beyond 28 days after BMT.

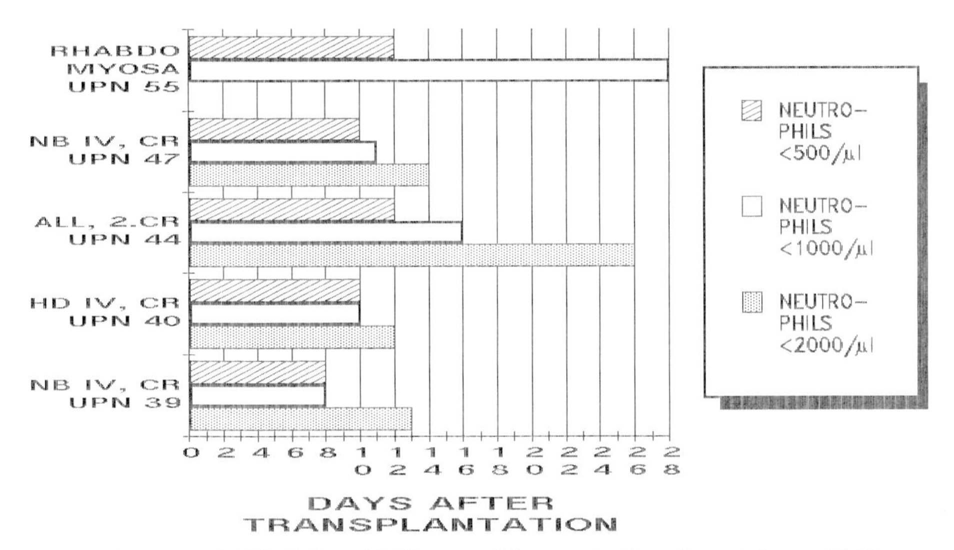

Fig. 1. Time to reach 500, 1000, and 2000 neutrophils per microliter after autologous BMT

Results

Protocol Patients

The clinical courses in five of the six patients were evaluable. One patient died of veno-occlusive liver disease, obviously due to very intensive previous cytostatic chemotherapy. The time to recovery from neutropenia after BMT is shown in Fig. 1. The kinetics of leukocyte regeneration in a patient with ALL is depicted in Fig. 2.

Treatment for Lack of Bone Marrow Regeneration After Autologous BMT

One patient with NHL derived from T cells (T-NHL) stage IV (UPN 28; male; age, 26 years) in 1st CR received an autologous BMT (2.0×10^8 mononuclear cells per kilogram after fTBI and VP-16 (etoposide) conditioning. His bone marrow failed to recover (Fig. 3). By day 71 after BMT, he received rhGM-CSF in the form of a daily, continuous infusion of 500 µg on days 71-75, 200 µg on days 76-78, 100 µg on days 79-86, and 50 µg on days 87-89. By day 75, his differential count of 300 leukocytes/µl showed 13% neutrophils, 16% bands, 31% monocytes, 1% basophils, 1% metamyelocytes, 2% promyelocytes, and 36 lymphocytes. After day 88, leukocytes were 1700-2000 µl, with 60%-70% granulocytes. The absolute number of granulocytes was 200-500 until day 132, when he died of cytomegalovirus pneumonia.

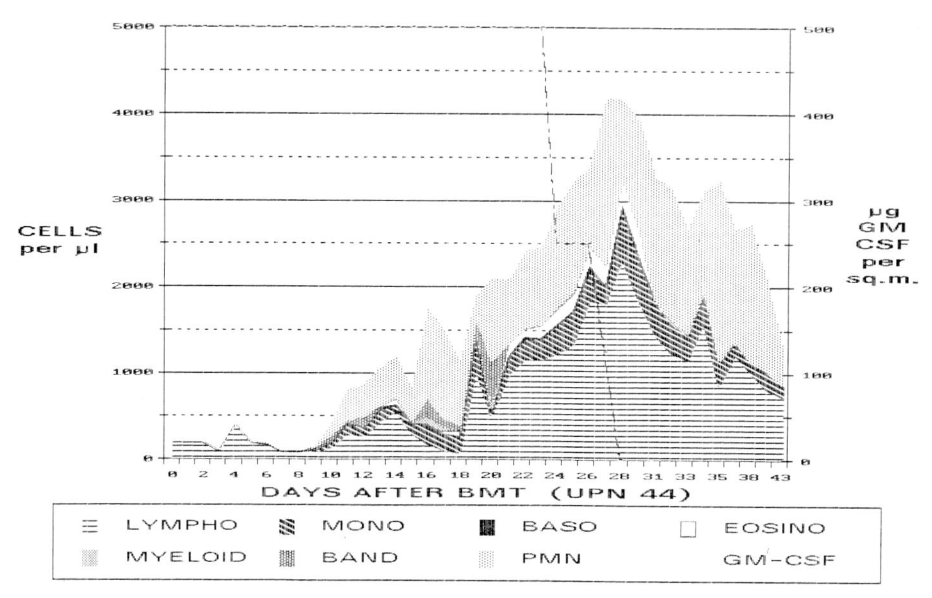

Fig. 2. Regeneration of leukocytes after autologous BMT in a patient with ALL in 2nd CR (UPN 44). Neutrophils rose by day 9, monocytes by day 10, and band forms by day 11. Eosinophils were elevated between day 21 and 31 and disappeared 3 days after discontinuation of the drug

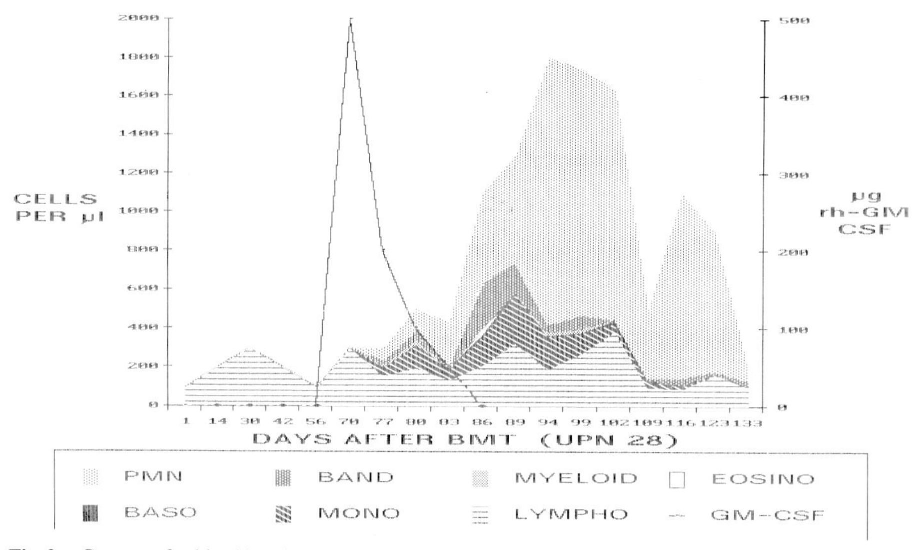

Fig. 3. Course of white blood count in a patient (UPN 28) who failed to recover bone marrow function after fTBI, high-dose VP-16 (etoposide), and autologous BMT; response to treatment with rh-GM-CSF. *PMN*, polymorphonuclear neutrophils; *BASO*, basophils; *BAND*, band forms; *MONO*, monocytes; *MYELOID*, myeloid precursors; *LYMPHO*, lymphocytes; *EOSINO*, eosinophils

Side Effects

In some patients, a slight skin rash was observed. Fever of unknown origin and weight gain occurred in all patients. None of these observations was clearly attributable to treatment with rhGM-CSF.

Discussion

Despite the limited number of patients, it was possible to show in this study that the duration of severe and dangerous neutropenia is very short after autologous BMT with rhGM-CSF. In five patients, the time to reach 500 neutrophils per microliter was 8–12 days. This seems to be 7–10 days less than expected without rhGM-CSF. However, in a phase I/II study with rhGM-CSF as a continuous infusion over a period of 15 days after BMT, the duration of neutropenia ($<500/\mu l$) was only reduced from 17 to 15 days after high-dose chemotherapy and autologous BMT for melanoma and breast cancer patients [4]. Therefore, our results should be confirmed in a larger study with equivalent conditioning regimens. We have initiated a multicenter trial in Europe with 15 transplantation centers. Only patients with ALL and NHL who receive an autologous bone marrow graft after total-body irradiation with at least 10 Gy in combination with high-dose chemotherapy will be included in this randomized double-blind study with rhGM-CSF. Patients without bone marrow recovery after autologous BMT have a very poor prognosis owing to imminent severe infections and bleeding. Even if there is a minimal chance of bone marrow regeneration, it seems advisable to use rhGM-CSF in such a situation to stimulate hemopoiesis, as has been shown in our study. There was no toxicity clearly attributable rhGM-CSF administration. Our preliminary results show that rhGM-CSF stimulates and accelerates the regeneration of granulopoiesis after BMT. Further studies are urgently needed to evaluate the potential of this promising new drug in the field of bone marrow transplantation.

References

1. Appelbaum FR, Sullivan KM, Thomas ED (1985) Marrow transplantation as a treatment for patients with recurrent malignant lymphoma. Int J Cell Cloning 4: 216–217
2. Appelbaum FR, Thomas ED (1983) Review of the use of marrow transplantation in the treatment of non-Hodgkins lymphomas. J Clin Oncol 7: 440–447
3. Barrett AJ, Kendra JR, Lucas CF, Joss DV, Joshi R, Desai M, Hugh-Jones K, Phillips RH, Rogers TR, Tabara Z, Williamson S, Hobbs Jr (1982) Bone marrow transplantation for acute lymphoblastic leukemia. Br J Haematol 52: 181–188
4. Brandt SJ, Kurtzberg J, Atwater SK, Borowitz MJ, Jones RB, Shpall EJ, Gilbert CJ, Bast RC jr, Oette DH, Peters WP (1987) Effect of recombinant human granulocyte-macrophage colony-stimulating factor (rHuGM-CSF) on hematopoietic reconstitution following high-dose chemotherapy and autologous bone marrow transplantation (ABMT). Blood 70 [Suppl 1]: 131
5. Cantrell MA, Anderson D, Cerretti DP, Price V, McKereghan K, Tushinski RJ, Mochizuki DY, Larsen A, Grabstein K, Gillis S, Cosman D (1985) Cloning, sequence, and expression of a human granulocyte/macrophage colony-stimulating factor. Proc Nat Acad Sci USA 82: 6250–6254

6. Carella AM, Congiu A, Santini G, Martinengo M, Frassoni F, Nati S, Giordano D, Sessarego C, Raffo MR, Lamparelli T, Marmont AM (1986) High-dose chemotherapy (HDC) and autologous BMT in advanced highly treated Hodkin's disease (AHT-HD). Bone Marrow Transplantation [Suppl] 1: 293-296
7. Dicke KA, Spitzer G (1986) Clinical studies of autografting in acute lymphocytic leukaemia. Clin Haematol 15 (1): 85-103
8. Dinsmore RE, Kirkpatrick D, Flomenberg N, Gulati S, Kapoor N, Shauk B, Reid A, Groshen S, O'Reilly RJ (1983) Allogeneic bone marrow transplantation for patients with lymphoblastic leukemia. Blood 62: 381-388
9. Gasson JC, Weisbart RH, Kaufman SE, Clark SC, Hewick RM, Wong GG, Golde DW (1984) Purified human granulocyte-macrophage colony-stimulating factor: direct action on neutrophils. Science 226: 1339-1342
10. Gerson SL, Talbot GH, Hurwitz S (1984) Prolonged granulocytopenia: The major risk factor for invasive pulmonary aspergillosis in patients with acute leukemia. Ann Intern Med 100: 345-351
11. Gorin NC (1987) Autologous bone marrow transplantation: a review of recent advances in acute leukemia. In: Gale RP, Champlin RE (eds) Progress in bone marrow transplantation. Liss, New York, pp 723-750
12. Link H, Ostendorf P, Wernet P, Reinhart U, Walter E, Fischbach H, Niethammer D, Waller HD (1984) Pulmonary complications after allogeneic bone marrow transplantation. The Tuebingen experience. Exp Hematol 12 [Suppl 15]: 21-22
13. Metcalf D (1984) The haematopoietic colony stimulating factors. Elsevier, Amsterdam
14. Metcalf D (1986) The molecular biology and functions of the granulocyte macrophage colony-stimulating factors. Blood 67: 257
15. Philip T, Bernard JL, Bordigoni P, Paris A, Philip I, Pinkerton R, Favrot MC, Zucker JM (1986) Vincristine, melphalan, fractionated TBI, with purged ABMT as consolidation for an unselected group of patients with stage IV neuroblastoma. Bone Marrow Transplantation 1 [Suppl 1]: 319
16. Phillips GL, Herzig RG, Lazarus HM, Fay JW, Griffith R, Herzig GP (1986) High-dose chemotherapy, fractionated total body irradiation, and allogeneic marrow transplantation for malignant lymphoma. J Clin Oncol 4: 480-488
17. Van der Meer JWM, Guiot HFL, Van den Broek PJ, Van Furth R (1984) Infections in bone marrow transplant recipients. Semin Hematol 21: 123-140

A Phase Ib Evaluation of Recombinant Human Granulocyte-Macrophage Colony-Stimulating Factor*, **

R. G. STEIS,[1] J. CLARK,[1] D. L. LONGO,[1] J. SMITH,[1] R. MILLER,[1] F. RUSCETTI,[1] J. HURSEY,[2] and W. URBA[3]

Introduction

Colony-stimulating factors (CSFs) are glycoproteins that were originally characterized as agents capable of enhancing myeloid stem cell growth and differentiation and mature myeloid cell function. With the availability of large quantities of these agents in recombinant form [1-4], it was soon demonstrated that they could as well increase the rate of myeloid cell proliferation in vivo and increase blood myeloid cell numbers [5-8]. The most obvious potential application of these agents in cancer therapy would be in the restoration of myeloid cell number and function in patients following myelosuppressive chemotherapy regimens [7, 8]. If effective in this regard, the CSFs might allow the administration of more dose-intense chemotherapy regimens, which might result in higher tumor response rates than those obtained at conventional doses. Because CSFs can also stimulate granulocyte and monocyte function [9-13], and such activated cells can specifically recognize and lyse tumor cells [14-17], another potential application of these agents might be as antitumor drugs which mediate their antitumor effects through activation of effector cell function. To evaluate the potential of CSFs in this regard, we conducted a phase Ib study of recombinant human GM-CSF (rHuGM-CSF) in patients with a variety of malignancies. We evaluated not only the hematopoietic and toxic effects of this agent, but also its effects on granulocyte and monocyte function. This preliminary report summarizes our experience with rHuGM-CSF in doses of up to 50 mcg/kg.

* This project has been funded at least in part with Federal funds from the Department of Health and Human Services under contract number N01-Co-74102. The content of this publication does not necessarily reflect the views or policies of the Department of Health and Human Services, nor does mention of trade names, commercial products, or organizations imply endorsement by the U.S. Government.

[1] Biological Response Modifiers Program, Division of Cancer Treatment, National Cancer Institute, Frederick Cancer Facility, Frederick, MD 21701, USA.
[2] Frederick Memorial Hospital, Frederick, MD 21701, USA.
[3] Clinical Immunology Services, Program Resources, Inc., National Cancer Institute, Frederick Cancer Research Facility, Frederick, MD 21701, USA.

H. G. Beger et al. (Eds.), Cancer Therapy

Materials and Methods

Study Outline

To be eligible for this trial, patients must have had a histologically confirmed diagnosis of a solid tumor; for those tumors for which effective standard therapy is available, this therapy must have been previously administered. Patients with a history of myelodysplastic syndromes or with myeloproliferative disorders were excluded from this study. Also excluded were patients with a performance status of less than 70% on the Karnofsky scale, a diffusion capacity for carbon monoxide of less than 70% of the predicted value, a serum creatinine level greater than 2 mg/dl and a serum bilirubin level greater than 2 mg/dl. Patients must not have received radiation therapy to more than 50% of their axial skeleton and must have baseline granulocyte counts of more than 1500/mm^3, platelet counts of more than 100000/mm^3, and an untransfused hematocrit of 25% or greater. Chemotherapy must have been excluded for 4 weeks prior to study entry (6 weeks for nitrosoureas) and patients must not have had CNS metastases. All patients gave written informed consent, and this study was approved by the investigational review boards of both the Clinical Oncology Program, NCI, and the Frederick Cancer Research Facility. Prior to administration of rHuGM-CSF, patients were evaluated for tumor extent by standard clinical and radiologic means. Unilateral iliac crest bone marrow biopsy and aspiration were performed prior to and 1 day after the last day of administration of rHuGM-CSF.
The rHuGM-CSF used in this trial was produced and supplied by Immunex Corporation. It was prepared from genetically engineered yeast into which the human gene for GM-CSF had been inserted. The material was supplied as a lyophilized powder and was reconstituted with saline prior to infusion. Consecutive groups of three patients each received rHuGM-CSF as a 1- to 2-h intravenous infusion on day 0 of the study. If toxic effects were deemed acceptable, patients subsequently received daily infusions of rHuGM-CSF at the same dose for 21 consecutive days. The dose levels evaluated included 1, 10, 25, and 50 mcg/kg. Limitations in drug supply prevented further dose escalations. Dose-limiting toxicity was not reached. At the completion of rHuGM-CSF and 1 months later, patients returned to the clinic for re-evaluation of their tumor status.

Laboratory Evaluations

Serial blood samples were obtained throughout the course of the study to evaluate the hematologic and biologic response-modifying effects of rHuGM-CSF in those patients. Laboratory tests included complete blood counts with differential cell counts, levels of colony-forming units-granulocyte, erythrocyte, monocyte, megakaryocyte (CFU-GEMM) and colony-forming units-granulocyte, monocyte (CFU-GM) in peripheral blood and bone marrow, HLA-DR, Fc receptor and CD11b expression on peripheral blood monocytes, and superoxide anion induction and CD11b expression on granulocytes. Peripheral blood monocytes were also evaluated serially for cytotoxic activity against the melanoma cell line A375 and for changes in hydrogen peroxide generation.

Results

In all, 12 patients were admitted to this study, of whom 11 are evaluable for response and toxicity. One patient suffered a pathologic fracture of the left femoral neck shortly after receiving her first dose of rHuGM-CSF. Disease rapidly progressed elsewhere after treatment of this fracture, and the patient was removed from study. Table 1 provides a summary of the clinical characteristics of the 11 evaluable patients entered in this study. Five patients had colon carcinoma, four melanoma, one hepatocellular carcinoma, and one a small-bowel adenocarcinoma. All patients except for one had received prior therapy.

Toxic effects included fatigue (eight patients), bone pain (seven patients), nausea with anorexia (eight patients), fever (six patients), and myalgias (five patients). Occasional patients also complained of a chill during the infusion of the GM-CSF, pruritus, flushing, rash, and diarrhea. Three patients, including two patients treated at the 50 mcg/kg-dose level, had a transient reduction in blood pressure, with the lowest blood pressure reading being 80/50. The hypotensive episodes reversed spontaneously in two patients and with intravenous fluid administration in the third. Bone pain generally manifested as pain in the lower lumbar and posterior iliac crest areas. This bone pain was observed in patients shortly after the infusion of GM-CSF was begun and was not associated with bone tenderness. This phenomen was observed even in patients receiving the lowest dose of rHuGM-CSF (1 mcg/kg), for whom this agent had no apparent effect on marrow cellularity or peripheral blood counts. When pain developed during the infusion of rHuGM-

Table 1. Patient characteristics

Patient number	Dose level (mcg/kg)	Age/sex (years)	Diagnosis	Prior therapy
1	1	44/F	Hepatocellular carcinoma	AF, PBV, ^{131}I-labeled monoclonal antibody
2	1	48/F	Colon cancer	5-FU, TNF + IFN-gamma
3	1	70/M	Melanoma	BCG, IFN-alfa, TNF + IFN-gamma
4	10	55/M	Colon cancer	5-FU, TNF + IFN-gamma
5	10	65/M	Melanoma	None
6	10	56/M	Colon cancer	TNF + IFN-gamma
7	25	30/F	Melanoma	IFN-alfa
8	25	62/M	Colon cancer	TNF + IFN-gamma
9	25	73/M	Melanoma	IFN-alfa
10	50	57/F	Small-bowel adenocarcinoma	LAK + IL-2, TNF + IFN-gamma
11	50	67/M	Colon cancer	None

F, female; *M*, male; *A*, doxorubicin; F or *5-FU*, 5-fluorouracil; *P*, cisplatin; *B*, bleomycin; *V*, vinblastine; *TNF*, tumor necrosis factor; *IFN*, interferon; *BCG*, bacillus Calmette-Guérin; *LAK*, lymphokine-activated killer cells; *IL-2*, interleukin-2.

CSF, its severity could be reduced by slowing the rate of infusion. Except for hypotension, none of the toxic effects were dose related.

The effects of rHuGM-CSF on peripheral blood counts are shown in Table 2. There were dose-dependent increases in total white blood cell count, segmented neutrophil and neutrophilic band counts, eosinophil counts, and monocyte counts. There were slight increases in lymphocyte counts that were not definitely dose related. Peripheral blood counts tended to increase steadily and progressively during the 21 days of daily injections of rHuGM-CSF. After discontinuation of GM-CSF, there was a rapid fall of peripheral blood counts to baseline within 2–3 days. Peripheral blood counts were normal on evaluation 1 month after the last injection. GM-CSF had no appreciable effect on platelet or reticulocyte counts.

The granulocytes in these patients developed toxic granulations during the course of the study. No other morphologic changes were observed in the peripheral blood cells.

Unilateral bone marrow biopsies were obtained just prior to the first dose and 1 day after the last of rHuGM-CSF. Table 3 summarizes the changes observed in these marrow specimens. Cellularity tended to increase in a dose-dependent fashion, as did the ratio of myeloid to erythroid cells. In conjunction with the development of a peripheral eosinophilia, patients receiving GM-CSF also developed a marrow eosinophilia. Numbers of CFU-GMs and CFU-GEMMs, either in the bone marrow or peripheral blood, did not change appreciably at ony dose level. Although marrow stem cell numbers did not change, in one patient treated with 50 mcg/kg, there was a progressive increase in peripheral blood CFU-GM numbers from one colony to 24 colonies per 10^5 cells plated during administration of rHuGM-CSF.

Table 2. Effects of rHuGM-CSF on peripheral blood counts

Dose level (mcg/kg)	Total WBC	Segmented neutrophils	Neutrophilic bands	Eosinophils	Monocytes	Lymphocytes
1	0.3	−0.4	0.4	0.2	−0.5	0.5
10	12.9	6.9	1.4	2.4	0.5	1.5
25	23.6	8.3	4.3	8.4	0.8	1.6
50	48.1	14.7	14.6	16.9	1.0	0.9

Numbers represent the mean maximal change $\times 10^3/mm^3$ in absolute counts from baseline.

Table 3. Bone marrow effects of rHuGM-CSF

Dose level (mcg/kg)	Increase in cellularity	Increase in M:E ratio	Increase in eosinophils
1	1/3	0/3	0/3
10	2/2	1/2	1/2
25	2/3	3/3	3/3
50	2/2	2/2	2/2

M, myeloid; *E*, erythroid.
Number of patients with the effect/number of patients treated at that dose level.

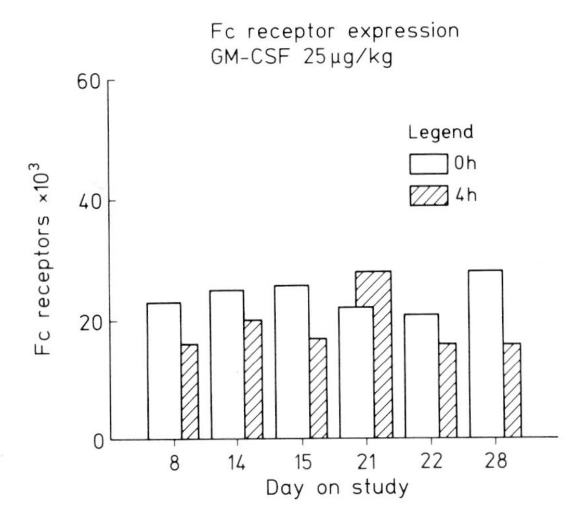

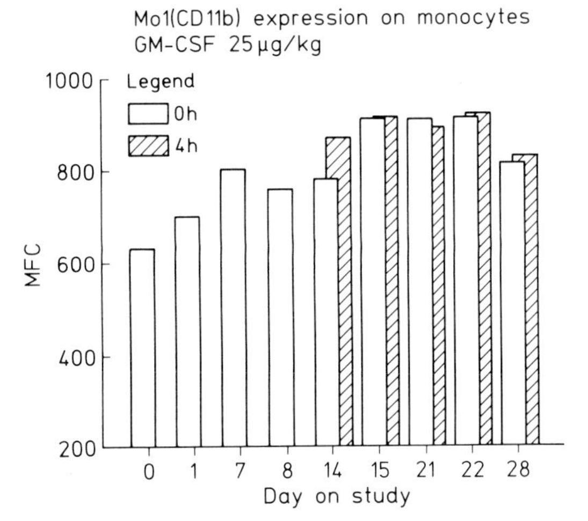

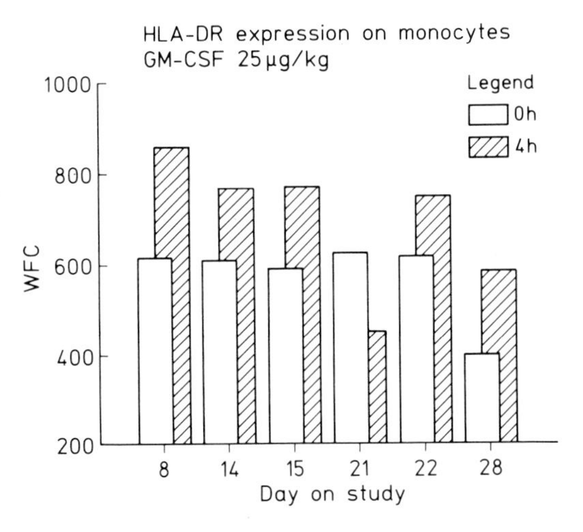

Fig. 1. Effects of rHuGM-CSF on monocyte expression of the Fc receptor for IgG, CD11b, and HLA-DR. Results are shown for a single patient treated at the 25 mcg/kg-dose level. *Open bars* represent blood samples obtained just prior to drug administration, and *hatched bars* represent results obtained from samples drawn 4 h after administration of GM-CSF

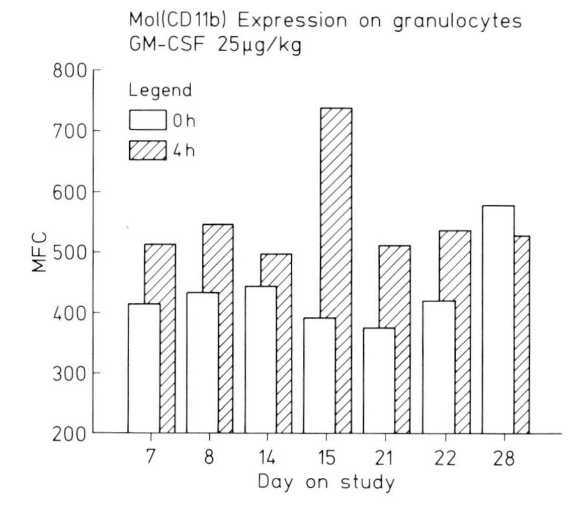

Fig. 2. Effect of rHuGM-CSF on granulocyte expression of CD11b. Results are from a single patient treated at the 25 mcg/kg-dose level. *Open bars* are the results obtained from samples drawn just prior to drug administration, and *hatched bars* from samples obtained 4 h after GM-CSF administration

The effect of rHuGM-CSF on monocyte function was evaluated by serial measurements of the production of hydrogen peroxide by these cells, by killing of A375 melanoma cells in vitro, and by the cell surface expression on monocytes of Fc receptors, CD11b, and HLA-DR. At no dose level was hydrogen peroxide production or lysis of A375 cells by monocytes enhanced by the administration of rHuGM-CSF. Cell surface expression of the receptor of the Fc portion of IgG was not significantly affected by rHuGM-CSF. In fact, there seemed to be a slight suppression of Fc receptor expression within 4 h of administration of this drug. However, both HLA-DR expression on monocytes and expression of the adhesion molecule, CD11b, were enhanced. Figure 1 is a composite of representative flow cytometric analyses performed on monocytes from one patient treated at the 25 mcg/kg-dose level.
Activation of peripheral blood granulocytes by the administration of rHuGM-CSF was assessed by serial measurements of phorbol myristic acetate (PMA)-induced superoxide anion production. In our hands, the marked variability from assay to assay within and between patients made it difficult to discern any reproducible change in this parameter following the administration of GM-CSF. This was observed when peripheral blood samples were collected 4 and 24 h after administration of GM-CSF. However, the cell surface expression of CD11b on granulocytes was reproducibly enhanced within 4 h of administration of the drug (Fig. 2).

Discussion

Through their demonstrated ability to stimulate myeloid cell proliferation and differentiation, CSFs will undoubtedly influence the design of studies using myelosuppressive drugs in that regimens with the potential to cause significant myelosuppression might be given with less concern for this toxic effect and its associated morbidity. Limited information in this regard has already been published for granulocyte CSF [7, 8]. The CSFs however are also biological response modifiers (BRMs) in that they have the capacity to enhance monocyte-mediated cytotoxicity [12, 14, 15], antibody-dependent cellular cytotoxicity mediated by neutrophils and eosinophils [11, 16, 17], augment the antigen-presenting capacity of splenic adherent cells [18], and enhance monocyte production of tumor necrosis factor and hydrogen peroxide [12–14]. Clinical and laboratory studies have demonstrated that doses of BRMs that optimally augment immune function might be substantially different from the maximally tolerated dose [19]. We undertook an evaluation of rHuGM-CSF given over a 50-fold dose range to determine not only the hematopoietic and toxic effects of this agent but also its BRM effects in patients with a variety of solid tumors.

At doses above 10 mcg/kg, we observed reproducible increments in peripheral blood granulocyte, monocyte, and eosinophil counts without significant associated toxic effects. rHuGM-CSF was capable of increasing total peripheral white blood cell counts to as high as 72000/mm^3 at doses of 50 mcg/kg. White blood cell increments occurred progressively throughout the duration of rHuGM-CSF administration; there was no apparent plateau in the maximum white blood cell count at this dose level. This increase in peripheral white blood cell counts was associated with an increase in marrow cellularity and the ratio of myeloid to erythroid cells. However, using superoxide anion generation in response to PMA and hydrogen peroxide production and killing of A375 melanoma cells in vitro as indicators of activation of granulocytes and monocytes, we were unable to demonstrate activation of either of these cell types as has been observed in vitro [12, 13, 15]. However, rHuGM-CSF was clearly exerting effects on monocytes as assessed by the surface expression on these cells of CD11b and HLA-DR. Unfortunately, limitations in drug supply did not permit us to escalate the dose beyond 50 mcg/kg and, thus the ability of rHuGM-CSF to augment monocyte and granulocte functions in vivo have not been fully assessed. Nonetheless, it is possible to conclude that, at the dose levels tested, no enhancement of monocyte and granulocyte function was observed.

We did not determine whether granulocyte in our patients retained the capacity to migrate to sites of tissue injury. However, migration of granulocytes into skin chambers was markedly reduced by rHuGM-CSF in the study of Peters et al. [20]. This observation is important, as its suggests that the ability of granulocytes to localize to sites of inflammation might be impaired in these patients, rendering them less able to control infections. Perhaps this observation can be explained by the enhanced expression of CD11b on granulocytes observed in our study. Expression of this leukocyte adhesion molecule should be correlated with the ability of granulocytes to migrate into tissues in future studies of rHuGM-CSF.

We thus conclude that rHUGM-CSF has potent effects on granulocyte, eosinophil, and monocyte numbers in the peripheral blood of patients with various solid tumors. Although there was enhancement of cell surface expression of various monocyte- and granulocyte-associated markers, there was no obvious effect of this agent, at the doses tested, on functional properties of mature neutrophils and monocytes. Furthermore, we did not observe any antitumor effects in any of our patients. Because higher doses were not tested, the possibility exists that higher doses might be associated with antitumor effects or with demonstrable in vivo activation of granulocytes and monocytes. At least in the doses tested, rHuGM-CSF is capable of increasing effector cell numbers, and perhaps by combining this agent with more traditional monocyte-activating agents, such as interferon-gamma [19], induction of tumor cell cytotoxicity might be achievable in vivo.

Acknowledgement. The authors wish to acknowledge the expert nursing care provided by the 2B nursing staff of the Frederick Memorial Hospital, the administrative and laboratory assistance provided Program Resources, Inc., and the secretarial skills of Sharon Lewis.

References

1. Cantrell MA, Anderson D, Cerretti DP et al. (1985) Cloning, sequence, and expression of a human granulocyte/macrophage colony-stimulating factor. Proc Natl Acad Sci 82: 6250–6254
2. Kaushansky K, O'Hara PJ, Berkner K et al. (1986) Genomic cloning, characterization, and multilineage growth-promoting activity of human granulocyte-macrophage colony-stimulating factor. Proc Natl Acad Sci 83: 3101–3105
3. Lee F, Yokota T, Otsuka T et al. (1985) Isolation of cDNA for a human granulocyte-macrophage colony-stimulating factor by functional expression in mammalian cells. Proc Natl Acad Sci 82: 4360–4364
4. Wong GG, Witek JS, Temple PA et al. (1985) Human GM-CSF: Molecular cloning of the complementary DNA and purification of the natural and recombinant proteins. Science 228: 810–815
5. Donahue RE, Wang EA, Stone DK et al. (1986) Stimulation of haematopoiesis in primates by continuous infusion of recombinant human GM-CSF. Nature 321: 872–875
6. Mayer P, Lam C, Obenaus H et al. (1987) Recombinant human GM-CSF induces leukocytosis and activates peripheral blood polymorphonuclear neutrophils in nonhuman primates. Blood 70: 206–213
7. Morstyn G, Campbell L, Souza LM et al. (1988) Effect of granulocyte colony stimulating factor on neutropenia induced by cytotoxic chemotherapy. Lancet 1: 667–672
8. Gabrilove JL, Jakubowski A, Scher H et al. (1988) Effect of granulocyte colony-stimulating factor on neutropenia and associated morbidity due to chemotherapy for transitional-cell carcinoma of the urothelium. New Eng J Med 318: 1414–1422
9. Fleischmann J, Golde DW, Weisbart RH et al. (1986) Granulocyte-macrophage colony-stimulating factor enhances phagocytosis of bacteria by human neutrophils. Blood 68: 708–711
10. Villalta F, Kierszenbaum F (1986) Effects of human colony-stimulating factor on the uptake and destruction of a pathogenic parasite *(Trypanosoma Cruzi)* by human neutrophils. J Immunol 137: 1703–1707
11. Lopez AF, Williamson DJ, Gamble JR et al. (1986) Recombinant human granulocyte-macrophage colony-stimulating factor stimulates in vitro mature human neutrophil and eosinophil function, surface receptor expression, and survival. J Clin Invest 78: 1220–1228
12. Reed SG, Nathan CF, Pihl DL et al. (1987) Recombinant granulocyte/macrophage colony-stimulating factor activates macrophages to inhibit *Trypanosoma cruzi* and release hydrogen peroxide. J Exp Med 166: 1734–1746
13. Weisbart RH, Golde DW, Clark SC et al. (1985) Human granulocyte-macrophage colony-stimulating factor is a neutrophil activator. Nature 314: 361–363
14. Cannistra SA, Vellenga E, Groshek P et al. (1988) Human Granulocyte-monocyte colony-stimulating factor and interleukin 3 stimulate monocyte cytotoxicity through a tumor necrosis factor-dependent mechanism. Blood 71: 672–676
15. Grabstein KH, Urdal DL, Tushinski RJ et al. (1986) Induction of macrophage tumoricidal activity by granulocyte-macrophage colony-stimulating factor. Science 232: 506–508
16. Vadas MA, Nicola NA, Metcalf D (1983) Activation of antibody-dependent cell-mediated cytotoxicity of human neutrophils and eosinophils by separate colony-stimulating factors. J Immunol 130: 795–799

17. Metcalf D, Begley CG, Johnson GR et al. (1986) Biologic properties in vitro of a recombinant human granulocyte-macrophage colony-stimulating factor. Blood 67: 37–45
18. Morrissey PJ, Bressler L, Park LS et al. (1987) Granulocyte-macrophage colony-stimulating factor augments the primary antibody response by enhancing the function of antigen-presenting cells. J Immunol 139: 1113–1119
19. Maluish AE, Urba WJ, Longo DL et al. (1988) The determination of an immunologically active dose of interferon-gamma in patients with melanoma. J Clin Oncol 6: 434–445
20. Peters WP, Brandt SJ, Atwater SK et al. (1988) Effect of recombinant human granulocyte macrophage colony-stimulating factor (rHuGM-CSF) on hematopoietic reconstitution and granulocyte function following high dose chemotherapy (HDC) and autologous bone marrow transplantation (ABMT). Proc ASCO 7: 160 (abstract 616)

The Role of Interferon in the Management of Patients with Hairy Cell Leukemia and Multiple Myeloma

N. NIEDERLE[1] and G. KUMMER[1]

Interferons (IFNs) were first described in 1957 [35]. During the last two decades, these cytokines have received increasing attention in the treatment of cancer, particularly since in 1981 highly purified material produced by recombinant DNA technology has become available in addition to natural IFNs [25, 51, 59]. So far, the most impressive clinical results have been achieved in hematologic disorders, especially in hairy cell leukemia [26, 41, 54].

Hairy Cell Leukemia

Hairy cell leukemia (HCL) is a rare lymphoproliferative disorder, which usually appears during the fourth to fifth decade of life, predominantly in men [6, 18, 50]. It is characterized by the proliferation of mononuclear cells, usually of the B-phenotype, which in most cases test positive with tartrate-resistant acid phosphatase staining [9, 37, 72, 82]. These hairy cells infiltrate predominantly the spleen, liver, and bone marrow and characteristically result in splenomegaly, varying degrees of pancytopenia, and a deficiency in cell-mediated immunity. Infections are the main cause of morbidity and mortality, followed by hemorrhage. Median survival after diagnosis is in the range of 3-4 years [27].

Splenectomy has generally been the initial treatment, resulting in a rapid improvement of cytopenia and attendant symptoms in 60%-80% of the patients. Complete disappearance of the leukemic cells from peripheral blood or bone marrow, however, almost never occurs, and most patients relapse after a period of months or years [36, 46, 55]. Once a relapse has occurred, or when there is no initial response to splenectomy, different therapeutic approaches are tried (Table 1). Most of these treatment modalities are of limited success and often are complicated by severe adverse reactions [7, 10, 28, 48, 77, 83]. Therapy has changed significantly since the introduction of alfa-IFNs and, later, 2′-deoxycoformycin [11, 24].

Since the first reports by Quesada and coworkers [64], several hundred patients have been treated with IFNs. Both natural and recombinant alfa-IFNs are effective in HCL. The remission rates are between 70% and 90%, including 10%-30% complete remissions (Table 2). Only approximately 5%-10% of the patients do not respond to alfa-IFN. So far, response rates are similar in previously untreated,

[1] University Clinic for Internal Medicine (Tumor Research), West German Tumor Center, Essen, Hufelandstraße 55, 4300 Essen 1, FRG.

H. G. Beger et al. (Eds.), Cancer Therapy

Table 1. Treatment modalities in hairy cell leukemia

Treatment modalities
Splenectomy (60%–80% improvement)
Cytostatic chemotherapy - Chlorambucil - Doxorubicin - Vinca-alkaloids
Corticosteroids
Androgens
Bacillus Calmette-Guérin (BCG)
Leukapheresis
Bone marrow transplantation
Natural and recombinant alfa-interferons
2′-deoxycoformycin (pentostatin)

splenectomized or cytostatically pretreated patients, although some investigators have reported a higher incidence of complete remissions in the previously untreated group, probably due to an earlier stage of the disease with lower levels of bone marrow infiltration.

During the first weeks of IFN therapy, most patients develop transient myelosuppression [8, 52, 70]. The initial improvement observed is the reduction in spleen size and the disappearance of hairy cells from peripheral blood. This occurs during the first month of treatment. An increase in platelets - often within 2–3 weeks after initiation of treatment, which return to normal values after about 2 months of treatment - usually precedes the rise in hemoglobin values, monocytes, or neutrophil leukocyte counts. Neutrophil values do no return to normal until 3–5 months after the start of IFN therapy (Fig. 1). The eradication of hairy cells from the bone marrow, however, requires a more prolonged period of treatment and does not result in complete elimination in most patients. Although alfa-IFNs have a significant impact on the course of the disease, they do not seem to be curative, since responses are not durable, and patients tend to relapse within 9–12 months after cessation of treatment or even during weekly administration of low-dose alfa-IFN [4, 39, 66, 70].

In contrast to the positive results with alfa-IFNs, there is still no evidence of significant efficacy of gamma-IFN in hairy cell leukemia. In our department, six patients with hairy cell leukemia were treated with gamma-IFN for 9–35 weeks [53]. After a short, therapy-free interval, all of them received approximately the same doses of alfa-2b-IFN. While there was no clinical or hematologic improvement during the application of gamma-IFN, alfa-2b-IFN led to a gradual normalization of the hemoglobin values and of the platelet and granulocyte counts in all patients.

These differing clinical effects of alfa- and gamma-IFNs on the proliferation of hairy cells have been confirmed by laboratory investigations [58]. After stimulating the growth of hairy cells with B-cell growth factor (interleukin 4/5), the HC prolif-

Table 2. Results of interferon therapy in hairy cell leukemia

Interferon (type)	Dose ($\times 10^6$)	Route/ Schedule	Patients (*n*) entered (evaluated)	Pretreatment		Response (*n*)				References
				Systemic	No splenectomy	CR	PR	MR	NR	
Leuko	0.5 (1.5)	s.c. 5/week	4	2	1		1	2	1	Porzolt, 1985 [60]
Alfa-2b	$2/m^2$	s.c. 3/week	13	1	6			9	4	Hofmann, 1985 [30]
Lympho	3 (6)	i.m. daily i.m. 2nd day	17	7	5	2	12	3		Worman, 1985 [80]
Alfa-2c	5	s.c. daily	26			3	15	4	4	Huber, 1985 [32]
Leuko	3	i.m. daily	22			5	13	4		Quesada, 1986 [66]
Alfa-2a	3–12	i.m. daily	30	11	7	9	17	4		Quesada, 1986 [67]
Alfa-2b	$2/m^2$	s.c. 3/week	64 (60)	39	3	3	45	9	3	Golomb, 1986 [29]
Alfa-2a Alfa-2b Leuko	3 $2/m^2$ 3	s.c. daily s.c. 3/week s.c. daily	37 (17)	1	6	1	14	1	1	Flandrin, 1986 [19]
Alfa-2b	$4/m^2$ (2)	s.c. 2nd day	19 (17)	4	6	2	13	2		Niederle, 1986 [52]
Alfa-2a	3	i.m. daily	15 (14)	3	5	1	12		1	Foon, 1986 [20]
Alfa-2b	$2/m^2$	s.c. 3/week	11 (10)	7	9	2	7		1	Ehman, 1986 [17]
Lympho	$0.2/m^2$ $2/m^2$	s.c. daily (3/week) s.c. daily (3/week)	24 (22) 24 (22)			5	9 4	17	6	Smalley, 1986 [74]
Alfa-2b	1	s.c. daily	19 (16)	2	13	2	10	2	2	v. Wussow, 1986 [81]
Alfa-2c	5 0.1–0.8	s.c. daily s.c. daily	10 11		8	2 1	5 4	2 5	1 1	Huber, 1987 [33]
Alfa-2c	$2.0/m^2$ (0.2)	s.c. daily (s.c. 2nd day)	97 (73)	4	39					Pralle, 1987 [63]
Gamma	$4/m^2$	s.c. 2nd day	6	1					6	Niederle, 1987 [53]
Alfa-2b	$2/m^2$	s.c. 3/week	212	94	46	8	159	23	22	Thompson, 1987 [79]
Alfa-2b	$2/m^2$ $4/m^2$	s.c. 3/week s.c. 7/week	34 (33) 29 5	7	12		23 5	4	1	Hofmann, 1988 [31]

CR, complete remission; *PR*, partial remission; *MR*, minor response; *NR*, no response.

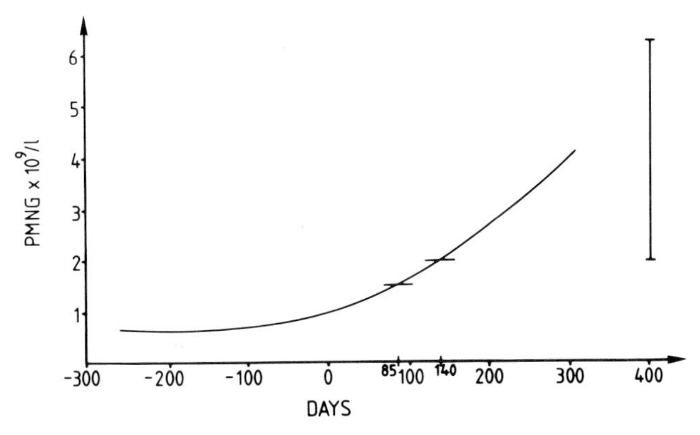

Fig. 1. Median granulocyte counts prior to and during treatment with alfa-2b-IFN. *PMNG*, polymorphonuclear leukocytes

eration was inhibited by alfa-IFN but not by gamma-IFN. The different antiproliferative activities of the two cytokines might be due to the fact that exogenously administered alfa-IFN is able to interrupt an autocrine loop created by the synthesis of interleukin 4 in hairy cells [22, 73]. This is supported by the fact that in active HCL the production of alfa-IFN, but not of gamma-IFN seems to be depressed [30, 43, 62, 78]. Clinically observed recurrences after cessation of treatment are easily explained by this model. There might also be a direct antiproliferative effect of IFN on hairy cells, since alfa-IFN is able to modulate oncogene expression and to induce synthesis of specific proteins which have a different pattern from those seen after gamma-IFN exposure [42, 71]. The effectiveness of alfa-IFN treatment in HCL, however, does not appear to be mediated by natural killer (NK) cells [23, 73]. The increase of NK activity in HCL patients treated with alfa-2b-IFN follows rather than precedes the clinical improvement in peripheral blood counts and even bone marrow histology.

Although an impressive body of data has accumulated over the past few years concerning the effectiveness of alfa- but not of gamma-IFNs in inducing remission in HCL, some questions remain to be answered. The optimal doses and schedules of interferon therapy still have to be defined. Recently published data indicate that the minimal effective doses of alpha-IFN should be used, for instance in the range of 500000–1 million units every day or 2 million units every second day. Our own experience with more than 30 patients seems to support this concept (Fig. 2), although in the 1-million-unit group, it appears to take somewhat longer to achieve normalization of all hematologic parameters.

Since treatment with alfa-IFN causes in vivo down-regulation of IFN receptors on hairy cells, further trials should investigate whether intermittent application of alfa-IFN provides as good clinical results as continuous administration [5, 12]. The question remains whether there is any survival advantage in complete remission over partial remission. Furthermore, it should be clarified whether there is any need for maintenance therapy beyond 12 months [39], especially since a second response can be induced in almost all relapsing patients by the renewed application of alfa-IFN.

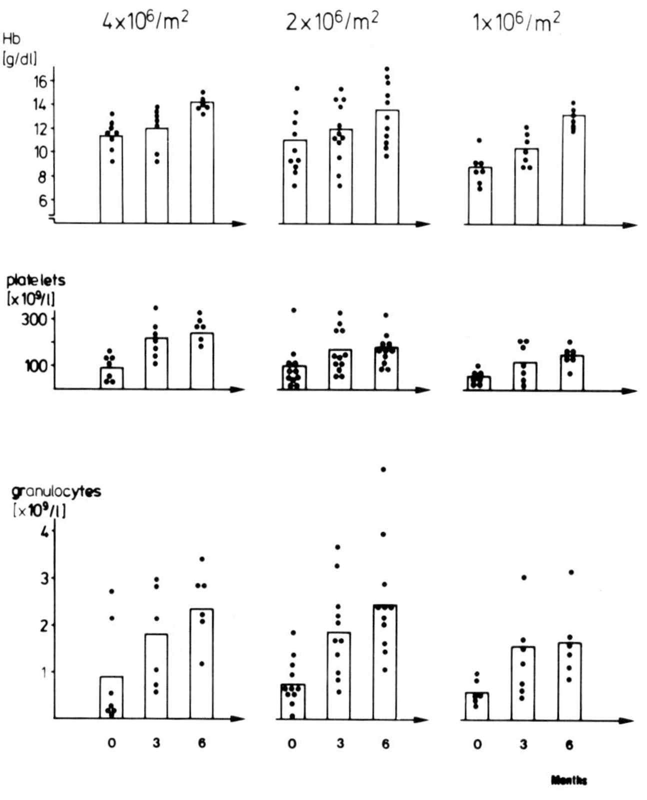

Fig. 2. Treatment results in 27 patients with progressive hairy cell leukemia who were treated with alfa-2b-IFN subcutaneously every second day at an initial dose of 4×10^6 U/m² ($n=7$), 2×10^6 U/m² ($n=12$), and 1×10^6 U/m² ($n=8$)

A major remaining question is whether IFN therapy should be used as initial treatment instead of splenectomy [61]. Since more than 50% of splenectomized patients have a prolonged, treatment-free survival, splenectomy continues to be advocated for patients with splenomegaly and symptomatic cytopenias. IFN may become the initial therapy, however, in all other cases, especially in patients with packed marrow, no splenomegaly, severe infections, and hemorrhage, or a leukemic phase of the disease [69]. Finally, the place of deoxycoformicin or other purine metabolism inhibitors in the treatment of HCL have to be determined [21, 38, 40, 75, 76].

Multiple Myeloma

In contrast to HCL, the potential role of IFN in multiple myeloma is controversial. Early clinical studies demonstrated antitumor activity of partially purified alfa-IFNs in patients with multiple myeloma (Table 3). Subsequent trials with a larger number of patients have confirmed the effectiveness of both natural and

Table 3. Results of interferon treatment in multiple myeloma

Interferon (type)	Units ($\times 10^6$)	Route/ schedule	Patients (*n*) entered (evaluated)	Prior therapy		Response (*n*)					Duration (months)	Reference
				yes	no	CR	PR	MR	NC	PD		
Leuko	3	i.m. daily	4		4	2	2					Mellstedt, 1979 [49]
Leuko	3	i.m. 2× daily	1	1			1					Ideström, 1979 [34]
Leuko	3–9	i.m. daily	21	9	12		5	3	13		16	Alexanian, 1982 [3]
Leuko	6	i.m. 5/week	9	9			1		1	7		Rapson, 1984 [68]
Alfa-2b	3–100/m²	i.v. 3/week s.c.	49 (38)	38		1	6				5	Costanzi, 1985 [15]
Alfa-2a	3–50	i.m. daily	64 (47)	39	8		10	5			2	Ohno, 1986 [57]
Alfa-2a	12/m²	i.m. daily	32 (27)	13	 14		2 7		7 5	4 2	14	Quesada, 1986 [65]
Leuko	10 (20–30)	i.m. 7 days/3rd week i.m. daily	50		50		18					Åhre, 1988 [2]

CR, complete remission; *PR*, partial remission; *MR*, minor response; *NC*, no change; *PD*, progressive disease.

Table 4. Prospective randomized studies comparing interferon treatment and standard chemotherapy in non-pretreated patients with multiple myeloma

Interferon (type)	Units ($\times 10^6$)	Route/Schedule	Patients (*n*) entered (evaluated)	Response (*n*)					Duration (months)	Referene
				CR	PR	MR	NC	PD		
< Leuko	3–(6)	i.m. daily	75 (74)		10*				13**	Ahre, 1984 [1]
MP			55 (54)		24*				35**	
< Alfa-2c	10 (20)	i.m. 5–7/week	21 (14)		2	4	7	1		Ludwig, 1986 [44]
VMCP			21 (19)		11	6	2			
< VMCP + alfa-2c	2	i.m. 5/week	15 (14)		7	3	3	1		Ludwig, 1987 [45]
VMCP			17 (15)		5	5	4	1		
< MP + leuko	7/m^2	i.m. 5/3rd week	95 (34)		27***					Österborg, 1987 [56]
MP			(29)		15***					
CTx < alfa-2b	3–10/m^2	s.c. 3/week	29						19+***	Mandelli, 1988 [47]
0			31						11***	

MP, melphalan/prednisone; *VMCP*, vincristine/melphalan/cyclophosphamide/prednisone.
* $P<0.001$; ** $P<0.05$; *** $P<0.01$.

recombinant alfa-IFNs. The results can be summarized as follows: Remissions (usually partial) can be induced in about 20% of the patients with a median time to response of 1.5 months [2, 65]. After IFN, but not cytostatic treatment, some of the responding patients showed a normalization of their serum immunoglobulin levels [15, 65] and a healing of lytic bone lesions [14, 57]. Objective response rates following IFN treatment among patients relapsing after chemotherapeutically induced remission seem to be superior to those of patients who are primarily resistant to conventional treatment [15]. Moreover, a significant number of patients relapsing after initial chemotherapy and receiving subsequent treatment with IFN will apparently respond to the reapplication of chemotherapy [16]. Low tumor mass, no specific pretreatment, and IgA myeloma have turned out to be further positive prognostic factors [1, 2, 44, 57, 65].
Melphalan/prednisone or the more intensive vincristine/melphalan/cyclophosphamide/prednisolone combination were compared with alpha-IFN in two prospective randomized trials (Table 4). In both studies, combination chemotherapy induced significantly more and longer-lasting remissions than the IFN monotherapy. Overall survival, however, was similar in both groups [1, 44].
Since additive or even synergistic antiproliferative effects were noted in vitro on tumor colony cell reduction with combinations of alfa-IFN plus cyclophosphamide or melphalan or prednisone, clinical trials were started combining IFN with standard chemotherapy [14]. The combinations were demonstrated to be safe, and the response rates approached 75% [13]. Prospective randomized studies are now being conducted to compare standard drug regimens with or without alfa-IFNs [45, 56]. Another question is whether IFN can prolong remission once a response to a multiagent drug regimen has been achieved [47]. Further follow-up is needed, however, before any conclusions can be drawn on the efficacy of alfa-IFN in this adjuvant setting. All in all, the role of IFNs in multiple myeloma is still controversial and requires further clinical verification.

References

1. Ahre A, Björkholm M, Mellstedt H, Brenning G, Engstedt L, Gahrton G, Gyllenhammar H, Holm G, Johansson B, Järnmark M, Karnström L, Killander A, Lerner R, Lockner D, Lönnqvist B, Nilsson B, Simonsson B, Stalfelt A-M, Strander H, Svedmyr E, Wadman B, Wedelin C (1984) Human leukocyte interferon and intermittent high-dose melphalan-prednisone administration in the treatment of multiple myeloma: A randomized clinical trial from the Myeloma Group of Central Sweden. Cancer Treat Rep 68: 1331–1338
2. Åhre A, Björkholm M, Österborg A, Brenning G, Gahrton G, Gyllenhammar H, Holm G, Johansson B, Juliusson G, Järnmark M, Killander A, Lerner R, Lockner D, Nilsson B, Simonsson B, Stalfelt A-M, Strander H, Smedmyr B, Svedmyr E, Uden A-M, Wadman B, Wedelin C, Mellstedt H (1988) High doses of natural α-interferon (α-IFN) in the treatment of multiple myeloma – a pilot study from the Myeloma Group of Central Sweden (MGCS). Eur J Haematol 41: 123–130
3. Alexanian R, Gutterman J, Levy H (1982) Interferon treatment for multiple myeloma. Clin Haematol 11: 211–220
4. Aulitzky W, Gastl G, Tilg H, v. Lüttichau I, Flener R, Huber C (1986) Recurrence of hairy cell leukemia upon discontinuation of IFN treatment. Blut 53: 215

5. Billard C, Sigaux F, Castaigne S, Valensi F, Flandrin G, Degos L, Falcoff E, Aguet M (1986) Treatment of hairy cell leukemia with recombinant alpha-interferon: II. In vivo down-regulation of alpha interferon receptors on tumors cells. Blood 67: 821-826
6. Bouroncle BA, Wiseman BK, Doan CA (1958) Leukemic retriculoendotheliosis. Blood 13: 609-630
7. Calvo F, Castaigne S, Sigaux F, Marty M, Degos L, Boiron M, Flandrin G (1985) Intensive chemotherapy of hairy cell leukemia in patients with aggressive disease. Blood 65: 115-119
8. Castaigne S, Sigaux F, Cantell K, Falcoff E, Boiron M, Flandrin G, Degos L (1986) Interferon alpha in the treatment of hairy cell leukemia. Cancer 57: 1681-1684
9. Catovsky D, Pettit JE, Galetto J, Okos A, Galton DAG (1974) The B-lymphocyte nature of the hairy cell of leukaemic reticuloendotheliosis. Br J Haematol 26: 29-37
10. Cheever MA, Fefer A, Greenberg PD, Appelbaum FR, Armitage JO, Buckner CD, Sale GE, Storb R, Witherspoon RD, Thomas ED (1984) Identical twin bone marrow transplantation for hairy cell leukemia. Semin Oncol 11 (suppl 2): 511-513
11. Cheson BD, Martin A (1987) Clinical trials in hairy cell leukemia. Ann Intern Med 106: 871-878
12. Clark RH, Dimitrov NV, Axelson JA, Oviatt DL, Penner JA, Charamella LJ, Walker W (1986) Intermittent alpha-leukocyte interferon in the treatment of hairy cell leukemia. Blood 68 (suppl 1): 220a
13. Cooper MR, Fefer A, Thompson J, Case DC, Kempf R, Sacher R, Neefe J, Bickers J, Scarffe JH, Spiegel R, Bonnem E (1986) Alpha-2-interferon/melphalan/prednisone in previously untreated patients with multiple myeloma: A phase I-II trial. Cancer Treat Rep 70: 473-476
14. Cooper MR, Welander CE (1987) Interferons in the treatment of multiple myeloma. Cancer 59: 594-600
15. Costanzi JJ, Cooper MR, Scarffe JH, Ozer H, Grubbs SS, Ferraresi RW, Pollard RB, Spiegel RJ (1985) Phase II study of recombinant alpha-2 interferon in resistant multiple myeloma. J Clin Oncol 3: 654-659
16. Costanzi JJ, Pollard RB (1987) The use of interferon in the treatment of multiple myeloma. Semin Oncol 14 [Suppl 2]: 24-28
17. Ehmann WC, Silber R (1986) Recombinant alpha-2 interferon for treatment of hairy cell leukemia without prior splenectomy. Am J Med 80: 1111-1114
18. Flandrin G, Sigaux F, Sebahoun G, Bouffette P (1984) Hairy cell leukemia: Clinical presentation and follow-up of 211 patients. Semin Oncol 11 [Suppl 2]: 458-471
19. Flandrin G, Sigaux F, Castaigne S, Billard C, Aguet M, Boiron M, Falcoff E, Degos L (1986) Treatment of hairy cell leukemia with recombinant alpha interferon: I. Quantitative study of bone marrow changes during the first months of treatment. Blood 67: 817-820
20. Foon KA, Maluish AE, Abrams PG, Wrightington S, Stevenson HC, Alarif A, Fer MF, Overton WR, Poole M, Schnipper EF, Jaffe ES, Herberman RB (1986) Recombinant leukocyte A interferon therapy for advanced hairy cell leukemia. Am J Med 80: 351-356
21. Foon KA, Nakano GM, Koller CA, Longo DL, Steis RG (1986) Response to 2'-deoxycoformycin after failure of interferon-alfa in nonsplenectomized patients with hairy cell leukemia. Blood 68: 297-300
22. Ford RJ, Kwok D, Quesada J, Sahasrabuddhe CG (1986) Production of B cell growth factor(s) by neoplastic B cells from hairy cell leukemia patients. Blood 67: 573-577
23. Gastl G, Aulitzky W, Leiter E, Flener R, Huber C (1986) Alpha-interferon induces remission in hairy cell leukemia without enhancement of natural killing. Blut 52: 273-279
24. Glaspy JA, Jacobs AD, Golde DW (1987) Evolving therapy of hairy cell leukemia. Cancer 59: 652-657
25. Goeddel DV, Yelverton E, Ullrich A, Heyneker HL, Miozzari G, Holmes W, Seeburg PH, Dull T, May L, Stebbing N, Crea R, Maeda S, McCandliss R, Sloma A, Tabor JM, Gross M, Familletti PC, Pestka S (1980) Human leukocyte interferon produced by *E. coli* is biologically active. Nature 287: 411-416
26. Goldstein D, Laszlo J (1986) Interferon therapy in cancer: From imaginon to interferon. Cancer Res 46: 4315-4329
27. Golomb HM (1983) Hairy cell leukemia: Lessons learned in twenty-five years. J Clin Oncol 1: 652-656
28. Golomb HM, Schmidt K, Vardiman JW (1984) Chlorambucil therapy of twenty-four post-splenectomy patients with progressive hairy cell leukemia. Semin Oncol 11 [Suppl 2]: 502-506

29. Golomb HM, Jacobs A, Fefer A, Ozer H, Thompson J, Portlock C, Ratain M, Golde D, Vardiman J, Burke JS, Brady J, Bonnem E, Spiegel R (1986) Alpha-2 interferon therapy of hairy-cell leukemia: A multicenter study of 64 patients. J Clin Oncol 4: 900-905
30. Hofmann V, Fehr J, Sauter C, Ottino J (1985) Hairy cell leukemia: an interferon deficient disease? Cancer Treat Rev 12 [Suppl B]: 33-37
31. Hofmann V, Frey B (1988) Long-term treatment of hairy cell leukemia with interferon alfa-2b. Cancer Treat Rev 15 [Suppl A]: 7-13
32. Huber C, Flener R, Gastl G (1985) Interferon-alpha-2c in the treatment of advanced hairy cell leukaemia. Results of a phase II trial. Oncology 42 [Suppl 1]: 7-9
33. Huber C, Aulitzky W, Tilg H, v. Lüttichau I, Troppmair J, Nachbauer K, Gastl G (1987) Studies on the optimal dose and the mode of action of alpha-interferon in the treatment of hairy cell leukemia (HCL). Leukemia 1: 355-357
34. Ideström K, Cantell K, Killander D, Nilsson K, Strander H, Willems J (1979) Interferon therapy in multiple myeloma. Acta Med Scand 205: 149-154
35. Isaacs A, Lindenmann J (1957) Virus interference. I. The interferon. Proc R Soc Ser B 147: 258-267
36. Jansen J, Hermans J (1981) Splenectomy in hairy cell leukemia: A retrospective multicenter analysis. Cancer 47: 2066-2076
37. Jansen J, den Ottolander GJ, Schuit HRE, Waayer JLM, Hijmans W (1984) Hairy cell leukemia: Its place among the chronic B cell leukemias. Semin Oncol 11: 386-393
38. Johnston JB, Glazer RI, Pugh L, Israels LG (1986) The treatment of hairy-cell leukaemia with 2′-deoxycoformycin. Br J Haematol 63: 525-534
39. Kloke O, Niederle N, May D, Kruse H, Bartsch H, Wandl U, Osieka R, Schmidt CG (1988) The effect of two schedules of low-dose interferon alfa on remission maintenance in hairy cell leukemia. J Cancer Res Clin Oncol 114 [Suppl]: 110
40. Kraut EH, Bouroncle BA, Grever MR (1986) Low-dose deoxycoformycin in the treatment of hairy cell leukemia. Blood 68: 1119-1122
41. Krown SE (1986) Interferons and interferon inducers in cancer treatment. Semin Oncol 13: 207-217
42. Lehn P, Sigaux F, Grausz D, Loiseau P, Castaigne S, Degos L, Flandrin G, Dautry F (1986) c-myc and c-fos expression during interferon-alfa therapy for hairy cell leukemia. Blood 68: 967-970
43. Lepe-Zuniga JL, Quesada JR, Gutterman JU (1986) Deficiency of production of alpha interferon in patients with active hairy cell leukemia and its restoration after complete remission. Blood 68 [Suppl 1]: 202a
44. Ludwig H, Cortelezzi A, Scheithauer W, van Camp BGK, Kuzmits R, Fillet G, Peetermans M, Polli E, Flener R (1986) Recombinant interferon alfa-2c versus polychemotherapy (VMGP) for treatment of multiple myeloma: A prospective randomized trial. Eur J Cancer Clin Oncol 22: 1111-1116
45. Ludwig H, Cortelezzi A, Fritz E, Kührer I, Polli E, Scheithauer W, Flener R (1987) Combined interferon-polychemotherapy versus polychemotherapy in multiple myeloma: A phase-III study. In: Cantell K, Schellekens H (eds) The Biology of the interferon system 1986. Martinus Nijhoff, Dordrecht
46. Magee MJ, McKenzie S, Filippa DA, Arlin ZA, Gee TS, Clarkson BD (1985) Hairy cell leukemia. Durability of response to splenectomy in 26 patients and treatment of relapse with androgens in six patients. Cancer 56: 2557-2562
47. Mandelli F, Tribalto M, Avvisati G, Cantonetti M, Petrucci MT, Boccadoro M, Pileri A, Marmont F, Resegotti L, Lauta V, Dammacco F (1988) Recombinant interferon alfa-2b (INTRON A) as post-induction therapy for responding multiple myeloma patients. M84 protocol. Cancer Treat Rev 15 [Suppl A]: 43-48
48. McCarthy D, Catovsky D (1978) Response to doxorubicin in hairy cell leukaemia. Scand J Haematol 21: 445-447
49. Mellstedt H, Ahre A, Björkholm M, Holm G, Johansson B, Strander H (1979) Interferon therapy in myelomatosis. Lancet 1: 245-247
50. Mende S, Fülle H-H, Weißenfels I (1975) Diagnose und Differentialdiagnose der Haarzell-Leukämie ("Hairy cell leukaemia"; "Leukämische Retikuloendotheliose"). Blut 30: 163-174
51. Nagata S, Taira H, Hall A, Johnsrud L, Streuli M, Ecsödi J, Boll W, Cantell K, Weissmann C (1980) Synthesis in *E. coli* of a polypeptide with human leukocyte interferon activity. Nature 284: 316-320

52. Niederle N, Kloke O, Nowrousian MR, Kruse H, Schmidt CG (1986) Efficacy of gamma and alpha interferon in the treatment of hairy cell leukemia. J Cancer Res Clin Oncol 111 [Suppl]: 40
53. Niederle N, Doberauer C, Kloke O, Höffken K, Schmidt CG (1987) Zur Wirksamkeit von IFN-γ und IFN-α bei der Haarzellenleukämie. Klin Wochenschr 65: 706-712
54. Niederle N (1988) Aspekte und Ergebnisse der Therapie mit Interferonen. Arzneim Forsch/ Drug Res 38 (I): 449-453
55. van Norman AS, Nagorney DM, Martin JK, Phyliky RL, Ilstrup DM (1986) Splenectomy for hairy cell leukemia. A clinical review of 63 patients. Cancer 57: 644-648
56. Österborg A, Björkholm M, Gahrton G, Grimfors G, Gyllenhammar H, Hast R, Holm G, Juliusson G, Järnmark M, Killander A, Kimby E, Lerner R, Paul C, Simonsson B, Smedmyr B, Stalfelt A-M, Strander H, Svedmyr E, Uden A-M, Wadman B, Wedelin C, Ösby E, Mellstedt H (1987) Melphalan/prednisone (MP) therapy vs melphalan/prednisone + human alfa-interferon (MP/IFN) in patients with multiple myeloma, stage II and III. A randomized study from the Myeloma Group of Central Sweden (MGCS). An interimistic report. Abstract of the annual meeting of the Swedish Medical Society, 2-4 Dec 1987, p 169
57. Ohno R, Kimura K (1986) Treatment of multiple myeloma with recombinant interferon alfa-2a. Cancer 57: 1685-1688
58. Paganelli KA, Evans SS, Han T, Ozer H (1986) B cell growth factor-induced proliferation of hairy cell lymphocytes and inhibition by type I interferon in vitro. Blood 67: 937-942
59. Pestka S (1986) Interferon: A decade of accomplishments, foundations of the future in research and therapy. Semin Hematol 23: 27-37
60. Porzsolt F, Thomä J, Unsöld W, Wolf W, Obert HJ, Kubanek B, Heimpel H (1985) Platelet-adjusted IFN dosage in the treatment of advanced hairy cell leukemia. Blut 51: 73-82
61. Porzsolt F (1986) Primary treatment of hairy cell leukemia: Should IFN-therapy replace splenectomy? Blut 52: 265-272
62. Porzsolt F, Janik R, Heil G, Brudler O, Raghavachar A, Scholz S, Papendick U, Heimpel H (1986) Deficient IFN alfa production in hairy cell leukemia. Blut 52: 185-190
63. Pralle H, Zwingers T, Boedewadt S, Bross K, Dörken B, Gamm H, Ho AD, Parwaresch RM, Schmitz N, Papendick U, Asshoff D, Bremer K, Euler H, Fischer T, Ganser A, Goldmann A, Hartlapp J, Hayungs J, Heinen U, Heyll A, Kraft J, Lohmeyer J, Meier P, Neubauer A, Nowicki L, Pflüger K, Saß R, Schmidt W, Schuster D, Straif K, Westerhausen M (1987) A prospective multicenter trial with human recombinant alpha-2c-interferon in hairy cell leukemia before and after splenectomy. Leukemia 1: 337-340
64. Quesada JR, Reuben J, Manning JT, Hersh EM, Gutterman JU (1984) Alpha interferon for induction of remission in hairy-cell leukemia. N Engl J Med 310: 15-18
65. Quesada JR, Alexanian R, Hawkins M, Barlogie B, Borden E, Itri L, Gutterman JU (1986) Treatment of multiple myeloma with recombinant alfa-interferon. Blood 67: 275-278
66. Quesada JR, Gutterman JU, Hersh EM (1986) Treatment of hairy cell leukemia with alpha interferons. Cancer 57: 1678-1680
67. Quesada JR, Hersh EM, Manning J, Reuben J, Keating M, Schnipper E, Itri L, Gutterman JU (1986) Treatment of hairy cell leukemia with recombinant alfa-interferon. Blood 68: 493-497
68. Rapson C, Scholnik A, Stoutenborough K, Schwartz K (1984) Treatment of patients with lymphoma and myeloma with human leukocyte interferon. Proc Am Soc Clin Oncol 3: 252
69. Ratain MJ, Vardiman JW, Golomb HM (1986) Prognostic variables in hairy cell leukemia following splenectomy as initial therapy. Blood 68 [Suppl 1]: 205 a
70. Ratain MJ, Golomb HM, Bardawil RG, Vardiman JW, Westbrook CA, Kaminer LS, Lembersky BC, Bitter MA, Daly K (1987) Durability of responses to interferon alfa-2b in advanced hairy cell leukemia. Blood 69: 872-877
71. Samuels BL, Golomb HM, Brownstein BH (1987) Different proteins are induced by alpha- and gamma-interferon in hairy cell leukemia. J Biol Resp Mod 6: 268-274
72. Schaefer H-E, Hellriegel K-P, Zach J, Fischer R (1975) Zytochemischer Polymorphismus der sauren Phosphatase bei Haarzell-Leukämie. Blut 31: 365-370
73. Sigaux F, Chapuis F, Castaigne S, Degos L, Flandrin G, Gluckman JC (1987) Hairy-cells are not lysed by NK-cells. Blut 54: 319-320
74. Smalley RV, Tuttle RL, Whisnant JK, Anderson SA, Huang AT, Robinson WA, and Other Participating Clinical Investigators at 26 Centers (1986) Effectiveness of Wellferon at a dose of 0.2 MU/m^2 in the treatment of hairy cell leukemia. Blood 68 [Suppl 1]: 233 a

75. Spiers ASD, Parekh SJ, Bishop MB (1984) Hairy-cell leukemia: Induction of complete remission with pentostatin (2′-deoxycoformycin). J Clin Oncol 2: 1336–1342
76. Spiers ASD, Moore D, Cassileth PA, Harrington DP, Cummings FJ, Neiman RS, Bennett JM, O'Connell MJ (1987) Remissions in hairy-cell leukemia with pentostatin (2′-deoxycoformycin). N Engl J Med 316: 825–830
77. Stewart DJ, Benjamin RS, McCredie KB, Murphy S, Keating M (1979) The effectiveness of rubidazone in hairy cell leukemia (leukemic reticuloendotheliosis). Blood 54: 298–304
78. Stryckmans PA, Huygen K, Vanhaelen C, Dorval C, Bondue H, Bron D, Debusscher L (1986) In vitro production of alpha and gamma interferon by blood cells of patients with hairy cell leukemia. Blood 68 [Suppl 1]: 181 a
79. Thompson JA, Fefer A (1987) Interferon in the treatment of hairy cell leukemia. Cancer 59: 605–609
80. Worman CP, Catovsky D, Bevan PC, Camba L, Joyner M, Green PJ, Williams HJH, Bottomley JM, Gordon-Smith EC, Cawley JC (1985) Interferon is effective in hairy-cell leukaemia. Br J Haematol 60: 759–763
81. von Wussow P, Hill W, Diedrich H, Freund M, Poliwoda H, Deicher H (1986) Low-dosage interferon-alpha therapy of hairy cell leukemia. Blut 53: 214
82. Yam LT, Li CY, Lam KW (1971) Tartrate-resistant acid phosphatase isoenzyme in the reticulum cells of leukemic reticuloendotheliosis. N Engl J Med 284: 357–360
83. Yam LT, Klock JC, Mielke CH (1984) Therapeutic leukapheresis in hairy cell leukemia: Review of literature and personal experience. Semin Oncol 11 [Suppl 2]: 493–501

Possible Mechanism of Interferon Action in Hairy Cell Leukemia*

F. PORZSOLT[1, 2], W. DIGEL[2], C. BUCK[2], A. RAGHAVACHAR[3], M. STEFANIC[2], and W. SCHÖNIGER[2]

Introduction

Recently, we described that peripheral blood mononuclear cells (MNC) from patients with hairy cell leukemia (HCL) can be induced in vitro to produce higher levels of interferon-gamma (IFN-γ) but lower levels of IFN-α than in healthy controls [7]. The reduced IFN-α production has been explained by the lack of monocytes in this disease. The increased production of IFN-γ suggests an increased release of cytokines by T cells. This assumption has been confirmed by Ford et al. [2], who described that a conditioned medium of T4-lymphocytes from patients with HCL contains a cytokine that stimulates the growth of activated, normal B cells. Kehrl et al. [5] demonstrated tumor necrosis factor alpha (TNF-α) to be a stimulator of activated normal B cells, and we (Digel et al. 1988) have shown recently that recombinant TNF-α stimulates the growth of purified B cells from patients with B-chronic lymphocytic leukemia (B-CLL). Based on these findings, we hypothesize that TNF is produced in B-cell disorders like HCL and that TNF may stimulate the growth of hairy cells (HC).

Material and Methods

Blood Donors

Heparinized peripheral blood was drawn from healthy controls and from patients with HCL. The diagnoses of HCL were confirmed in peripheral blood by bi- or tricytopenia, demonstration of HC in smears, and binding to monoclonal antibodies HD6 and HD39. Bone marrow biopsies showed the typical architecture and morphology of HCL. In splenectomized patients, the diagnoses were confirmed by typical spleen histology.

* This work was supported by Grant No. 164/3-1 from the *Deutsche Forschungsgemeinschaft*.

[1] Tumor Center, University of Ulm, Steinhövelstraße 9, 7900 Ulm, FRG.
[2] Department of Internal Medicine III, University of Ulm, Steinhövelstraße 9, 7900 Ulm, FRG.
[3] Department of Transfusion Medicine, University of Ulm, Oberer Eselsberg, 7900 Ulm, FRG.

H. G. Beger et al. (Eds.), Cancer Therapy

Separation of Cells

Mononuclear cells from peripheral blood (PB) were obtained by Ficoll-Hypaque (Pharmacia, Freiburg, FRG) density centrifugation. Further separation was done by a discontinuous Percoll gradient. The densities of fractions FI-FVI (1.050 g/ml-1.070 g/ml) were adjusted by using density marker beads (Pharmacia). A quantity of 6×10^7 MNC was suspended in 3 ml of the 50% Percoll solution. Aliquots of 3 ml of the other fractions were overlayered. The gradient was centrifuged for 45 min at 300 *g*. Harvested fractions were washed with Hanks' balanced salt solution (HBSS) three times.

Surface Markers

Cells were stained with specific monoclonal antibodies using the indirect immunofluorescence method in suspension. Cells were incubated for 30 min with the respective reagents and stained with fluorescence isothiocyanate (FITC)-conjugated goat anti-mouse IgG or IgM (Medac, Hamburg, FRG) for 30 min.

Reagents

RPMI culture medium (Gibco, Karlsruhe, FRG) was supplemented with 2 m*M* L-glutamine, 100 U/ml penicillin, 100 μg/ml streptomycin (Flow Laboratories, Meckenheim, FRG), and 10% heat-inactivated fetal bovine serum (Seromed, Berlin, FRG). For induction of cytotoxic activity, PHA (Wellcome, Burgwedel, FRG) and/or 4β-phorbol 12β-myristate 13-acetate (TPA) (Sigma Chemicals, Heidelberg, FRG) was added. Purified rTNFα and rTNFβ was provided by BASF/Knoll, Mannheim, FRG. Polyclonal and monoclonal antibodies against TNFα and a polyclonal antibody against TNFβ were donated by G. Adolf, Ernst Boehringer Institut für Arzneimittelforschung, Vienna.

Cytotoxic Activity (TNF Assay)

Cytotoxic activity was monitored by a L929 fibroblast lytic assay. Briefly, murine L929 cells (5×10^4 per well) were cultured with serially diluted test samples in 96-well, flat-bottom microtiter plates (Nunc, Wiesbaden, FRG) for 18 h at 39.5 °C in the presence of actinomycin D (2 μg/ml). The plates were washed and stained with crystal violet (0.5%). One unit of cytotoxic activity was defined to lyse 50% of the L929 target cells. Standards for TNFα and TNFβ were included.

Proliferation Assay

DNA synthesis was measured by ^{3}H-labeled (TdR) uptake. Triplicates of 6×10^5 cells were seeded in flat-bottom microtiter plates in a total volume of 200 μl. Cultures were incubated up to 144 h at 37 °C and were pulsed with 1 μCi ^{3}H-labeled

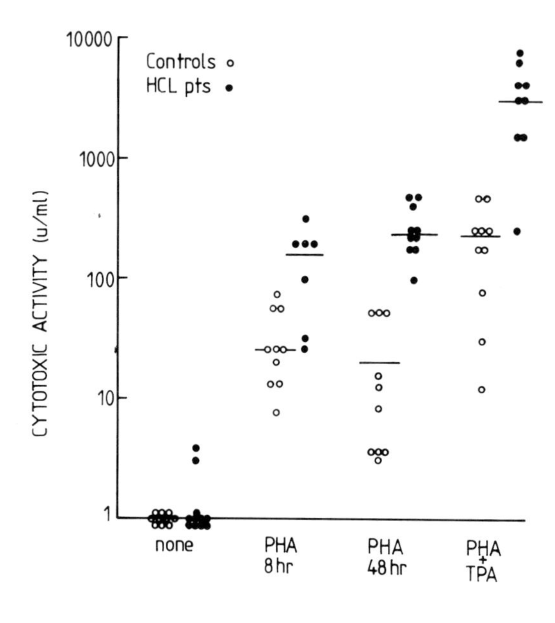

Fig. 1. In vitro induction of cytotoxic factors by PHA or PHA plus TPA in MNC from healthy controls and HCL patients. Supernatants of inducing cultures were tested on L929 cells for cytotoxic activity. Cytotoxic activity is expressed in U/ml

thymidine residue (^{3}H-TdR) (6.7 Ci/mmol, Amersham, Braunschweig, FRG) 7 h prior to cell harvesting (Scatron, Norderstedt, FRG). Incorporated radioactivity was measured by liquid scintillation counting (Packard Tricorb 1500).

Results

Production of Cytotoxic Factors

Ficoll-separated mononuclear cells from both healthy donors and untreated patients with HCL produced cytotoxic factors upon phythemagglutinin (PHA) stimulation in vitro. Figure 1 shows that the mean level of cytotoxic factor production after both culture periods (8 h and 48 h) was about tenfold higher in patients with HCL than in controls.

Neutralization of Cytotoxic Factors

Cytotoxic activity, which was produced by MNC from patients with HCL in an 8-h PHA culture, was neutralized almost completely by anti-TNFα but not by anti-TNFβ. In contrast, factors produced in a 48-h culture were neutralized by anti-TNFβ but not by anti-TNFα (Fig. 2).

TNF-Producing Cells

We found in previous experiments that HC can be separated from other lymphocytes by Percoll gradient centrifugation. Hairy cells are enriched up to 99% in the low-density fraction (FI) while small lymphocytes are enriched in high-density

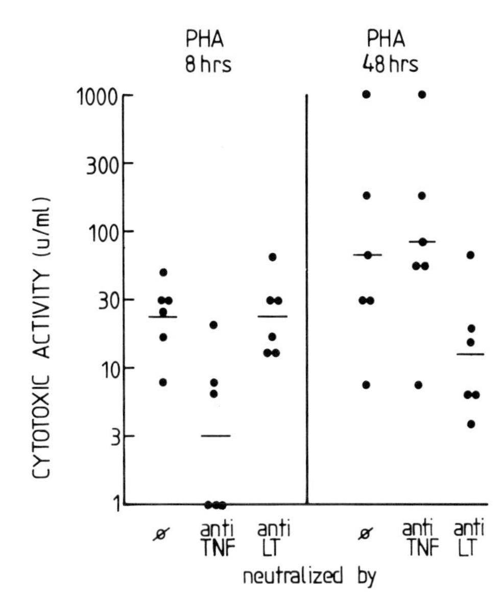

Fig. 2. Neutralization of cytotoxic activity by antibodies against TNFα or TNFβ. MNC from HCL patients were induced by PHA for 8 h or 48 h. Antibodies against TNFα (2000 U/ml anti-TNF) or TNFβ (2000 U/ml anti-lymphotoxin) were added before testing the supernatants on L929 cells

Table 1. Cytotoxic activity (as measured by TNF in U/ml) of Percoll-separated cells from a patient with HCL after in vitro culture without or with PHA

	No PHA		PHA	
	8 h	48 h	8 h	48 h
Fraction F I	0	0	0	0
Fraction F III	0	0	0	64
Fraction F V	0	0	6	512

fractions (FIV-VI). In the experiment shown in Table 1, Percoll-separated cells from a patient with HCL were induced with PHA. In unstimulated cells, no cytotoxic activity could be detected. Cytotoxic activity in enriched HC could not be induced by PHA. However, cytotoxic activity (512 U/ml) was found in FV, which contains non-HC lymphocytes. In this experiment, cytotoxic activity was induced only in the 48-h but not in the 8-h PHA culture.

Stimulation of the Growth of Hairy Cells

To test whether or not a PHA-conditioned medium (PHA-CM) of MNC from patients with HCL will stimulate the growth of HC, we cultured Percoll-enriched HC (fraction I/II) with cell-free PHA-CM of MNC from the same patient. The results summarized in Table 2 demonstrate that PHA-CM increased the ^{3}H-labeled TdR uptake of purified HC tenfold. This stimulatory activity of PHA-CM could be completely inhibited by the addition of antibodies against TNFβ but not by

Table 2. Stimulation of hairy cell proliferation. HC purified by Percoll gradient centrifugation were stimulated with a conditioned medium of PHA-stimulated MNC from the same HCL patients

Inducer	^{3}H-TdR (cpm) x ± SD	Stimulation index
None	957 ± 218	1.0
PHA-CM	9472 ± 669	9.9
PHA-CM + anti-TNFα	7790 ± 1418	8.1
PHA-CM + anti-TNFβ	87 ± 218	0.1

PHA-CM, PHA-conditioned medium; *TNF*, tumor necrosis factor.

antibodies against TNFα. Since anti-TNFβ completely abrogated the ^{3}H-labeled TdR incorporation, it is unlikely that PHA directly induced the ^{3}H-labeled TdR incorporation.

Inhibition of TNFβ-induction by Interferon

Figures 1 and 2 show that stimulation of MNC with PHA for 8 h resulted in the production of TNFα. When MNC from healthy donors were stimulated with PHA in the presence of IFNα (100 U/ml), a marginal increase in cytotoxic activity was seen (Fig. 3). In contrast, PHA-stimulation of cells for 48 h resulted in the induction of mainly TNFβ (Figs. 1 and 2). In the presence of IFNα, induction of this cytotoxic activity was reduced by 85% in cells of fraction IV–VI. This data suggests that IFNα can inhibit the production of TNFβ but not the production of TNFα.
A similar effect has been observed after treatment of patients with HCL either by splenectomy or therapy with IFNα. MNC from patients with HCL before therapy produced tenfold higher levels of cytotoxic activity upon PHA stimulation in vitro than did MNC from controls (Table 3). However, after splenectomy or therapy with IFNα, levels of cytotoxic activity similar to those in controls were induced in MNC from patients with HCL.

Discussion

Our data demonstrates that peripheral blood cells from patients with HCL can be induced in vitro to produce higher levels of TNFα and TNFβ than controls. Not HC but probably activated T cells, produce these factors. Supernatants of PHA-induced MNC contain factor(s) which stimulate the DNA synthesis of purified HC. It is likely that the stimulatory activity in the experiment shown in Table 2 was only TNFβ since it was possible to inhibit ^{3}H-labeled TdR incorporation completely by anti-TNFβ. The production of TNFβ but not of TNFα is inhibited by IFNα in vitro, and the production of cytotoxic activity (TNF) is inhibited after in vivo treatment with IFNα or splenectomy.

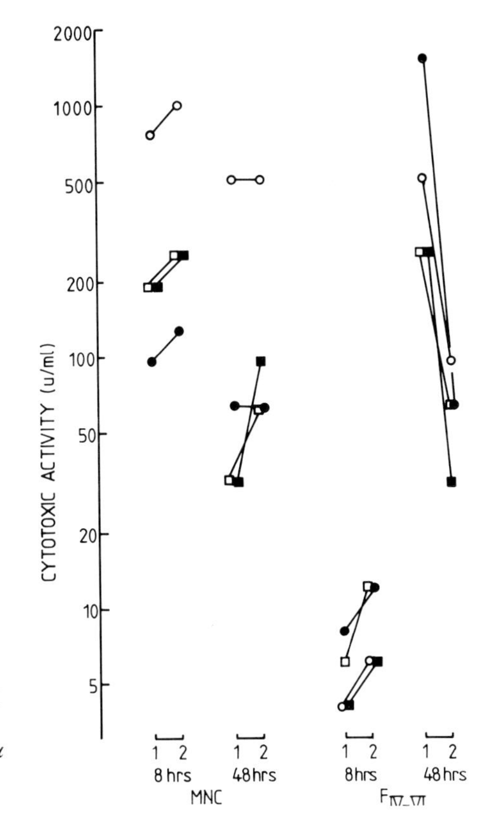

Fig. 3. Inhibition of TNFβ induction by IFNα. Mononuclear cells *(MNC)* and FIV-VI cells from four healthy donors were induced for 8 h or 48 h by PHA [1] or PHA plus IFNα [2]. The cytotoxic activity of supernatants was tested as described

Table 3. Induction of cytotoxic activities by PHA in MNC from healthy controls and patients before and after therapy. Mean values ± standard deviations of cytotoxic activity (U/ml) are shown

	n	Cytotoxic activity (U/ml) $\bar{x} \pm SD$
Controls	10	23 ± 20
HCL before therapy	11	212 ± 153
HCL after IFN-α	9	48 ± 32
HCL after splenectomy	7	29 ± 23

HCL, hairy cell leukemia; *IFN*, interferon.

Recently, Vilcek et al. [10] observed that the growth of FS-4 fibroblasts is stimulated by recombinant TNFα, and the authors assumed that this stimulation of growth might be a physiologic function of TNFα. This assumption has been supported by Kehrl et al. [5] and Jelinek et al. [4], who found that TNFα stimulated the proliferation of anti-μ activated [5] or *Staphylococcus aureus*-activated [4] B cells but not of unstimulated B cells. We found in previous experiments that ^{3}H-labeled TdR incorporation of purified B-CLL cells is increased in vitro up to 100-fold by recombinant TNFα. As CLL and HCL show a similar clonal rearrangement of genes coding for κ- and λ-immunoglobulin light chains, CLL and HCL were thought to be related diseases [3]. Therefore, it is possible that the growth of both CLL and HCL cells, might be regulated by related cytokines, TNFα or TNFβ. According to our results, IFNα inhibits the PHA-induced production of TNFβ but not of TNFα in healthy controls. If this is also true in B-cell disorders, patients with CLL and HCL can be expected to respond favorably to IFNα therapy if TNFβ but not TNFα is the major stimulator of tumor cells in a particular patient.

Our data shows that splenectomy reduces the level of PHA-induced TNF in MNC from patients with HCL, whose disease status remains stable after this therapy. This observation suggests an in vivo relevance of TNF in HCL because long-lasting remissions are known in HCL following splenectomy [1]. There are several possible explanations for the induction of remissions in HCL by splenectomy. First, it is possible that the majority of cells that produce TNF are located in the spleen; in this case, splenectomy could reduce the number of TNF-producing cells. Second, if HC are produced mainly in the spleen and if they stimulate peripheral blood cells to produce TNF, the spleen could be the best place for activation of TNF-producing cells by tumor cells. In this case, splenectomy would prevent the stimulation of T cells by HC.

Here, we demonstrate that not the tumor cell itself but probably activated T cells produce cytotoxic factors. These factors, e.g., TNFα and TNFβ, stimulate the growth of tumor cells and inhibit normal hemopoiesis, as shown previously for IFNγ and TNF [6]. If the cells producing cytotoxic factors respond to a signal provided by the tumor cells, an endocrine loop (Fig. 4) may exist, which is interrupted either by splenectomy or by IFNα therapy in most patients with HCL.

Our results do not contradict those of others [6], which describe an autocrine B cell growth factor (BCGF) loop in HCL, which is interrupted by IFNα. It is possible that an endocrine loop mediated by TNF triggers an autocrine BCGF loop of HC. Since IFNα has been found [6] to inhibit the autocrine loop, it might be postulated that IFNα can inhibit the production of cytokines that are produced by non-HC (e.g., TNF) and by HC (e.g., BCGF). These data suggest that not one but several effects of interferon are responsible for its efficacy in the treatment of HCL. Since HCL presents with varying symptoms (e.g., small or enlarged spleen, leukopenia

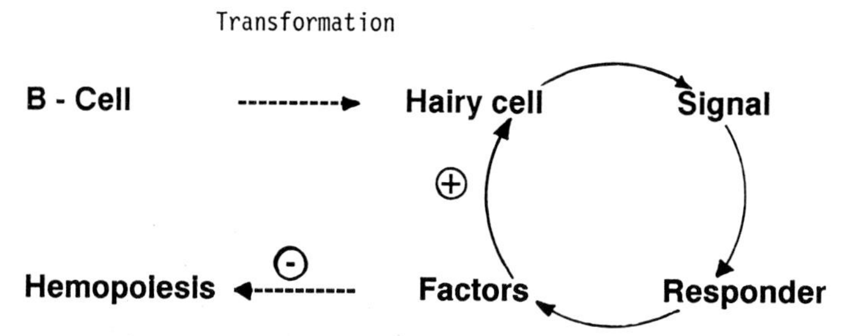

Fig. 4. Postulated endocrine loop in HCL. Responder cells other than HC produce cytokines (factors). These factors are potential inhibitors of normal hemopoiesis and stimulate the growth of HC. Since only activated responder cells produce cytokines, it is assumed that a stimulatory signal is necessary, which may be provided by HC in this model

or leukocytosis) and responses of HCL to splenectomy vary considerably among different patients, it should be kept in mind that different cytokines may be involved in the pathology of different HCL.

These findings also show that lymphocytes do not necessarily inhibit the growth of tumor cells but may even produce factors which stimulate the proliferation of tumor cells. Since HCL is currently the only disease that responds favorably to IFNα therapy, it is unlikely that the regulation of tumor growth in HCL is comparable to regulation of tumor growth in other malignancies.

Acknowledgements. The skillfull technical assistance of S. Scholz and A. Roepke is appreciated. We thank I. Brand for typing the manuscript.

References

1. Bouroncle BA (1984) The history of hairy cell leukemia: characteristics of long-term survivors. Semin Oncol 11 [Suppl 2]: 479-485
2. Ford RJ, Mehta S, Sharma S (1987) In vitro studies on leukemia cells and T-lymphocytes in hairy cell leukemia. Leukemia 4: 386-389
3. Foroni L, Catovsky D, Luzzatto L (1987) Immunoglobulin gene rearrangements in hairy cell leukemia and other chronic B-cell lymphoproliferative disorders. Leukemia 4: 389-392
4. Jelinek DF, Lipsky PE (1987) Enhancement of human B-cell proliferation and differentiation by tumor necrosis factor and interleukin 1. J Immunol 139: 2970-2976
5. Kehrl JH, Miller A, Fauci AS (1987) Effect of tumor necrosis factor on mitogen-activated human B-cells. J Exp Med 166: 786-791
6. Paganelli KA, Evans SS, Han T, Ozer H (1986) B-cell growth factor-induced proliferation of hairy cell lymphocytes and inhibition by type I interferon in vitro. Blood 67: 937-942
7. Peetre C, Gullberg U, Nilsson E, Olsson I (1986) Effects of recombinant tumor necrosis factor on proliferation and differentiation of leukemic and normal hemopoietic cells in vitro. J Clin Invest 78: 1694-1700
8. Porzsolt F, Janik R, Heil G, Brudler O, Raghavachar A, Scholz S, Papendick U, Heimpel H (1986) Deficient IFNα production in hairy cell leukemia. Blut 52: 185-190
9. Raghavachar A, Digel W, Frickhofen N, Porzsolt F, Adolf GR, Heimpel H (1986) Studies of recombinant-DNA-derived interferon and tumor necrosis factor as regulators of hematopoietic cell proliferation. Blut 53: 258
10. Vilcek J, Palombella VJ, Henriksen-DeStefano D, Swenson C, Feinman R, Hirai M, Tsujimoto M (1986) Fibroblast growth enhancing activity of tumor necrosis factor and its relationship to other polypeptide growth factors. J Exp Med 163: 632-643

Tumor Vaccination in the Treatment of Colorectal Cancer

R. SCHIESSEL[1]

The prognosis of colorectal cancer following curative surgery has remained unchanged over the past 40 years. In a patient collective comprising all Dukes stages, the 5-year-survival rates never exceeded 50% [1, 2]. Surgical progress has been restricted to the development of sphincter-saving procedures for rectal cancer at low levels [3-6]. However, an improvement in the prognosis of colorectal cancer patients should not be expected from surgery alone. The value of perioperative radiation therapy is as yet uncertain, and its use is confined to rectal cancer [7]. At present, chemo- and immunotherapy are the essential modalities in trials of adjuvant treatment of colorectal cancer. However, most of the therapy schemes published so far have not led to significantly improved, long-term survival times following either radical or palliative surgery of colorectal cancer [8, 9]. Nonetheless, the sporadic reports of successes with respect to the improvement of survival time [10-12] have encouraged us to investigate the effect of chemotherapy and immunotherapy as adjunctive treatment in a prospective randomized study of patients operated on in one medical center.

Materials and Methods

Patient Selection

From 1 April 1978 to 31 March 1983, patients in the First University Clinic of Surgery who had undergone radical surgery for colorectal cancer (Dukes B and C) were accepted for the trial. Informed consent was obtained from every patient. Age above 80 years, evidence or suspicion of distant metastases, synchronous second malignancy of another organ, and patient's or referring doctor's refusal to participate in the trial all resulted in exclusion from the trial.

Randomization

Patients were randomly assigned to one of three groups: (A) controls, (B) chemotherapy, and (C) immunotherapy. Prerequisites for randomization were the histopathology report and thorough patient knowledge about the therapy. To achieve an adequate balance of the distribution of important variables, the adaptive ran-

[1] 1. Surgical Clinic, University of Vienna, Alser Straße 4, 1090 Vienna, Austria.

H. G. Beger et al. (Eds.), Cancer Therapy

domization procedure by Pocock and Simon [13] and a corresponding computer program by Schemper [14] were used. The following variables were taken into account: patient's age and sex, Dukes stage ($B/C_1/C_2$) and degree of differentiation (hig/average/low) of the primary tumor, location of the primary tumor (colon/rectum), and the operative procedure (colonic resection/anterior resection/abdominoperineal excision of the rectum).

Schemes of Therapy

Group A. Controls: Patients received no adjuvant treatment but were followed up by the same blood tests and clinical and endoscopic examinations as the patients in groups B and C.

Group B. Chemotherapy: Patients received three courses of cytostatic polychemotherapy 6, 12, and 18 weeks after surgery with 12 mg/kg 5-fluorouracil (5-FU) i.v. on days 1–4, 2 mg mitomycin C (MMC) i.v. on days 1–4, and 100 mg cytosine-arabinoside (ARA-C) per os on day 1.

Group C. Immunotherapy: Patients received three courses of vaccination with inactivated allogenic tumor cells (DETA-cells) 6, 18, and 30 weeks after surgery. Our cheme of immunotherapy is based on data from animal experiments [15] and was administered in a modification as described by Rainer [16]. After incubation with mitomycin C, increasing concentrations of DETA-cells (0, 10^5, 10^6, 10^7, 10^8 cells) were mixed with different dilutions (0, 3, 10, 30, 100 IU) of *Vibrio cholerae* neuraminidase (VCN), which increases the immunogenicity and reduces the oncogenicity of tumor cells. The mixtures of various concentrations were injected subcutaneously in doses of at least 0.2 ml in a chessboard pattern in the clavicular and inguinal regions. A positive reaction (reactivity) at the vaccination site was defined as an infiltration with a diameter of 5 mm within 72 h. After vaccination, reactivity was assessed three times in 24-h intervals.

Follow-up

The following blood tests were repeatedly monitored during adjuvant therapy: blood sedimentation rate (BSR), red and white blood cell count, differential blood count, blood urea nitrogen (BUN), serum creatinine, electrolytes, alkaline phosphatase, serum glutamic oxaloacetic transaminase (SGOT), serum glutamic pyruvic transaminase (SGPT), lactic dehydrogenase (LDH), leukin amino peptide (LAP), γ-glutamyl transpeptidase total blood protein, and carcinoembryonic antigen (CEA) level. Side effects of the adjuvant therapy were evaluated according to the grades defined by the WHO [17].
All patients in the trial were examined regularly for follow-up in the surgical outpatient department (years 1 and 2, every 3 months; years 3–5, every 6 months; thereafter, annually). Every check-up included a clinical examination, blood tests (red and white blood cell count, liver function tests, CEA level), sigmoidoscopy of

anastomoses at low level (20 cm above the anus), and colonoscopy or barium enema respectively in more proximal anastomoses (20 cm above the anus). Pulmonary X-ray films were taken, and a colonoscopy or a barium enema was performed usually to rule out metachronous tumors of the large bowel. If tumor recurrence was suspected, additional special investigations, such as computed tomography of the pelvis, sonography of the liver and, if necessary, second-look surgery were carried out to locate a possible local recurrence and/or distant metastases [18, 19]. If not stated otherwise, the term "recurrence" in this series always means locoregional tumor recurrence and/or distant metastases.

Statistical Methods

The probability of survival and expected incidence of recurrences were described by Kaplan-Meier survival functions [20]. Statistically significant differences between the Kaplan-Meier survival functions were calculated with the Breslow test [21]. The mean of monotonic responses to the vaccination at different sites (reactivity) in the immunotherapy group was evaluated with the mean Kendall's tau [22]. The Mann-Whitney test [23] served to investigate possible differences in reactivity.

Results

A total of 178 patients aged 33–80 years completed the study. Although originally 274 patients had fulfilled the conditions of the protocol, altogether 35% of the patients or their doctors withdrew their consent to additional treatment after randomization and before the onset of therapy. As they were evenly distributed among the three groups, this did not lead to accidental selection of randomization criteria. Because of the comparatively small number of patients with a primary Dukes C_2 tumor, both stages Dukes C_1 and C_2 were categorized as stage Dukes C for further analyses.

Randomization

The first statistical analysis was completed after a median observation time of at least 28 months. The distribution of the randomization criteria over the three groups was extremely homogenous (Figs. 1–3). Occasional major surgery, e.g. concomitant small-bowel resection or simultaneous hysterectomy, did not produce irregularities in randomization.

Side Effects

Among the side effects, nausea with 31% in group B and allergic reactions with 12% in group C prevailed. However, side effects never exceeded grade 3 of the

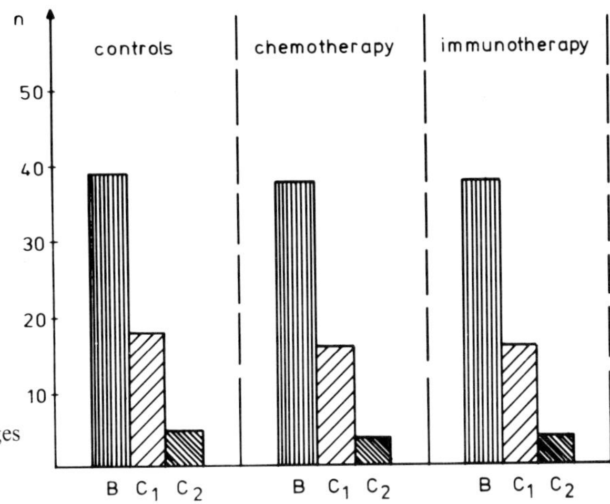

Fig. 1. Distribution of Dukes stages within the three groups

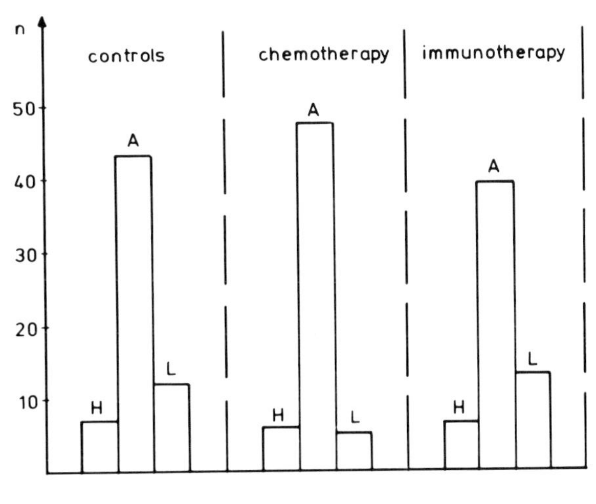

Fig. 2. Distribution of degree of differentiation

WHO scale, and chemotherapy had to be stopped for only one patient because of attacks of angina pectoris.

Effect of Therapy on Survival and Recurrences

Evaluation After 3 Years

There is no difference in the survival functions among the three groups including all tumor stages studied (Fig. 4). This is also true when controls, chemotherapy, and immunotherapy are compared with respect to subgroup Dukes B only. How-

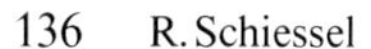

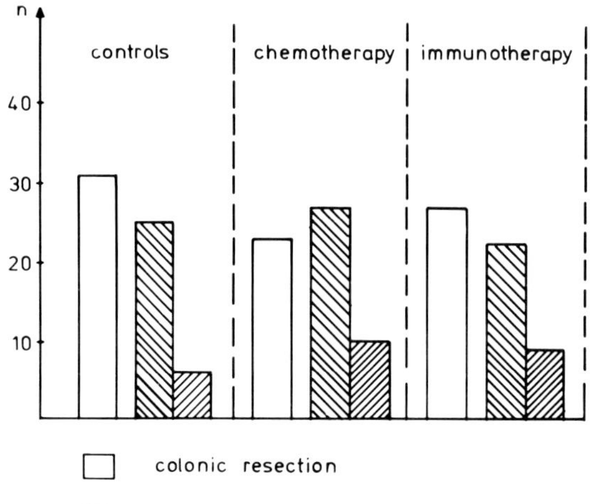

Fig. 3. Distribution of operative procedures

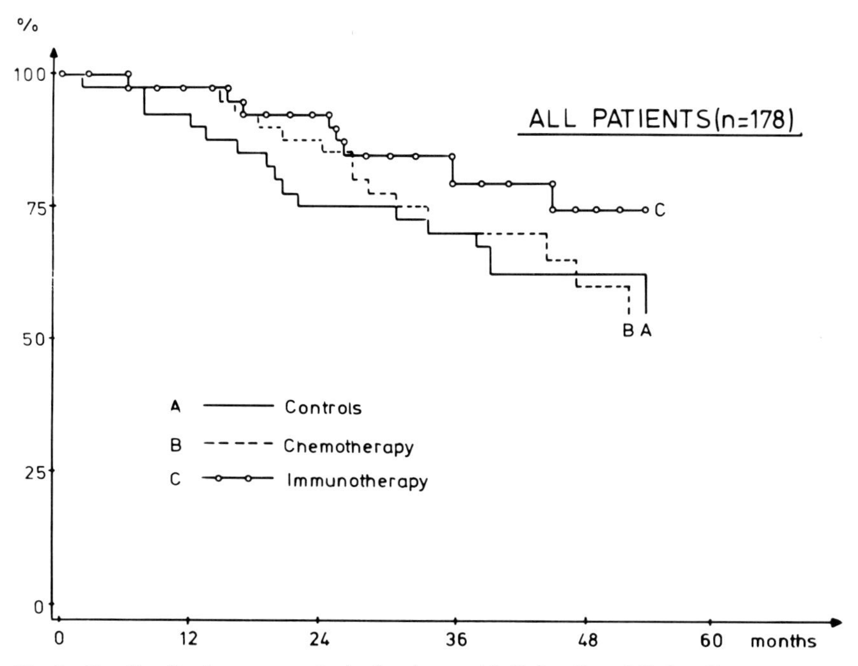

Fig. 4. Results after 3 years: survival of patients with Dukes B and Dukes C tumors

ever, for patients with primary tumor stage Dukes C, there are obvious differences among the three groups: at 40 months after surgery, the probability of survival is 72% for group C, 51% for group B, and 39% for group A (Fig. 5). The differences between the groups with adjuvant therapy on the one hand and the control group on the other are statistically significant. The difference between groups B and C is not significant.

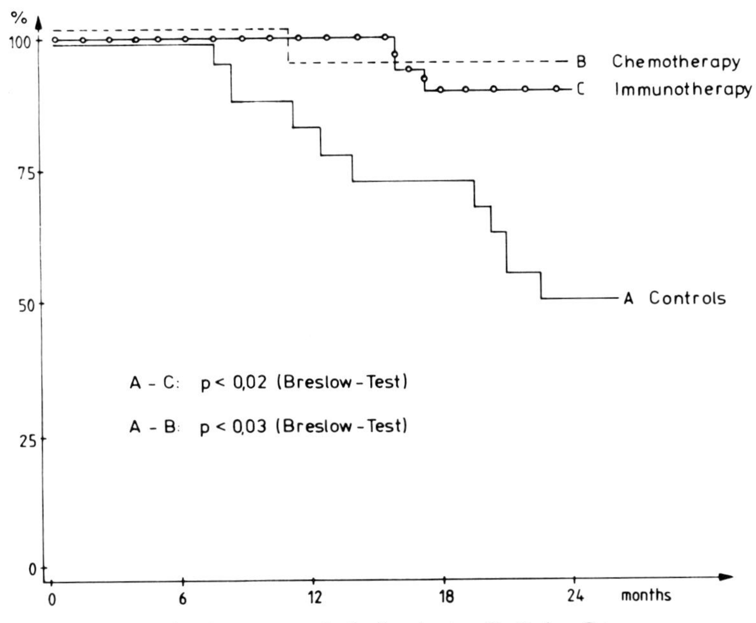

Fig. 5. Results after 3 years: survival of patients with Dukes C tumors

There seems to be no difference among the three complete groups concerning the effect of adjuvant therapy on the probability of tumor recurrence. This is also true for stages Dukes B and C if analyzed as separate subgroups. In stage Dukes B, there is no difference among the control group, chemotherapy group, and the immunotherapy group in the incidence of local recurrences, of distant metastases, and of liver metastases only, if these types of recurrence are analyzed separately. In stage Dukes C, the probability to be free of local recurrences is virtually the same for all three therapy groups. However, there is a marked difference in the incidence of distant metastases and of liver metastases only (Fig. 6) in stage Dukes C. Thirty months after surgery, the probability to be free of distant metastases is 80% for group B, 68% for group C, and over 52% for group A. The difference between group A and group B is statistically significant, but the difference between group A and group C is not. At 21 months after surgery, the probability to be free of liver metastases is 83% for group B, 81% for group C, and 54% for group A. The differences are significant between group A and B and between group A and C [24].

Evaluation After 7 Years

At this point, the survival data for Dukes B and C show no difference between the treatment groups and the control group. The separate evaluation of the Dukes C patients does not confirm the previous result, since many patients in groups B and C died during the third year of the trial. This, at 48 months there was no difference between groups B and C and the control group: group A = 47%, group B = 55%,

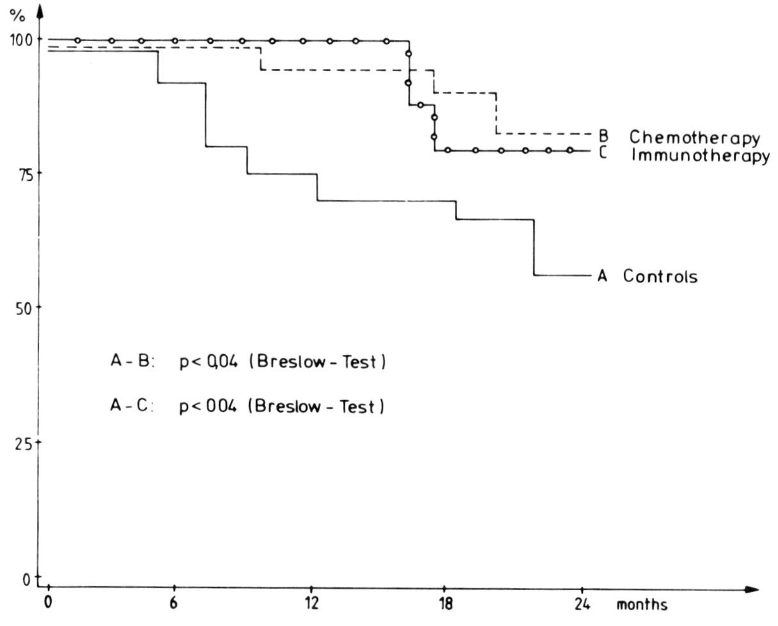

Fig. 6. Results after 3 years: incidence of liver metastases

group C = 55% surviving patients (Mantel Test $P = 0.15$). There was, however, still a measurable effect on the incidence of distant metastases at 48 months: 70% in group A and 50% in groups B and C (Mantel test $P < 0.03$). The incidence of liver metastases at 48 months was 53% in group A, 30% in group C, and 15% in group B (Mantel test $P < 0.05$).

Discussion

The present trial has shown that patients with Dukes C tumors benefit from adjuvant therapy. Although the 7-year evaluation did not show an effect on survival, this is one of the few clinical studies to show any effect of chemo- or immunotherapy on colorectal cancer.

Currently, we are performing a multicenter trial investigating the effect of a simplified immunotherapy scheme with lyophilized tumor cells as an adjuvant therapy in Dukes C cancers. In addition, we plan to investigate whether the prolongation of the therapy can improve the survival time.

Acknowledgements. This work was performed in cooperation with Doz. Dr. M. Wunderlich, Doz. Dr. R. Rauhs, Doz. Dr. M. Schemper, Dr. E. Kovats (1st University Clinic of Surgery, Vienna), Prof. Dr. H. Rainer, Dr. C. Dittrich (University Clinic of Chemotherapy, Vienna), Prof. Dr. M. Micksche (Institute for Applied and Experimental Oncology, University of Vienna), and Dr. H. H. Sedlacek (Behring Company, Marburg, Germany).

References

1. Dukes CE (1944) The surgical pathology of rectal cancer. Proc Roy Soc Med 37: 131-144
2. Goligher JC (1975) Surgery of the anus, rectum and colon. Baillière Tindall, London
3. Dixon CF (1939) Surgical removal of lesions occurring in the sigmoid and rectosigmoid. Am J Surg 46: 12
4. Localio SA, Eng K, Gouge TH, Ranson JHC (1978) Abdomino-sacral resection for carcinoma of the midrectum: 10 years' experience. Ann Surg 188: 475-480
5. Parks AG, Percy JP (1982) Resection and sutured colo-anal anastomosis for rectal carcinoma. Br J Surg 69: 301-304
6. Heald RJ, Leicester RJ (1981) The low-stapled anastomosis. Dis Colon Rectum 24: 437-444
7. Scherer E, Schulz U (1981) Die Stellung der Strahlentherapie bei der Behandlung des Rektumkarzinoms. In: Eigler FW, Beersiek F (eds) Aktuelle Probleme der kolorektalen Tumorchirurgie. Schattauer, Stuttgart
8. Carter SK (1976) Large-bowel cancer - The current status of treatment. JNCI 56: 3-10
9. Rosato FE, Brown SA, Miller EE, Rosato EF, Mullis WF, Johnson J, Moskovitz A (1974) Neuraminidase immunotherapy of tumors in man. Surg Gyn Obstet 139: 675-682
10. Moertel CG (1975) Clinical management of advanced gastrointestinal cancer. Cancer 36: 675-682
11. Mavligit GM, Gutterman JV, Malahy MA, Burgess MA, McBride CM, Iubert A (1977) Adjuvant immunotherapy and chemoimmunotherapy in colorectal cancer (Dukes class C). Cancer 40: 2726-2730
12. Taylor I, Brooman P, Rowling JT (1977) Adjuvant liver perfusion in colorectal cancer: initial results of a clinical trial. Br Med J 2: 1320-1322
13. Pocock SJ, Simon R (1975) Sequential treatment assignment with balancing for prognostic factors in the controlled clinical trial. Biometrics 31: 103-116
14. Schemper M (1986) Randomisierung für kontrollierte Therapiestudien. Wien Klin Wschr 94: 604-609
15. Seiler FR, Sedlacek HH (1978) Chessboard vaccination: A pertinent approach to immunotherapy of cancer with neuraminidase and tumor cells. In: Rainer H, Borberg H, Mishler JM, Schäger U (eds) Immunotherapy of malignant diseases. Schattauer, Stuttgart
16. Rainer H, Kovats E, Lehmann HG, Micksche M, Rauhs R, Sedlacek HH, Seide W, Schemper M, Schiessel R, Schweiger B, Wunderlich M (1981) Effectiveness of postoperative adjuvant therapy with cytotoxic chemotherapy (cytosine arabinoside, mitomycin C, 5-fluorouracil) or immunotherapy (neuraminidase-modified allogenic cells) in the prevention of recurrence of Dukes B and C colon cancer. In: Klein HO (ed) Chemotherapy and radiotherapy of gastrointestinal tumors (Recent results in cancer research, vol 79). Springer, Berlin Heidelberg New York, pp 41-47
17. WHO Handbook for reporting results of cancer treatment. WHO offset publication Nr 48. World Health Organisation, Geneva 1979
18. Schiessel R, Wunderlich M, Kovats E, Rath T, Rauhs R (1983) Die Therapie des Lokalrezidivs nach kolorektalem Karzinom. Wien Klin Wschr 95: 295-297
19. Wunderlich M, Schiessel R, Kovats E, Rauhs R, Seidl W, Imhof H, Hajek P (1983) Der Wert der Computertomographie des kleinen Beckens zur frühzeitigen Diagnose von Lokalrezidiven nach operiertem Rektumkarzinom. Wien Klin Wschr 95: 291-294
20. Kaplan EL, Meier P (1958) Nonparametric estimation from incomplete observations. J Am Statist Ass 53: 457-481
21. Breslow NE (1970) A generalized Kruskal-Wallis test for comparing K samples subject to unequal patterns of censorship. Biometrika 57: 579-594
22. Kendall MG (1962) Rank correlation methods. Griffin, London
23. Mann HB, Whitney DR (1947) On a test of whether one of two random variables is stochastically larger than the other. Ann Math Statist 18: 50-60
24. Wunderlich M, Schiessel R, Rainer H, Rauhs R, Kovats E, Schemper M, Dittrich C, Micksche M, Sedlacek HH (1985) Effect of adjuvant chemo- or immunotherapy on the prognosis of colorectal cancer operated for cure. Br J Surg 72: 107-110

NEW APPROACHES IN SURGICAL ONCOLOGY

New Developments in Surgical Oncology

R. BITTNER[1] and H. G. BEGER[1]

Introduction

Only surgical therapy can influence decisively the course of a solid malignant tumor of the gastrointestinal tract and cure the patient. Today, the results of standard operative procedures have reached an extremely high standard that will hardly be surpassed even in the future. However, only little improvement has been achieved with regard to cure rates, because more than half of the patients admitted for surgery present with an advanced stage of systemic disease, rendering curative surgery impossible.

At present, numerous new therapeutic possibilities that are employed as adjuvants or after exhaustion of surgical therapy are being developed and clinically tested. A great deal of attention is being directed toward biotherapy, which, after surgical therapy and radio- and chemotherapy, promises to become the forth modality in the treatment of malignant tumors.

The goals of surgical oncology are (a) eradication of the tumor, (b) low morbidity and mortality due to the surgical procedure, and (c) few long-term side effects following resection. In short, the aim is to heal the patient or, at least, to achieve a long survival time without diminishing the quality of life. Achieving progress in surgical oncology involves painstaking endeavor. The problem is that, even today, more than half of the patients with a cancer of the gastrointestinal tract are in a stage of systemic disease at admission, prohibiting cure even with maximum local radicality of the surgical intervention. Therefore, it is urgently necessary to develop adjuvant or alternative methods of cancer treatment with systemic effects.

In attempting to improve the overall results, three steps should be considered. The first step includes the reduction of morbidity and mortality resulting from standard operative procedures. Surgical mortality must not be higher than the anticipated 5-year survival for the respective type of carcinoma. The second step is to verify whether or not a benefit for the patient can be obtained by means of radical surgical resection. And, finally, the third step is the development and clinical implementation of new methods that are effective in inoperable patients or palliatively resected patients or are suitable as adjuvant measures following surgery for which the curative value is questionable. Since malignant neoplasms of the stomach, colon, rectum, and pancreas, with their 61000 deaths per

[1] Department of General Surgery, University of Ulm, Steinhövelstraße 9, 7900 Ulm, FRG.

H. G. Beger et al. (Eds.), Cancer Therapy

Table 1. Carcinoma of the pancreas – Surgical mortality of the Whipple procedure

		n	Mortality (%)
	1970–1983 [1][a]	1378	17.0
Trede	1985 [2]	91	1.1
Crist et al.	1987 [3]	47	2.1
Ulm	1982–1987	69	2.9

[a] Collective review.

Table 2. Cancer of the stomach – Surgical mortality of the total gastrectomy

	n	Mortality (%)
1950–1978 [4][a]	2726	23.7
1970–1980 [5][a]	106	26.4
Herfarth et al. 1987 [6]	144	6.9
Siewert et al. 1987 [7]	241	7.1
Bittner et al. 1987 [8]	164	2.4
Bittner 1988 [9] (in patients aged >70 years)	96	3.1

[a] Collective review.

year in Germany, present the predominant field of activity for the oncologically active surgeon, I will basically refer to these types of carcinomas in this chapter.

Present Trends in Morbidity and Mortality Relating to Standard Operative Procedures

It is incontrovertible that the only way to obtain cure in gastrointestinal cancer, if at all, is by surgical intervention. The first question to be answered is what progress has been made in the past years with respect to morbidity and mortality of standard operative procedures in the above-mentioned three types of carcinomas. Tables 1 and 2 show that, in the field of gastrointestinal surgery, rapid progress has been made during the past 10 years. While mortality related to the Whipple operation and total gastrectomy amounted to 25% in the late 1970s, nowadays surgical mortality of 2%–6% is taken for granted. This is also true in patients older than 70 years of age. A similar development can be seen in colorectal surgery (Table 3). In the mid-1970s, there was an operative mortality of 6%–19% for anterior resection of the rectum, whereas today mortality related to this procedure ranges between 1% and 7%. These data illustrate that present surgical techniques, supported by modern anesthesia and intensive care, have at tained an extraordinarily high level of expertise unlikely to be exceeded in the future.

Table 3. Carcinoma of the rectum – Surgical mortality of the anterior resection

		Before 1950 (%)	Between 1950 and 1975 (%)	Today (%)
Grundmann et al.	1984 [10]	33.3	19.7	5.2
Reifferscheid and Weishaupt ($n=213$)	1974 [11]		8.6	
Gall ($n=300/404$)	1986 [12]		6.3	7.2
Stelzner ($n=123$)	1981 [13]			4.8
Heberer et al. ($n=50/107$)	1982 [14]		10.0	1.9
Ulm ($n=81$)	1987			1.2

Table 4. Carcinoma of the stomach – 5-year survival rate following total gastrectomy

		Before 1950 (%)	Between 1950 and 1970 (%)	Today (%)
Lahey	[15]	24.0	23.0	
Harvard	[16]	24.0	15.0	
Diehl et al.	1983 [17]			25.6
Scott et al.	1984 [18]			15.0
Siewert et al.	1987 [7]			34.0[a]
Meyer et al.	1987 [19]			29.8
Bittner et al.	1987 [8]			26.7

[a] Three-year survival rate (with systemic lymph node dissection).

Survival After Standard Operative Procedures

Despite the enormous improvements in the operative results, no such gratifying developments can be observed with regard to rates of cure. Table 4 shows that, in the past 30 years in Germany and the USA, no major improvements in the results for gastric carcinomas or pancreatic carcinomas could be obtained [1]. With reference to pancreatic carcinoma, the cure of a patient is more attributable to a miracle than to a triumph of surgical technique.

What is the Benefit of an Extension of Standard Operative Procedures?

As shown in Table 5, immense efforts have been undertaken to improve the overall survival rates by an extension of local surgical radicality. Unfortunately, up to now only few proven data have been compiled. Neither Fortner's regional pancreatectomy [20], where high operative mortality must also be taken into account, nor total gastrectomy with radical lymph node dissection and combined pancreaticosplenectomy have been proven to prolong survival [23–25]. Only for gastric carcinomas with N1 lymph node invasion does lymph node dissection (R2 resection) seem advantageous. However, only Japanese clinics have been able to prove this

Table 5. Surgical oncology – Improvement of the results Via extension of radicality?

Carcinoma site	Method of treatment	Benefit
Pancreas	Regional pancreatectomy [20]	?
Colon	"No-Touch" Technique [21]	?
	Radical lymph node dissection [22]	
Stomach	Total gastrectomy [23]	?
	Combined splenectomy [24]	–
	Combined pancreaticosplenectomy [25]	–
	Radical lymph node dissection [26]	+ (N1) (+) (N2) ∅ (N3)

?, effect uncertain; ∅, no effect; –, negative effect; +, reasonably positive effect; (+), questionable effect.

[26, 27]. According to Koga et al. [25], "... that the course of the total gastrectomy for advanced gastric cancer is more affected by serosal invasion than lymph node metastasis." Once the organic wall is passed, in most cases the carcinoma has also passed the limits of local and, thus, surgically curable disease. This is equally true for pancreatic and colonic carcinoma. Commenting on the long-term results of colorectal surgery for carcinoma, B. G. Wolf of the Mayo Clinics said, "It would appear that we reached the anatomic limits for surgical cure on colon carcinoma a long time ago" [28].

New Therapeutic Strategies

The development of new and useful strategies adjuvant to surgical resection depends on precise knowledge of how metastases develop and where recurrences may appear. Today, we know that recurrences of colorectal carcinoma are located in the liver in approximately 40%–50% of all cases [29, 30], whereas gastric and pancreatic carcinomas recur locally or as peritoneal carcinosis in 60%–80% of the patients [26]. Based on this knowledge, a series of treatment strategies has been developed in the past few years to (a) prevent recurrence and (b) offer an effective presence of treatment in the metastases.

Intraportal Chemotherapy

The rationale for intraportal chemotherapy performed intraoperatively or immediately postoperatively adjuvant to surgery is, firstly, that micrometastases already exist even without any macroscopic and pathological evidence in the liver at the time of surgery, and, secondly, that the initial tumor dissemination occurs in the liver via the portal vein; here, the surgeon's manipulations on the bowel might be of potential importance. The preliminary results of two randomized studies of intraportal chemotherapy indicate an advantage for the treated group (Table 6). According to Taylor [31], particularly patients in the Dukes B stage benefit from this

Table 6. Prevention of liver metastasis in colorectal surgery by intraportal chemotherapy

	Agent	Patients (*n*)	Protocol	Deaths	
				(*n*)	(%)
Taylor et al. 1985 [31][a]	5-FU	247	ICT ($n=117$)	26	(22.0)
			Control ($n=127$)	54	(42.5)
Metzger et al. 1987 [32][a]	5-FU	378	ICT ($n=191$)	20	(10.5)
			Control ($n=187$)	30	(16.0)

[a] Randomized controlled trials.
ICT, intraportal chemotherapy; *5-FU*, 5-fluorouracil.

Table 7. Prevention of local recurrence by intraoperative radiation therapy

Carcinoma site	Institution	Patients (*n*)	Protocol (*n*)	Deaths	
				(*n*)	(%)
Rectosigmoid colon	Massachusetts General Hospital [36, 37][a]	50	27 (IORT)	7	(26.0)
			23 (no IORT)	16	(69.5)
Stomach	Kyoto University Hospital [33, 34][a]	194	84 (IORT)[b]	37	(44.0)
			110 (no IORT)[b]	50	(45.0)
Pancreas	Massachusetts General Hospital [35][a]	30	IORT[c]	Median survival: 15 months	

[a] No randomized study.
[b] Difference in stage IV: 20% vs 0%.
[c] Historical group: median survival 10 months.
IORT, intraoperative radiation therapy.

therapy. According to Metzger [32], however, patients in the Dukes C stage are the beneficiaries. Such a discrepancy demonstrates that a definite assessment of this kind of adjuvant therapy is still not possible.

Intraoperative Radiotherapy

Up to now, strictly randomized studies of the effectiveness of intraoperative radiotherapy do not exist. Only a few centers, such as the Massachusetts General Hospital and, especially, Abe and his co-workers at Kyoto University have gained extensive experience with this therapeutic modality [33-37].

The comparison with historical collectives without intraoperative radiotherapy reveals benefits for the irradiated group. The results gained at Kyoto University [33, 34] prove above all that patients with T4 gastric carcinoma benefit significantly from intraoperative irradiation. However, it should be emphasized that employing this kind of therapy requires considerable expenditures of personnel, time, space, and apparatus that restrict its use.

Continuous Intraperitoneal Chemotherapy

In comparison to intraoperative radiotherapy, intraperitoneal chemotherapy, which is applied in the same way as peritoneal dialysis in patients with renal insufficiency, may be performed with far fewer difficulties. A controlled study, by Koga and Hamazoe [38] is available. A continuous hyperthermic peritoneal perfusion with mitomycin C was performed postoperatively via two catheters subsequent to a radical surgical intervention. For patients with T3 gastric carcinoma, it was possible to achieve a 5-year survival rate of 62.2% with this therapy compared with only 39.3% among the control patients. However, some critics of this form of therapy fear that intra-abdominal adhesions could result, leading to a greater risk of postoperative ileus.

Regional Intra-arterial Chemotherapy

The most common topic concerning our efforts to improve the results of colorectal surgery in the past few years has been regional chemotherapy for liver metastases. While there has been a continuing interest for over two decades in drug delivery systems for treating liver metastases, the recent morbidity of totally implantable drug infusion pumps and access ports has greatly increased the research interest in this area [39]. The rationale for this kind of therapy is that the hepatic artery is the major source of blood supply to hepatic metastases. Continuous regional chemotherapy has the following advantages:
First, it delivers higher concentrations of the drug directly to the liver. Second, many antimetabolites are more effective when administered by a continuous infusion than by impulse injection. Third, there is significant hepatic extraction of many drugs when injected directly into the hepatic circulation, particularly fluorodeoxyuridine (FUDR) and, to a lesser extent, 5-fluorouracil (5-FU), mitomycin C, and adriamycin; this further increases the concentration of the drug at the site of the hepatic neoplasm. Fourth, continuous infusion has a lower peak serum concentration, thus decreasing systemic toxicity, such as bone marrow depression: The current results for this approach are shown in Table 8. Depending on the response parameters chosen, the literature shows response rates ranging from 33% to 91%. In spite of this considerably higher response rate in comparison to systemic chemotherapy, no significant prolongation of survival with regional chemotherapy has been shown. The problem in assessing the results of this new type of treatment is that, although many therapeutic comparisons with so-called historical collectives exist, no clinical study with a randomization related to an untreated group of patients is available.
Our own experience is based on the treatment of more than 64 patients with continuous regional perfusion of chemotherapy in the liver via an implantable pump

Table 8. Continuous regional chemotherapy – Results of non-randomized clinical trials

Author		patients (*n*)	Response rates (%)	Median survival (months)
Ensminger et al./Niederhuber et al. [40, 41]	1981/84	93	91[b]/79[c]	19
Barone et al. [42]	1982	18	56[c]	12
Cohen et al. [43]	1983	50	54[c]	12
Balch et al./Balch and Urist [44, 45]	1983/86	110	83[a]	18
Daly et al. [46]	1984	40	41[c]	unknown
Shepard et al. [47]	1985	62	33[c]	17
Kemeny et al. [48]	1986	42	69[b]	15
Patt et al. [49]	1986	29	52[c]	12
Hottenrott and Lorenz [50]	1987	52	75	16
Ulm	1987	64	54[b]	18

[a] Decrease in CEA >33%
[b] Decrease in CEA = 50%.
[c] 50% reduction in volume as determined by radiologic scans.

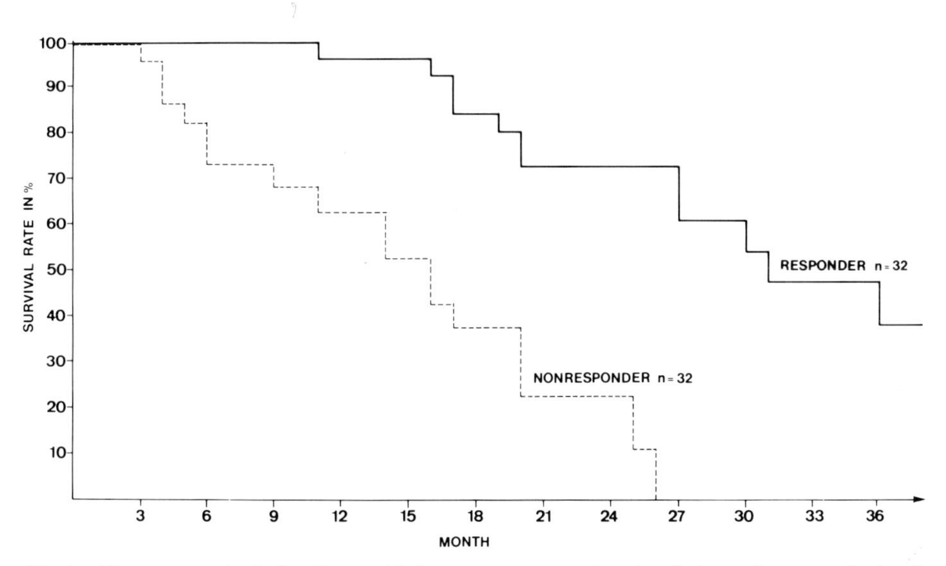

Fig. 1. Five-year survival of patients with liver metastases and regional chemotherapy, calculated according to Kaplan/Meier

system. The response rate was 54%. Figure 1 shows the survival curves of responders and nonresponders. The median survival time of the responders is 31 months, whereas the median nonresponders' survival time is as little as 14 months. The difference is significant. However, such a therapeutic success is achieved at the price of numerous side effects (Table 9). In this context, the high percentage of patients with biliary sclerosis (23%) needs to be mentioned. Another disadvantage of regional chemotherapy to the liver is that there is no systemic exposure to the drug so that metastases at other sites are not treated in the same degree.

Table 9. Hepatic metastasis – Continuous regional chemotherapy and accompanying hepatic and systemic toxicity (Ulm experience, $n=64$)

Side effects	Patients	
	(*n*)	(%)
Diarrhea	3	4.0
Ulcer	4	6.0
Stomatitis	8	12.0
Gastritis	10	15.6
Biliary sclerosis	15	23.0
Chemical hepatitis	37	57.0

Table 10. Surgical oncology – New treatment modalities

1. Laser therapy, hyperthermia, thermochemotherapy, and kryosurgery
2. Biological agents and biological response modifiers
   Immunomodulating agents (bacterial products)
   Interferons and interferon inducers
   Thymosins
   Lymphokines and cytokines (CSF, IL2, MGF, TNF)
   Antigens, effector cells
3. Radiolabelled antibodies
4. Monoclonal antibodies

CSF, colony-stimulating factor; *IL2*, interleukin 2; *MGF*, macrophage growth factor; *TNF*, tumor necrosis factor.

Summarizing, no study could prove an advantage for the patients, measured in survival time, for any one of the four discussed new adjuvant methods. Therefore, these methods must be considered experimental therapeutic modalities and thus far can only be justified on the basis of clinical studies.

New Perspectives in Cancer Treatment

The development of numerous new therapeutic approaches can be traced back to the general progress in technology (Table 10). However, only laser therapy for tumors in the neck and head and hyperthermia in perfusion of the extremities have acquired a firm position within the therapeutic concept of the oncologically active surgeon. A rapid development is presently taking place in the field of biological agents and biological response modifiers for their employment in tumor therapy. We therefore agree with Oldham [51], who stated "... that we are entering a new era in cancer treatment. Historically all efforts have been toward the eradication of cancer by cytotoxic modalities. Exstirpation [sic] by surgery, sterilisation by radiotherapy and eradication of the last cell by chemotherapy have been major approaches in cancer treatment thus far. With the advent of biologicals and biological response modifiers, several other approaches are now possible. These approaches represent a strategically different way of developing therapeutics. And biotherapy should be considered as a fourth modality of cancer treatment." In spite of this euphoric quotation, I cannot refrain from stating that, although a series of doors is indeed presently in sight for the successful treatment of cancer disease, the appropriate keys are still missing: We urgently hope to discover one or sine another of these keys within the shortest possible time.

References

1. Bittner R (1985) Das duktale Pankreaskopfkarzinom - Stagnation oder Fortschritt in der chirurgischen Therapie? Klinikarzt 14: 467-477
2. Trede M (1985) The surgical treatment of pancreatic carcinoma. Surgery 97 (1): 8-35
3. Crist DW, Sitzmann JV, Cameron JL (1987) Improved hospital morbidity, mortality, and survival after the Whipple procedure. Ann Surg 206, 3: 358-365
4. Peiper HJ, Siewert R (1978) Magenersatz. Chirurg 49: 81-88
5. Bittner R, Schirrow H, Butters M, Roscher R, Krautzberger W, Oettinger W, Beger HG (1985) Total gastrectomy. Arch Surg 120: 1120-1125
6. Herfarth C, Schlag P, Buhl K (1987) Surgical procedures for gastric substitution. World J Surg 11: 689-698
7. Siewert JR, Lange J, Böttcher K, Hölscher M, Weiser HF, Gössner W (1987) Magenkarzinom - Bestandsaufnahme aus chirurgischer Sicht. Dtsch Med Wochenschr 112: 622-628
8. Bittner R (1987) Gastrectomie de nécessité. Langenbecks Arch Chir 372: 577-582
9. Bittner R, Butters M, Roscher R, Schirrow H, Büchler M, Beger HG (1988) Gastrektomie - Gestern und Heute. 105th meeting of the German Association of Surgery, Munich 1988 Scientific Exhibition, 6-9 April 1988
10. Grundmann R, Blettenberg U, Pichlmaier H (1984) Behandlung des koloraktalen Karzinoms in den letzten 35 Jahren - perioperativer Aufwand und postoperatives Ergebnis. Leber Magen Darm 14 (4): 174-180
11. Reifferscheid M, Weishaupt W (1974) Die Chirurgie des Mastdarmkrebses in heutiger Sicht. Chirurg 45: 444-451
12. Gall FP (1986) Chirurgische Therapie des Rektumkarzinoms im mittleren Drittel "Anteriore Resektion". Leber Magen Darm 5: 325-330
13. Stelzner F (1981) Moderne Radikaloperationen und Ergebnisse - Bedeutung der Kontinenzerhaltung. Krankenhausarzt 54: 288-290
14. Heberer G, Denecke H, Pratschke E, Teichmann R (1982) Anterior and low anterior resection. World J Surg 6: 517-524
15. Cady B, Ramsden DA, Stein A, Haggitt RC (1977) Gastric cancer. Am J Surg 133: 423-429
16. Buchholtz TW, Welch CE, Malt RA (1978) Clinical correlates of resectability and survival in gastric carcinoma. Ann Surg 188: 711-715
17. Diehl JT, Hermann RE, Coopermann AM, Hoerr SO (1983) Gastric carcinoma. A ten-year review. Ann Surg 198: 9-12
18. Scott HW, Adkins RB, Sawyers JL (1985) Results of an aggressive surgical approach to gastric carcinoma during a twenty-three-year period. Surgery 97: 55-58
19. Meyer HJ, Jähne J, Pichlmayer R (1987) Magencarcinom: Gastrektomie de principe. Langenbecks Arch Chir 372: 571-576
20. Fortner JG (1981) Surgical principles for pancreatic cancer: Regional total and subtotal pancreatectomy. Cancer 47: 1712-1718
21. Turnbull RB, Kyle K, Watson FR, Spratt J (1967) Cancer of the colon: The influence of the no-touch isolation technique on survival rates. Ann Surg 166: 420-427
22. Pezim ME, Nicholls RJ (1984) Survival after high or low ligation of the inferior mesenteric artery during curative surgery for rectal cancer. Ann Surg 200: 729-733
23. Pichlmayr R, Meyer HJ (1979) Value of the gastrectomy "de principe". In: Herfarth C, Schlag P (eds) Gastric cancer. Springer-Verlag Berlin Heidelberg New York, pp 196-204

24. Yoshino K, Haruyama K (1983) Bedeutung der Splenektomie für die Lymphknotenausräumung bei Magenkarzinom. Akt Chir 18: 81-84
25. Koga S, Kaibara N, Kimura O, Nishidoi H, Kishimoto H (1981) Prognostic significance of combined splenectomy or pancreatico-splenectomy in total and proximal gastrectomy for gastric cancer. Am J Surg 142: 546-550
26. Maruyama K, Okabayashi K, Kinoshita T (1987) Progress in gastric cancer surgery in Japan and its limits of radicality. World J Surg 11: 418-425
27. de Aretxabala X, Konishi K, Yonemura Y, Ueno K, Yagi M, Noguchi M, Miwa K, Miyazaki I (1987) Node dissection in gastric cancer. Br J Surg 74: 770-773
28. Wolff BG (1987) Invited commentary. World J Surg 11: 809
29. Eder M (1984) Die Metastasierung - Fakten und Probleme aus humanpathologischer Sicht. Verh Dtsch Ges Pathol 68: 1-11
30. Kemeny N, Daly J, Reichman B, Geller N, Botet J, Oderman P (1987) Intrahepatic or systemic infusion of fluorodeoxyuridine in patients with liver metastases from colorectal carcinoma. Ann Int Med 107: 459-465
31. Taylor I, Machin D, Mullee M, Trotter G, Cooke T, West C (1985) A randomized controlled trial of adjuvant portal vein cytotoxic perfusion in colorectal cancer. Br J Surg 72: 359-363
32. Metzger U, Mermillod B, Aeberhard P, Gloor F, Bissat A, Egeli R, Luffer U, Martinoli S, Mueller W, Schroeder R, Weber W (1987) Intraportal chemotherapy in colorectal carcinoma as an adjuvant modality. World J Surg 11: 452-458
33. Abe M, Takahashi M (1981) Intraoperative radiotherapy: The Japanese experience. Int J Radiat Oncol Biol Phys 7: 863-868
34. Abe M, Shibamoto Y, Takahashi M, Manabe T, Tobe T, Inamoto T (1987) Intraoperative radiotherapy in carcinoma of the stomach and pancreas. World J Surg 11: 459-464
35. Wood CW, Shipley WU, Gunderson LL, Cohen AE, Nardi GL (1982) Intraoperative irradiation for unresectable pancreatic carcinoma. Cancer 49: 1272-1275
36. Dosoretz D, Gunderson LL, Hoskins B, Hedberg S, Blitzer PH, Shipley W, Cohen A (1983) Preoperative irradiation for unresectable rectal and rectosigmoid carcinomas. Cancer 52: 814-818
37. Gunderson LL, Cohen AM, Dosoretz DD, Shipley W, Hedberg S, Wood W, Rodkey G, Suit H (1983) Residual, unresectable or recurrent colorectal cancer: External beam irradiation and intraoperative electron beam boost resection. Int J Radiat Oncol Biol Phys 9: 1597-1606
38. Koga S, Hamazoe R (1986) Continuous hyperthermic peritoneal perfusion for cancer. In: Gastric cancer surgery (The latest therapy), vol 3. Igaku Kyoiku Shuppan, Tokyo, pp 525-529
39. Balch CM, Levin B (1987) Regional and systemic chemotherapy for colorectal metastases to the liver. World J Surg 11: 521-526
40. Ensminger W, Niederhuber J, Dakhil S, Thrall J, Wheeler R (1981) Totally implanted drug delivery system for hepatic arterial chemotherapy. Cancer Treat Rep 65: 393-400
41. Niederhuber JE, Ensminger W, Gyves J, Thrall J, Walker S, Cozzi E (1984) Regional chemotherapy of colorectal cancer metastatic to the liver. Cancer 53: 1336-1343
42. Barone RM, Byfield JE, Goldfarb PB, Frankel S, Ginn S, Greer S (1982) Intra-arterial chemotherapy using an implantable infusion pump and liver irradiation for the treatment of hepatic metastases. Cancer 50: 850-862
43. Cohen AM, Kaufman SD, Wood WC, Greenfield AJ (1983) Regional hepatic chemotherapy using an implantable drug infusion pump. Am J Surg 145: 529-533
44. Balch CM, Urist MM, Soong SJ, McGregor MA (1983) A prospective phase II clinical trial of continuous FUDR regional chemotherapy for colorectal metastases to the liver using a totally implantable drug infusion pump. Ann Surg 198: 567-573
45. Balch CM, Urist MM (1986) Intra-arterial chemotherapy for colorectal liver metastases and hepatomas using a totally implantable drug infusion pump. In: Herfarth C, Schlag P, Hohenberger P (eds) Therapeutic Strategies in primary and metastatic liver cancer. Springer-Verlag Berlin Heidelberg New York Tokyo, pp 234-247 (Recent results in cancer research, vol 100)
46. Daly JM, Kemeny N, Oderman P, Botet J (1984) Long-term hepatic arterial infusion chemotherapy; Anatomic considerations, operative technique and treatment morbidity. Arch Surg 119: 936-941
47. Shepard KV, Levin B, Karl RC, Faintuch J, DuBrow RA, Hagle M, Cooper RM, Beshorner J, Stablein D (1985) Therapy for metastatic colorectal cancer with hepatic artery infusion chemotherapy using subcutaneous implanted pump. J Clin Oncol 3: 161-169

48. Kemeny N, Reichman B, Oderman P, Daly J, Geller N (1986) Update of randomized study of intrahepatic (H) vs systemic (S) infusion of fluorodeoxyuridine (FUDR) in patients with liver metastases from colorectal carcinoma (CRC). Proc Am Soc Clin Oncol 5: 47
49. Patt YZ, Boddie AW, Charnsangavej C, Ajani JA, Wallace S, Soski M, Claghorn L, Mavligit GM (1986) Hepatic arterial infusion with floxuridine and cisplatin: Overriding importance of antitumor effect versus degree of tumor burden as determinants of survival among patients with colorectal cancer. J Clin Oncol 4: 1356-1364
50. Hottenrott C, Lorenz M (1987) Stellenwert der regionalen Chemotherapie der Leber. Z Gastroenterol 25: 364-373
51. Oldham RK, Smalley RV (1985) Newer methods of cancer treatment: Biologicals and biological response modifiers. In: DeVita Jr VT, Hellman S, Rosenberg SA (eds) Cancer 2nd edn. Lippincott, Philadelphia, pp 2223-2245

Cancer Surgery – Conservative or Radical?

P. SCHLAG[1]

The optimal goal of cancer surgery is to achieve local tumor control and definitive eradication of the disease. This can generally be realized only as long as no metastases have developed. In any other case, local surgical procedures have only a palliative effect, or constitute are part of a multidisciplinary approach.
Effective palliation can, however, sometimes only be obtained through an extensive resection of the tumor. Radical surgical procedures might result in mutilation and loss of body functions. The rationale of radical surgical tumor therapy is to excise completely the primary tumor and regional lymph nodes in order to prevent recurrent or metastatic tumor growth. Therefore, multicentricity of the tumor and possible lymph node metastases should be taken into consideration when excising the primary tumor. Morbidity and mortality incurred by different surgical procedures should also be kept in mind. Less extensive surgery, especially when the tumor is not advanced, is recommendable, but the risks of conservative surgery must be considered. Principal contraindications for radical or supraradical surgical procedures can be defined. Supraradical surgery is not justified when the surgical risks are higher than the chances of possible cure or when the quality of life following surgery will be significantly reduced. However, the realisation of these theoretical maxims is often difficult.

The Extent of Surgical Resection Margins

One of the main difficulties concerning conservative or radical surgery is to define adequate surgical margins. The importance of an adequate safety margin in the excision of malignant melanoma has been thoroughly examined [1]. Studies have demonstrated that a safety margin of 3 cm for small tumors has the same results as a margin of 5 cm [2]. Furthermore, removal of the tumor fascia during the treatment of the primary lesion does not influence the prognosis. It is much more difficult to obtain adequate surgical margins in the resection of malignant visceral tumors. Total pancreatectomy has been recommended because definition of sufficient resection margins in the treatment of pancreatic carcinoma is problematic, but this surgical technique is associated with an increase in postoperative complications and morbidity [6, 7]. It is therefore not surprising that total pancreatectomy does not positively influence the prognosis in comparison to subtotal

[1] Department of Surgical Oncology, Surgical Clinic, University of Heidelberg, Im Neuenheimer Feld 110, 6900 Heidelberg, FRG.

H. G. Beger et al. (Eds.), Cancer Therapy

pancreatic resection. Nevertheless, morbidity and mortality accompanying the Whipple procedure are high, and the prognosis of this kind of surgery in ductal carcinoma of the head of the pancreas is not very favorable. Generally, bypass procedures in ductal pancreatic carcinoma result in a median survival time similar to that of more radical surgical measures, and they have lower morbidity and post-operative mortality (Tables 1 and 2). General rejection of tumor resection for patients with pancreas head carcinoma is not reasonable because, in the individual patient, radical surgical procedures can have a curative effect, which is not the case with conservative operations, such as the cholecystojejunostomy. Also, the palliative effect of a pancreas resection on existing or future pain symptoms have to be taken into consideration. The best palliation can be achieved by tumor resection (Table 3).

In a prospective trial, we investigated different resection lines for surgery of gastric cancer [21]. In this study, we found that the prognosis for tumors located in the

Table 1. Supraradical (total pancreatectomy) surgery in ductal pancreatic carcinoma

Author	Patients (*n*)	Lethality (%)	Survival time	
			Median (months)	5-Year (%)
Cubilla et al. (1978)	19	26	4.0	0
Tryka and Brooks	25	21	24.0	19.0
Gall (1981)	21	29	7	
Van Heerden et al. (1981)	51	14	13.0	2.3
Own results (1984)	15	26	12.0	

Table 2. Radical surgery (Whipple procedure) in ductal pancreatic carcinoma

Author	Patients (*n*)	Lethality (%)	Survival time	
			Median (months)	5-Year (%)
Cubilla et al. (1978)	43	16	8.0	7.0
Tryka and Brooks	11	21	7.6	0
Gall (1981)	24	4	11.0	
Own results (1984)	12	8	18.0	8.0

Table 3. Whipple procedure versus biliodigestive bypass for treatment of carcinoma of the pancreas head

	Whipple (*n*=50)	Bypass (*n*=76)
Improvement of well-being	68%	28%
Improvement of symptoms	68%	39%
Median duration of improvement	7 months	5 months
Median survival	15 months	13 months

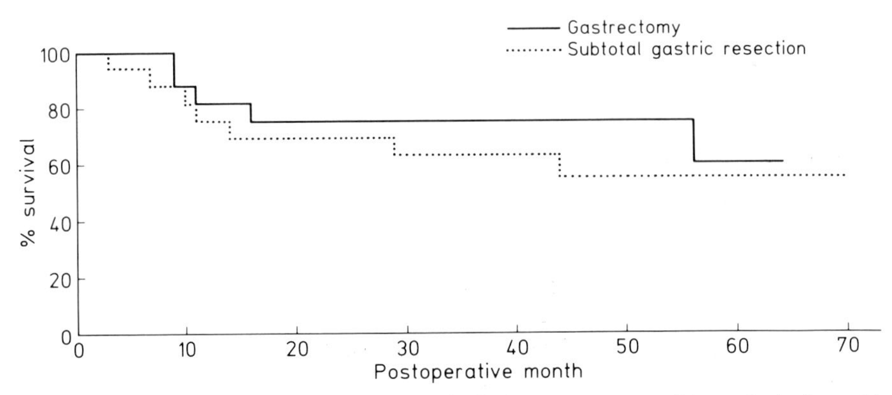

Fig. 1. Own prospective trial comparing survival after gastrectomy with survival after subtotal gastric resection in small, intestinal, differentiated tumors of the gastric antrum

prepyloric antrum of the stomach following subtotal gastrectomy is no worse than following total gastrectomy, provided that it is a small, well-differentiated tumor according to the Laurén classification (Fig. 1). Otherwise, especially for the diffuse type of gastric carcinoma, discontinuous tumor growth, which is not macroscopically visible, must be taken into consideration. Thus sufficient surgical margins can often be achieved only by total gastrectomy [9, 21]. Multicentricity and discontinuous tumor spread make the assessment of sufficient resection margins difficult.

This must not necessarily lead to complete removal of the organ in which the tumor arose. When deciding between conservative or radical surgery, the patient's age and tumor biology must be considered. This can be demonstrated in the treatment of papillary thyroid cancer. Total thyroidectomy in younger and female patients with intrathyroid lesions is not superior to subtotal resection because identical survival time and lower morbidity are achieved by the conservative procedure (Fig. 2). Since effective treatment is possible in the event of a local recurrence, this further supports a modified radical procedure in the treatment of small (i.e., diameter less than 1.5 cm) papillary thyroid carcinomas [16, 27].

The Extent of Lymph Node Resection

The risk of lymph node metastases also plays an important role in deciding on the extent of surgical therapy. This can be shown in the treatment of rectal carcinoma. The probability of lymph node involvement has to be weighed against the general surgical risk and, especially, the morbidity induced by the surgical procedure [8, 10]. Since the risk of lymph node metastases among patients with prognostically favorable tumors is no higher than the surgical mortality incurred by a radical surgical procedure (Tables 4 and 5), a more conservative treatment is indicated, i.e., local tumor excision [2, 10]. Most recent results indicate that by using endosonography a relatively firm diagnosis can be made regarding tumor penetration and

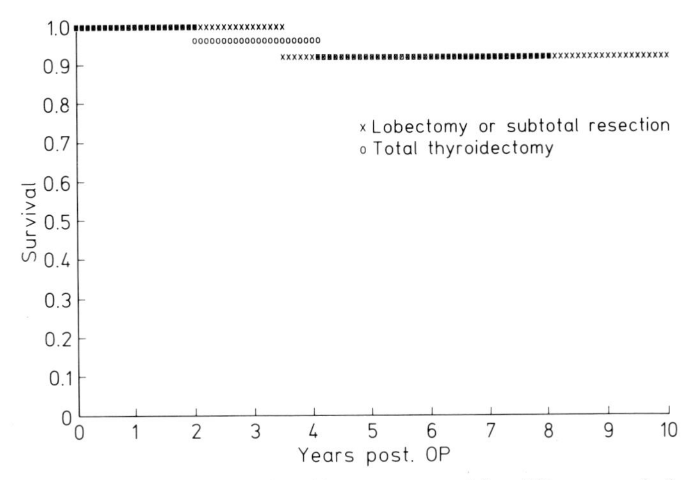

Fig. 2. Survival curves of patients with papillary thyroid cancer treated by different surgical procedures at the Department of Surgery, University of Heidelberg

Table 4. Lymph node metastases in pT1 colon cancer

Authors	Patients (*n*)	Lymph node metastases (*n*)	Lymph node metastases (%)
Haggilt (1985)	44	4	9.1
Wingard (1985)	48	5	10.4
Hermanek (1985)	130	4	3.1
Own material (1987)	22	1	4.5

Table 5. Postoperative mortality for radical surgery in colorectal cancer

Author	Patients (*n*)	Mortality (%)
Hermanek (1978–1983)	1194	6.5
Own results (1984–1987)	739	4.5

possible regional lymph node involvement [11]. This technique can facilitate decisions on the surgical procedure to be taken.
Adequate resection of involved lymph nodes is feasible by removing the mesenteric drainage area. The question is how large this area should be. Since exensive lymph node involvement generally implies systemic tumor dissemination, extensive resection of involved lymph node areas is usually not indicated. The crucial point is to define the level of lymph node involvement that still enables us to per-

form a curative resection. This question still cannot be definitively answered [13]. Most retrospective studies investigating the value of extended lymph node resection in colorectal cancer do not evince a significant benefit. The preliminary results of the only prospective trial confirmed the value of the „no touch technique" [25] for the surgical treatment of colonic cancer [28]. Interestingly enough, this study shows that not the local recurrence rate, but rather, the rate of liver metastases is significantly reduced.

Since even in early gastric cancer lymph node involvement has to be expected in about 20% of the patients, radical lymph node dissection has become more widely utilized for the treatment of gastric cancer [9, 21]. The recommendations are mainly based on Japanese experience [15]. However, by comparing the different operative procedures in relationship to survival time, we must consider a possible bias in the staging of the more aggressively treated patients. There are tumors for which primary radical surgery of lymph nodes is probably not indicated because the results are no more favorable than without lymph node resection.

In the treatment of malignant melanoma, for instance, it has been shown that prophylactic lymph node resection does not improve the expected survival time as compared with therapeutic resection of clincially suspicious lymph nodes [1].

The treatment of breast cancer also corresponds to these findings. Surgical removal of the lymph nodes is mainly carried out for diagnostic reasons [5]. A prerequisite for conservative surgical treatment is the combination with additive or adjuvant measures [5, 26]. Since breast cancer, even in the early stages, is a systemic disease, radical surgical procedures do not improve survival times but remain essential for local tumor control. Obviously, surgery plays an important role in the treatment of most solid tumors, but the decision concerning the extent of the surgical procedure must fit into a comprehensive treatment strategy in the modern concept of surgical oncology.

Combined Modality Therapy Reduces Radical Surgical Procedures

To prevent local tumor relapse, the concept of combining surgery with perioperative adjunctive measures is an attractive approach to circumvent radical surgery. There has been an increased use of combined modality therapy in a variety of solid tumors. Beside breast cancer, this concept is established in soft-tissue sarcomas. Pre- or postoperative radio- or chemotherapy [20] and isolated chemotherapeutic extremity perfusion can be indicated to reduce surgical radicality. By using this method in the treatment of soft-tissue sarcoma [12] as well as in the therapy of malignant melanoma and its intransit metastases [22], amputations can be avoided in many patients without shortening the survival time (Fig. 3).

By using radiotherapy [19] and chemotherapy [17] preoperatively in the treatment of anal cancer, surgery may become unnecessary or can be limited to a local excision of the lesion (Table 6), while the only other alternative would have been rectum exstirpation, resulting in definitive colostomy. Further combined modality treatment may increase the resection rate for some tumors which would otherwise not be suitable for surgery. Preoperative chemo- and radiotherapy increase the resectability of esophageal cancer [22]. Radical or supraradical surgical procedures

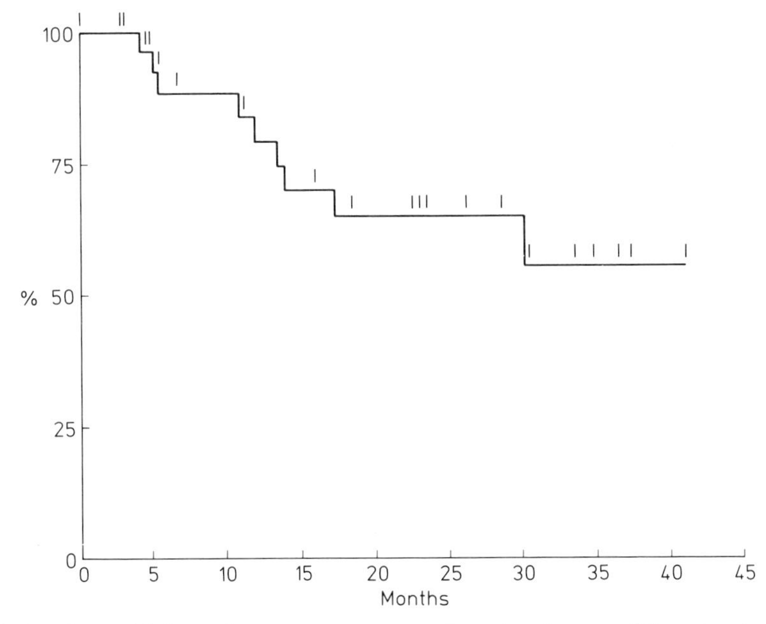

Fig. 3. Survival of patients with intransit metastases due to malignant melanoma of the extremities treated by isolated chemotherapeutic perfusion at the Department of Surgery, University of Heidelberg

Table 6. Results of radio-chemotherapy in anal carcinoma

Author	Patients (*n*)	Operated patients		
		Abdominoperineal resection (*n*)	Local excision (*n*)	No residual tumor (*n*)
Flam (1983)	12		12	12
Michaelson (1983)	37	18	19	22
Nigro (1983)	26	12	14	21
Own results (1986)	7	5	2	2
Total	82	35	47	57/82 (70%)

alone [4, 18, 24] have no significant influence on the survival time of patients with esophageal cancer (Fig. 4). This is why most recently conservative, nonsurgical treatment strategies have been investigated [3, 14]. First results have been encouraging.

In conclusion, radical or conservative surgical strategies are not in competition but mark different surgical procedures for a variety of tumors and tumor stages (Table 7). Less radical measures seem possible in the treatment of papillary carcinoma of the thyroid and in the management of malignant melanoma without any further treatment. A prerequisite is a macroscopically small tumor with prognosti-

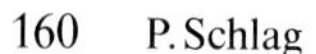

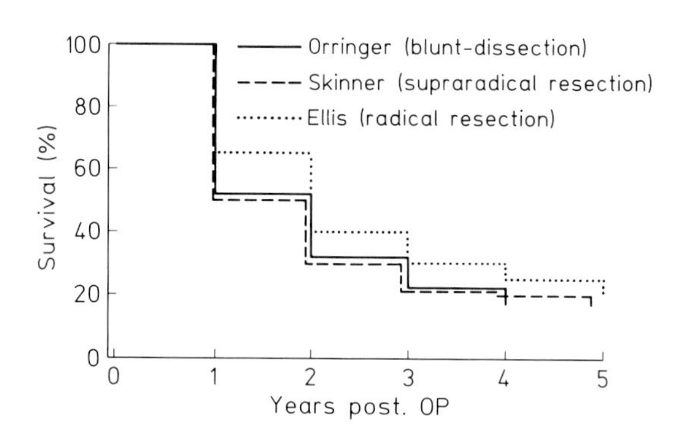

Fig. 4. Influence of different operative strategies on survival curves of patients with esophageal cancer (data from [4, 18, 24])

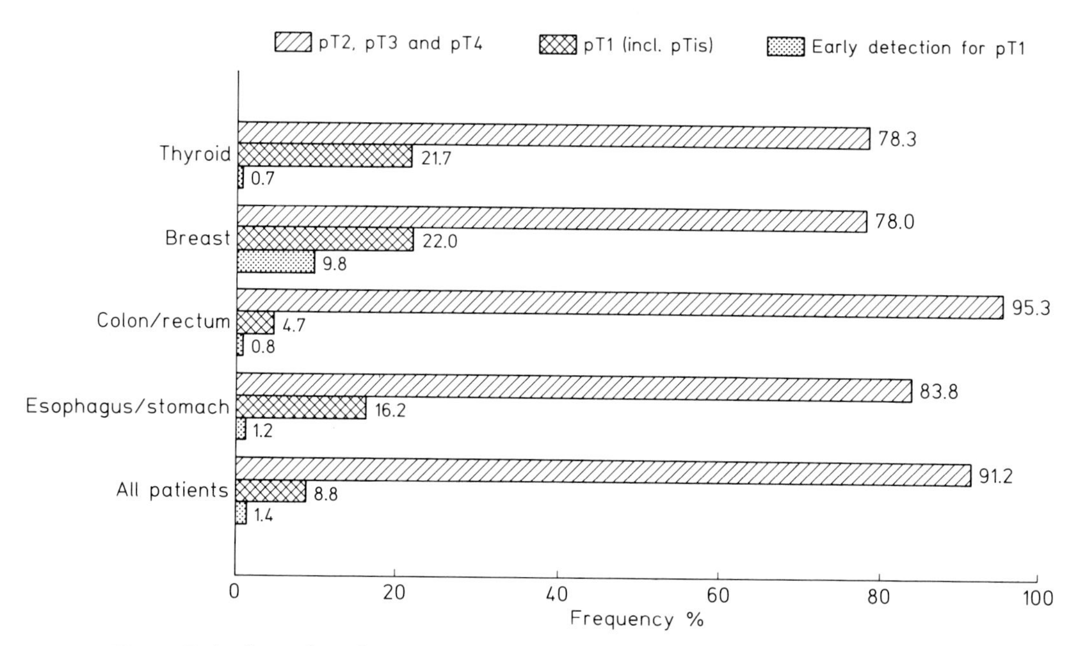

Fig. 5. Early diagnosis and pT categories out of about 5000 different malignant tumors seen at the Department of Surgery, University of Heidelberg (1982–1987)

Table 7. Some indications for conservative surgical procedures in cancer treatment

Operative treatment alone	Surgery and postoperative radiotherapy	Multimodality treatment
Papillary thyroid cancer	Breast cancer	Anal cancer
Malignant melanoma	Sarcoma of the extremity	Osteosarcoma
Liver tumors		Esophageal cancer?
pT1 rectal cancer?		

cally favorable histologic characteristics. Under these circumstances, conservative surgical procedure are indicated for microinvasive colorectal cancer. Conservative limited surgical treatment of breast cancer and soft-tissue sarcomas should be combined with postoperative radiation. Combined treatment modalities reduce the extent of surgery in anal carcinoma or osteosarcoma and improve the resectability of some other tumors, such as esophageal cancer.
The earlier the cancer can be diagnosed, the better the possibilities of conservative treatment methods. It should be mentioned that even today very few early diagnosed tumors are presented for surgical therapy. In our institute, we have had only 8.5% pT1 tumors out of about 5000 surgical cases (Fig. 5). This proportion must be improved in the future to increase the number of conservative surgical procedures for malignant tumors. We should not forget in our enthusiasm for less radical surgical intervention with its preservation of form and function that early diagnosis of cancer offers the best chance for cure. Let us to remember Max Schwaiger's words, "What has been neglected during primary surgery is lost forever."

References

1. Balch CM, Milton GW (eds) (1985) Cutaneous melanoma. Clinical management and treatment results worldwide. JB Lippincott, Philadelphia
2. Cascinelly N, van der Esch EP, Breslow A, Morabito A, Bufalino R (1980) Stage I melanoma of the skin: the problem of resection margins. Eur J Cancer 16: 1079-1085
3. Coia LR, Engstrom PF, Paul A (1987) Nonsurgical management of esophageal cancer: report of a study of combined radiotherapy and chemotherapy. J Clin Oncol 5: 1783-1790
4. Ellis FH, Gibb SP (1979) Esophagogastrectomy for carcinoma: current hospital mortality and morbidity rates. Ann Surg 190: 699-705
5. Fisher F, Redmond C, Evans J and participating NSABP investigators (1982) Adjuvant chemotherapy of breast cancer: An overview of NSABP findings. Adv Surg Oncol 5: 65-90
6. Gall FP, Hermanek P, Gebhardt C, Meier H (1981) Erweiterte Resektion der Pankreas- und perampullären Karzinome: Regionale, totale und partielle Duodenopancreatektomie. Leber Magen Darm 11: 179-184
7. Gudjonsson B (1987) Cancer of the pancreas. 50 years of surgery. Cancer 60: 2284-2303
8. Heberer G, Denecke H, Demmel N, Wirsching R (1987) Local Procedures in the Management of Rectal Cancer. World J Surg 11: 499-503
9. Herfarth C, Schlag P (eds) (1979) Gastric Cancer. Springer-Verlag, Berlin Heidelberg New York
10. Hermanek P, Gall FP (1986) Early (microinvasive) colorectal carcinoma. Pathology, diagnosis, surgical treatment. Int J Colorect Dis 1: 79-84
11. Hildebrandt U, Feifel G (1985) Preoperative staging of rectal cancer by intrarectal ultrasound. Dis Colon Rectum 28: 42
12. Hoekstra HJ, Schraffordt Koops H, Molenaar WM, Oldhoff J (1987) Results of isolated regional perfusion in the treatment of malignant soft tissue tumors of the extremities. Cancer 60: 1703-1707
13. Jeekel J (1987) Can radical surgery improve survival in colorectal cancer? World J Surg 11: 412-417
14. Leichman L, Herskovic A, Leichman CG, Lattin PB, Steiger Z, Tapazoglou E, Rosenberg JC, Arbulu A, Asfaw I, Kinzie J (1987) Nonoperative therapy for squamous-cell cancer of the esophagus. J Clin Oncol 5: 365-370
15. Maruyama K, Okabayashi K, Kinoshita T (1987) Progress in gastric cancer surgery in Japan and its limits of radicality. World J Surg 11: 418-425
16. Mazzaferri EL (1987) Papillary thyroid carcinoma: factors influencing prognosis and current therapy. Sem in Oncol 14: 315-332

17. Nigro ND (1987) Multidisciplinary Management of Cancer of the Anus. World J Surg 11: 446–451
18. Orringer MB, Sloan H, Arbor A (1978) Esophagectomy without thoracotomy. J Thorac Cardiovasc Surg 76: 643–653
19. Papillon J (1982) Rectal and anal cancers. Springer, Berlin Heidelberg New York
20. Rosenberg SA, Glatstein EJ (eds) (1981) Perspectives on the role of surgery and radiation therapy in the treatment of soft tissue sarcomas of the extremities. Sem Oncol 2: 190–200
21. Schlag P (1986) Considerations for surgical treatment of gastric carcinoma. Eur J Surg Oncol 12: 235–239
22. Schlag P, Hohenberger P, Metzger U (eds) (1988) Combined modality therapy of gastrointestinal tract cancer. (Recent results in cancer research, vol 110) Springer-Verlag, Berlin Heidelberg New York Tokyo
23. Schraffordt Koops H, Oldhoff J, Wolter Oosterhuis J, Beekhuis H (1987) Isolated regional perfusion in malignant melanoma of the extremities. World J Surg 11: 527–533
24. Skinner DB (1983) En bloc resection for neoplasms of the esophagus and cardia. J Thorac Cardiovasc Surg 85: 59–71
25. Turnbull RB, Kyle K, Watson FR, Spratt J (1967) Cancer of the colon: The influence of the no-touch isolation technic on survival rates. Ann Surg 166: 420–427
26. Veronesi U (1987) Rationale and indications for limited surgery in breast cancer: current data. World J Surg 11: 493–498
27. Vickery AL, Wang CA, Walker AM (1987) Treatment of intrathyroidal papillary carcinoma of the thyroid. Cancer 60: 2587–2595
28. Wiggers T, Jeekel J, Arends JW, Brinkhorst AP, Jörning PJG, Kluck HM, Luyk CI, Munting JDK, Povel AJ, Rutten APN, Greep JM (1987) The no-touch isolation technique in colon cancer – final report after 5-year follow-up. 4th European Conference on Clinical Oncology and Cancer Nursing (ECCO-4), Madrid, ECCO-4 proceedings abstracts, p 150

Regional Chemotherapy of the Liver and Hepatic Artery Occlusion

S. BENGMARK[1]

Introduction

Despite the fact that infusion chemotherapy has been used for almost 20 years, the indications for this treatment modality are far from clear. The attitude of physicians and surgeons varies between complete therapeutic nihilism and therapeutic overenthusiasm. Neither of these attitudes is right. The first denies some patients significant relief of symptoms and, possibly prolonged survival, and the second often leads to extensive, drug-related toxicity.

Cells seeded to the liver from an extrahepatic primary tumor multiply 30 times or more before the tumor becomes clinically detectable. Since most of the seeding occurs over the portal vein tumors in the very early stages derive their nutrients entirely the portal vein. As the tumor grows, it develops its own blood supply, mainly from the hepatic artery, by a very special neovascularization process. Although it has not been clearly documented, one can therefore assume that the portal vein is more useful for adjuvant chemotherapy while the hepatic artery is more useful in treating manifest hepatic tumors by infusion chemotherapy. There are, however, not much data in the literature indicating that portovenous infusion or intraperitoneal infusion is inferior to administration of chemotherapy via the hepatic artery.

Infusion Chemotherapy – Long-term versus Short-term

For prolonged infusion, mainly drugs active at a specific phase of the cell cycle (5-fluorouracil, methotrexate) are used. Drugs not active at a specific phase (such as nitrous and doxorubicin) are equally, if not more, effective when given as a bolus injection. When 5-fluorouracil is administered in colonic cancer, treatment has to continue for long periods of time, if not indefinitely, in order to be effective. One can calculate that a 14-day treatment will affect approximately 5% of the tumor cells and a 3-month treatment, approximately 85% of the tumor cells. This explains why so many studies have been ineffective in the past.

Table 1 illustrates the median survival time in the literature published between 1970 and 1985. The median survival time in these studies is generally not more than a year. It is clear that the median survival time is, to a great extent, affected by selection criteria.

[1] Department of Surgery, Lund University, 22185 Lund, Sweden.

H. G. Beger et al. (Eds.), Cancer Therapy

Table 1. Survival times after hepatic arterial infusion chemotherapy for colorectal liver metastases

Authors	Regimen	Patients (*n*)	Median survival time (months)
Watkins et al. (1970)	long-term FUDR	82	15
Cady and Oberfield (1974)	long-term FUDR	51	11
Pettavel and Morenthaller (1978)	long-term FUDR	57	10
Oberfield et al. (1979)	long-term FUDR	48	8
Petrek and Minton (1979)	3-week 5-FU	24	9
Reed et al. (1981)	long-term FUDR	88	10
Balch et al. (1983)	2-week FUDR	81	12
Patt et al. (1983)	5-day FUDR + mitomycin C	22	10
Weiss et al. (1983)	2-week FUDR	17	13
Fortner et al. (1984b)	short-term FUDR	109	12
Niederhuber et al. (1984)	2-week FUDR	50	18
Johnsson and Rivkin (1985)	2-week FUDR + cisplatin	40	13
Didolkar et al. (1985)	long-term 5-FU	30	17
Schwartz et al. (1985)	2-week FUDR + mitomycin C	25	10

FUDR, 5-fluoro-2-deoxyuridine; *5-FU*, 5-fluorouracil.

Table 2. Complications after hepatic arterial infusion of fluorinated pyramidines

	Mortality (%)	Morbidity (%)
Weiss et al. 1984	0	100
Kemeny et al. 1984	4	>50
Niederhuber et al. 1984	0	>50
Schwartz et al. 1985	0	>75

Table 2 shows the mortality and morbidity in some of the studies. As these are considerable, it is clear that quality of life is easily affected by overenthusiastic treatment.

Table 3 shows the uncontrolled studies in which implantable pumps have been tested. Although some authors report a rather high response rate, the median survival times do not seem to be significantly affected. The high response rate claimed can be explained on the basis of selection. One should however remember that toxicity to the liver (chemically induced hepatitis) and to the gastrointestinal and biliary tracts is high – a high price for limited success in cancer therapy.

Analysis of our early studies (Fig. 1) shows significantly prolonged survival time when long-term infusion therapy (3 weeks or more) is compared with short-term infusion therapy (about 2 weeks). Over the years, we have become increasingly convinced that there is an advantage to long-term treatment, if possible, for the rest of the patient's life.

Table 3. Studies evaluating the intra-arterial hepatic infusion pump (all uncontrolled)

	Patients (*n*)	Responses imaging (%)	Survival times		Toxicity	
			from pump implantation (months)	from diagnosis (months)	chemical hepatitis (%)	gastro-intestinal (%)
Balch 1983	81			26	90	17
Weiss 1983	17	29	13	17	53	38
Cohen 1983	17	59			24	18
Niederhuber 1984	93	76	18	25	32	56
Kemeny 1984	41	44			71	46
Johnson 1985	40	47	+13		50	10
Schwartz 1985	25	15	>10	(>15)		10
Shepard 1985	62	32	17		49	18

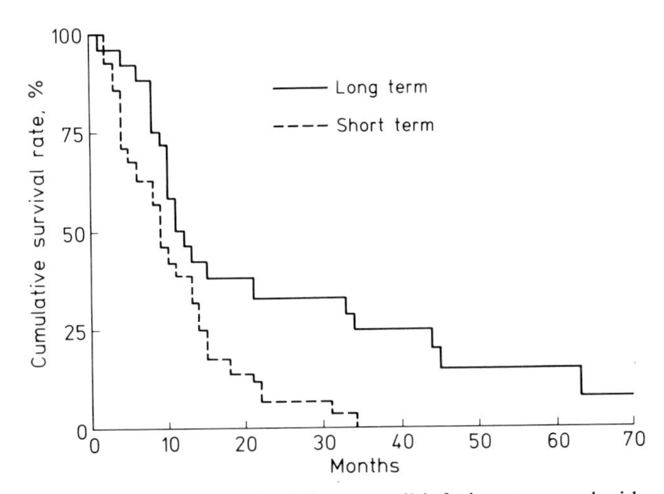

Fig. 1. Survival following long-term (more than 3 weeks) 5-fluorouracil infusion compared with short-term (less than 3 weeks) 5-fluorouracil infusion

Hepatic artery infusion and portovenous infusion are less likely to be successful as long-term therapy. Many complications, including thrombosis, occur rather early in this mode of treatment. For that reason, we are looking for alternative ways of treatment. In the last 2 years, we have developed an increasing interest in intraperitoneal administration of chemotherapy. There is no doubt that 5-fluorouracil (5-FU) and other oncolytic drugs can be administered with success and little toxicity over the peritoneum for long periods of time.

Hepatic Dearterialization

We have been interested in hepatic dearterialization for more than 25 years. With the exception of carcinoid disease, it has been difficult to document the value of hepatic dearterialization in the past.

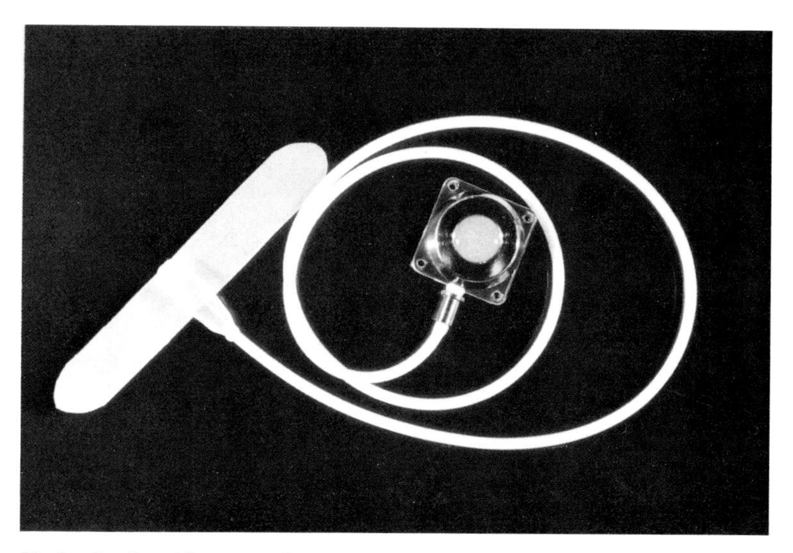

Fig. 2. Implantable port catheter and device for hepatic artery occlusion. Marketed by Baxter Travenol

The median survival times in published studies are about the same as those for infusion chemotherapy. This procedure also has a considerably high complication rate and, in the early days, resulted in significant mortality. However, in most patients with carcinoid tumors, a significant and long-lasting regression has been observed with this mode of treatment, and patients have often been free of symptom with normalized and stable levels of hydroxyindolacetic acid (HIAA) for long periods of time. The main reason for failure to respond after hepatic dearterialization has been the fact that there is very fast neoarterialization of hepatic tumors. This led us to test the effect of a short but repeated occlusion of the hepatic artery initially in experimental animals and then in patients. We were able to demonstrate that 1- or 2-h occlusion per day does not stimulate such a collateralization. With the aid of Nolato, Torekov, Sweden and Baxter Travenol, we have developed an implantable system (Fig. 2), which we use for daily occlusion of the hepatic artery. This has now been tried in more than a dozen patients with some very positive results. The patients have been able to occlude their hepatic arteries in the morning and the evening for months and years. This has often led to calcification of the tumors. Figure 3 shows a liver before (Fig. 3 a) and after (Fig. 3 b) 2 months of treatment.

Experimental studies have suggested that the surviving cells start to multiply immediately after occlusion (Fig. 4). This creates an ideal situation for chemotherapy. It is our hope that, by adapting a two-port concept (Fig. 5), we will be able to develop an effective treatment system that can be used on an outpatient basis – hopefully operated by the patients themselves. Such treatment should then include hepatic artery occlusion twice daily, as well as daily intraperitoneal infusions of 5-FU.

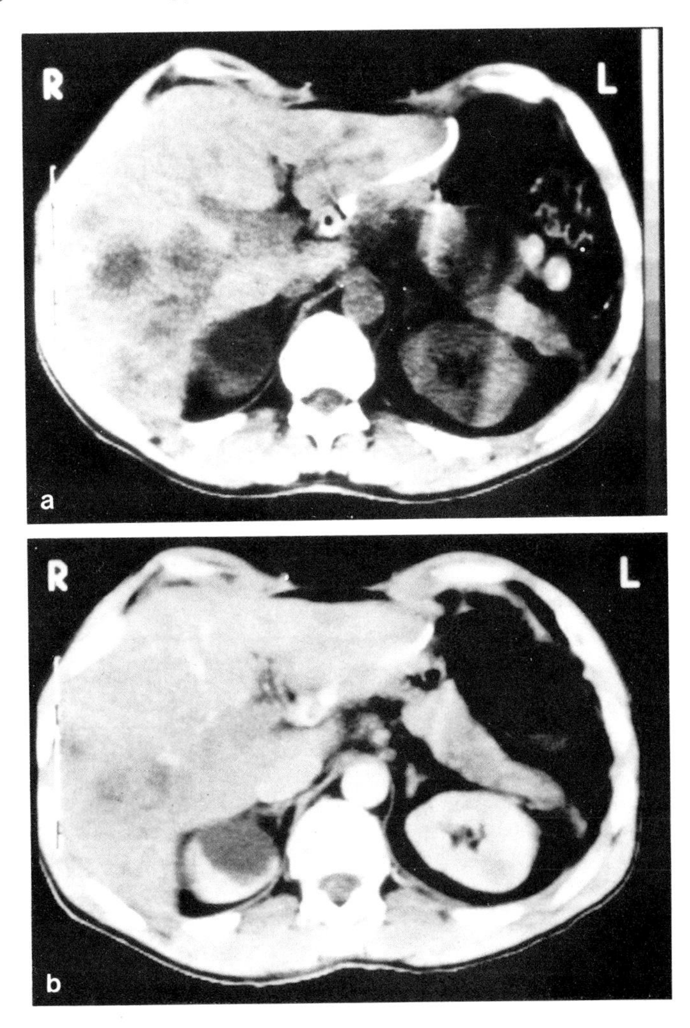

Fig. 3a, b. CT of a patient before (**a**) and 4 months after (**b**) the start of daily hepatic occlusions

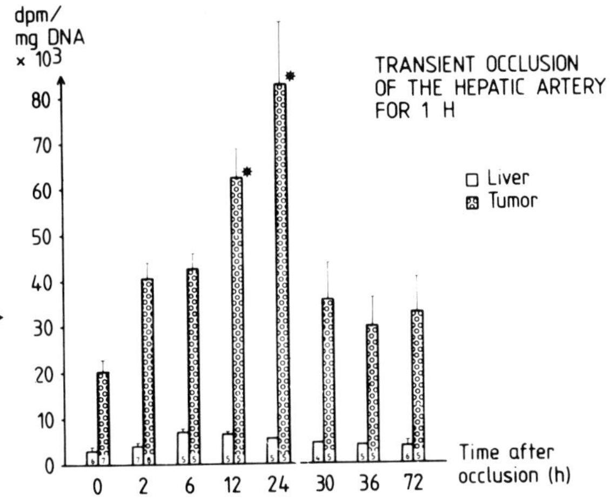

Fig. 4. Compensatory growth of tumor cells compared with that of liver cells after transient occlusion of the hepatic artery for 1 h as measured by DNA synthesis. *, statistically significant at the level <0.05 $P<0.001$

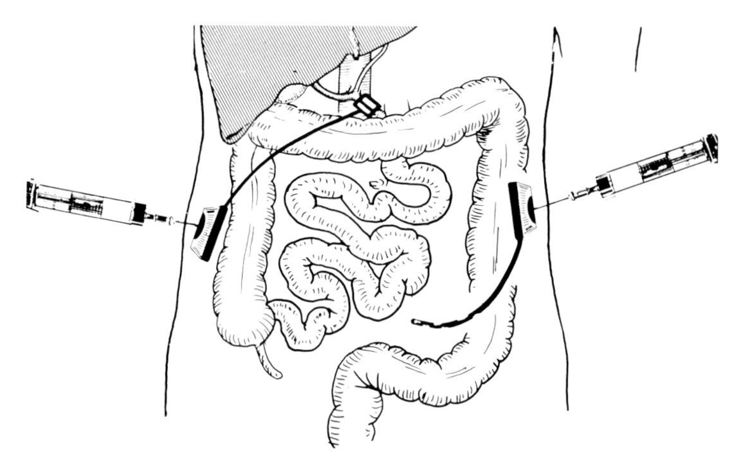

Fig. 5. Two-port concept, based on a combination of short-term hepatic artery occlusion and infusion of 5-fluorouracil via the peritoneum

References

1. Bengmark S, Jeppsson B (1987) Hepatische Desarterialisation bei der Behandlung von Lebertumoren. Chir Gastroenterolog mit Interdisziplinären Gesprächen 2: 65-70
2. Bengmark S, Jeppsson B (1988) Hepatic dearterialization. Surg Ann 4: 159-178
3. Bengmark S, Ekberg H, Tranberg K-G (1988) Metastatic tumours of the liver. In: Blumgart LH (ed) Surgery of the liver and biliary tract. Churchill Livingstone, Edinburgh
4. Bengmark S, Jeppsson B, Nobin A (1988) Arterial ligation and temporary dearterialization. In: Blumgart LH (ed) Surgery of the liver and biliary tract. Churchill Livingstone, Edinburgh
5. Hottenrott C, Lorenz M (1987) Lokale Chemoinfusionstherapie. Chir Gastroenterolog mit Interdiszipl Gesprächen 2: 73-90

Regional Chemotherapy of Hepatic Metastases

N. KEMENY[1]

Introduction

The rationale for the use of hepatic arterial infusion is to achieve higher drug levels in tumorous areas of the liver and lower systemic drug levels. This is possible because malignant lesions in the liver derive most of their blood supply from the hepatic artery, while normal hepatocytes derive most of their blood supply from the portal circulation. This observation was made on the basis of pathological data from animal tumors [1], and in a human study [2] using labeled 5-fluoro-2-deoxyuridine (FUDR). Ten patients were injected with tritium [^{3}H]-FUDR (1 μCi/kg) in either the hepatic artery or the portal vein. Liver biopsies obtained after injection demonstrated that the mean tumor FUDR levels following hepatic artery infusion were 12.4 nmol/g, while those following portal vein infusion were 0.8 nmol/g ($P < 0.01$). This clearly demonstrates that regional chemotherapy for hepatic metastases of colorectal carcinoma should be administered through the hepatic artery.

Chemotherapeutic drugs that would be most attractive for regional infusion are extracted by the liver during the first pass, leading to lower systemic drug levels and toxicity [3]. Ensminger et al. [4], by measuring drug levels from hepatic venous catheters, demonstrated that 94%–99% of FUDR was extracted in the first pass (Table 1). The ability to administer a higher dose locally exposes tumors to a higher drug concentration than can be achieved with systemic therapy. Since most

Table 1. Drugs for hepatic arterial infusion

Drug	Half-life (min)	Estimated increased exposure by hepatic arterial infusion
Fluorouracil (5-FU)	10	5–10-fold
5-Fluoro-2-deoxyuridine (5-FUDR)	< 10	100–400-fold
Bischlorethylnitrosourea (BCNU)	< 5	6–7-fold
Mitomycin C	< 10	6–8-fold
Cisplatin	20–30	4–7-fold
Adriamycin (doxorubicin hydrochloride)	60	2-fold
Dichloromethotrexate (DCMTX)		6–8-fold

[1] Associate Attending Physician, Solid Tumor Service, Department of Medicine, Memorial Sloan-Kettering Cancer Center, 1275 York Avenue, New York, NY 10021, USA.

H. G. Beger et al. (Eds.), Cancer Therapy

Table 2. Responses to hepatic arterial infusion of 5-fluoro-2-deoxyuridine with internal pump

Investigator	Patients (*n*)	Patients with prior chemotherapy (%)	Response rate (%)	Decrease in CEA (%)	Median survival time (months)
Niederhuber et al. [22]	70	45	83	91	25
Balch and Urist [23]	50	40		83	26
Kemeny, N. et al. [8]	41	43	42	51	12
Shepard et al. [24]	53	42	32		17
Cohen et al. [25]	50	36	51		
Weiss et al. [26]	17	85	29	57	13
Schwartz et al. [27]	23		15	75	18
Johnson et al. [28]	40		47		12
Kemeny, M. et al. [21]	31	50	52		22

CEA, carcinoembryonic antigen.

drugs have a steep dose-response curve, their antineoplastic efficacy should be increased by hepatic arterial infusion.

The first trials with hepatic artery infusion used external pumps and often required hospitalization and patient immobilization. The average response rate was 51%, with many of the studies including previously treated patients. Because of the hindrance to normal activity with external catheters, few oncologists advocated the use of hepatic arterial therapy, despite the apparently higher response rates [5].

The development of a totally implantable infusion device provided a new stimulus for the infusion advocates [6]. Use of an implantable pump delivery system offers several potential advantages: (a) reduction in catheter-related sepsis, (b) ease of drug administration, and (c) greater patient acceptance without bulky external devices [7]. Placement of the catheter at laparotomy eliminates the problem of catheter displacement and allows better determination of the presence of intra-abdominal, extrahepatic disease. The surgical technique has been described [8, 9].

The first study with the implantable pump and continuous FUDR therapy produced a response rate of 83% [10]. Despite the fact that other investigators using this method could not reproduce these results, the mean response rate of 44% (Table 2) in ten trials (where 42% of the patients had been previously treated) is higher than the mean response rate obtained with systemic chemotherapy [11].

Toxicity of Intrahepatic Chemotherapy via Implantable Pump

Although the operative and technical complications with the implantable pump have been minimal, there have been chemotherapy complications [8] (Table 3). Patients have developed endoscopically documented gastrointestinal ulcerations. The most likely mechanism for gastric toxicity from hepatic arterial infusion is inadvertent perfusion of the stomach and duodenum with drug via small vessels from the hepatic artery. Hohn et al. found no ulcers in their patients and feel this is related to their surgical technique, which involves very careful denuding of the

Table 3. Toxic side effects of hepatic arterial infusion of 5-fluoro-2-deoxyuridine with internal pump

Investigator	Patients (*n*)	Gastritis (%)	Ulcer (%)	SGOT elevations (%)	Bilirubin elevations (%)	Diarrhea (%)	Biliary sclerosis (%)
Niederhuber et al. [22]	70	56	8	32	24		
Balch and Urist [23]	50		6	23	23	0	
Kemeny, N. et al. [8]	41	29	29	71	22	0	5
Shepard et al. [24]	53		20	49	24		
Cohen et al. [25]	50		40	10	25		
Weiss et al. [26]	17	50	11	80	23	23	
Schwartz et al. [27]	23	53		77	20	10	
Johnson et al. [28]	40		8	50	13	0	5
Kemeny et al. [21]	31	17	6	47		8	19
Hohn et al. [18]	61	35	2	0	78	11	29

SGOT, serum glutamic oxaloacetic transaminase.

vessels arising from the hepatic artery (distal to the cannulation) that supply the stomach and duodenum [11]. Other attempts to modify this toxicity include careful reduction of the dose when any gastrointestinal symptoms or serum glutamic oxaloacetic transaminase (SGOT) elevation are noted. Drugs such as cimetidine, ranitidine, and antacids have been used but have failed to prevent the development of ulcers in these patients. However, they may decrease the incidence of ulcers.

Another frequent side effect is hepatic toxicity. In early stages of toxicity, elevations of hepatic enzymes will return to normal when the drug is withdrawn and the patient is given a rest period. In some patients, however, jaundice does not improve. These patients may develop biliary strictures, most commonly at the site of hepatic duct bifurcation, but also in the common bile duct or intrahepatic radicals. Radiographically, these lesions are similar to idiopathic sclerosing cholangitis. Since the ducts are sclerotic, sonograms are usually normal, and the diagnosis must be made by endoscopic retrograde cholangiopancreatography (ERCP) [8, 11].

Another side effect of hepatic arterial infusional chemotherapy is the development of cholecystitis. In a more recent series, the gallbladder was removed at the time of catheter placement to prevent this complication and to avoid the confusion of these symptoms with other hepatic side effects from pump treatment.

The usual side effects of chemotherapy are almost never seen with intrahepatic therapy. Myelosuppression does not occur with FUDR. While intrahepatic mitomycin or 1,3- bis 2-chlorethylnitrosourea (BCNU) may depress platelet counts, this occurs to a lesser degree than with systemic administration. Nausea and vomiting are not usually seen as a result of FUDR infusion, but if they are present, one should suspect that ulcerative disease or gastritis has developed. Diarrhea, which is frequently a problem with systemic FUDR infusion, is rarely seen with intrahepatic infusion. If it occurs, one should suspect high systemic drug levels caused by shunting either to the lung or to the bowel [12].

Randomized Studies

To understand the impact of hepatic infusional therapy on the natural history of patients with hepatic metastases, randomized studies were initiated in which patients were stratified for parameters known to affect response and survival. The strong influence of the percentage of liver involvement on survival has been shown by many investigators [13, 14]. At Memorial Sloan-Kettering Cancer Center (MSKCC), the median survival time for patients with less than 20% involvement (assessed medically or surgically) was greater than 29 months, while it was only 6 months for those with greater than 60% involvement [15]. Certain laboratory parameters also influence tumor response and patient survival. In one study, patients whose initial lactate dehydrogenase (LDH) and carcinoembryonic antigen (CEA) levels were normal had a median length of survival of 32 months versus only 8 months for those who originally had abnormal values [16].

There are presently a few completed randomized studies of patients with metastatic colorectal carcinoma. The study at MSKCC compared intrahepatic infusion with systemic infusion, applying the same chemotherapeutic agent (FUDR), drug schedule, and method of administration [17]. The dose of FUDR in the intrahepatic group was 0.3 mg/kg a day for 14 days, while the dose administereal systemically was 0.125 mg/kg a day for 14 days. All patients underwent exploratory laparotomy to assess the percentage of liver involvement and to confirm that there was no extrahepatic disease. At surgery, 33 of 162 patients were found to have disease outside the liver not detected by computed tomography and where thus excluded from analysis.

Patients randomized to the systemic group had the hepatic artery catheter connected to an Infus-a-port, and the pump was connected to an additional catheter placed in the cephalic vein. This allowed a crossover to intrahepatic therapy by a minor surgical procedure (ligation of the systemic catheter and Infus-a-port, followed by a connection of the pump to the intrahepatic catheter) in the event of tumor progression on systemic therapy.

This study demonstrated a significantly higher response rate (>50% reduction in measurable disease) with intrahepatic therapy (50%), versus 20% for systemic infusion ($P = 0.001$) (Table 4). Thirty-one of the patients receiving systemic therapy crossed over to intrahepatic therapy after tumor progression. Twenty-five percent showed a partial response, 22% stabilization of disease, and 50% a drop in CEA on intrahepatic therapy. The toxicity was quite different between the two groups. The toxicity from intrahepatic treatment was similar to the other intrahepatic studies described above, while the toxicity from systemic therapy was mostly evidenced in the form of diarrhea, occurring in 70% of the patients and requiring admission of 9% of the patients for intravenous hydration.

The median survival time for the intrahepatic and systemic groups was 17 and 12 months respectively ($P = 0.424$). Survival information is difficult to interpret because 60% of the patients in the systemic group crossed over and received intrahepatic therapy. The patients who were unable to cross over (usually for mechanical reasons, such as clotting of the Infus-a-port), had a median survival of 8 months, versus 18 months for those able to undergo the crossover.

A similar randomized study by the Northern California Cooperative Cancer

Table 4. Intrahepatic versus systemic infusion of 5-fluoro-2-deoxyuricidine (randomized study of Memorial Sloan-Kettering Cancer Center)

	Intrahepatic ($n=48$)	Systemic ($n=51$)	
Partial response	24 (50%)	10 (20%)	$P=0.001$
>50% decrease in CEA	29	13	
Extrahepatic metastases	27	19	$P=0.09$
Toxicity			
Ulcer	8	3	
Elevated enzymes	20 (42%)	12	
Bilirubin >3 mg/dl	9	2	
Diarrhea	1	36 (70%)	
Median survival (months)			
Total	17	12	$P=0.424$
Crossover		18	
No crossover		8	

CEA, carcinoembryonic antigen.

Group also used FUDR infusion in both the intrahepatic and systemic arms of the study and had response rates similar to those of the MSKCC study. They reported a 37% partial response rate in the intrahepatic infusion group and 12% in the systemic FUDR infusion group [18]. The dose of FUDR was lower in both arms: 0.2 mg/kg for the intrahepatic group and 0.075 mg/kg for the systemic group. The median survival was 15 months for both the intrahepatic and the systemic group. Although a crossover design was not built into the study, many patients received intrahepatic therapy after failing to respond to systemic therapy, and again there was a difference in the median survival times: 22 months for those who went on to receive intrahepatic therapy versus 12 months for those who did not receive intrahepatic therapy after failure to respond to systemic treatment.

A National Cancer Institute (NCI) study [19] also compared FUDR intrahepatic infusion and systemic FUDR infusion. They reported a significant increase in the response rates: 62% versus 17% respectively. If patients with positive lymph nodes are excluded, the 2-year survival was 47% versus 13% respectively, ($P=0.03$). Another randomized study conducted by a consortium of four institutions [20] was unable to enter enough patients and closed after 43 patients had entered. The response rates were 38%, 58%, and 56% for systemic 5-fluorouracil (5-FU) administration, intrahepatic FUDR infusion, and combined systemic and intrahepatic therapy, respectively (Table 5).

Conclusion

There are now five randomized trials demonstrating a significantly higher response rate with intrahepatic infusion as opposed to systemic infusion in the treatment of hepatic metastases from colorectal carcinoma. Because of the early successes with intrahepatic infusion, these studies allowed patients in the systemic arm to receive intrahepatic therapy after failure to respond to systemic therapy.

Table 5. Randomized studies of intrahepatic versus systemic chemotherapy for hepatic metastases

Group	Patients (*n*)	Intrahepatic		Systemic		
		Drug	Response (%)	Drug	Response (%)	
MSKCC (17)	163	FUDR	50	FUDR	20	$P=0.001$
NCOG (18)	143	FUDR	37	FUDR	10	$P=0.002$
NCI (19)	64	FUDR	62	FUDR	17	
Consortium (20)	43	FUDR	56	5FU	38	
City of Hope (21)	41	FUDR	56	5FU	0	

MSKCC, Memorial Sloan-Kettering Cancer Center; *NCOG*, Northern California Oncology Group; *NCI*, National Cancer Institute; *FUDR*, 5-fluoro-2-deoxyuridine; *5FU*, 5-fluorouracil.

Therefore, the impact of intrahepatic treatment on survival is difficult to evaluate. A longer survival has been observed for those who received intrahepatic therapy, whether administered originally or after ineffective systemic therapy. One might infer from this data that intrahepatic treatment is only needed after failure of systemic treatment. Two arguments against this viewpoint are: (a) the lack of systemic side effects and the ease in administering a continuous infusion via an implantable pump, and (b) the fact that if one waits until a patient fails on systemic treatment, the patient may then be too sick to undergo surgery for hepatic artery cannulation. Before hepatic infusional therapy via the hepatic pump becomes a standard treatment, more work is needed on: (a) clearly defining whether there is a survival advantage, (b) devising ways to decrease biliary sclerosis, and (c) developing ways to increase the response rate, particularly that of complete responses.

References

1. Breedis C, Young C (1954) The blood supply of neoplasms in the liver. Am J Pathol 30: 969
2. Sigurdson ER, Ridge JA, Kemeny N, Daly JM (1987) Tumor and liver drug uptake following hepatic artery and portal vein infusion. J Clin Oncol 5: 1836–1840
3. Chen HSG, Gross JF (1980) Intra-arterial infusion of anti-cancer drugs: theoretic aspects of drug delivery and review of responses. Cancer Treat Rep 64: 31–40
4. Ensminger WD, Rosowsky A, Raso V (1978) A clinical pharmacological evaluation of hepatic arterial infusions of 5-fluoro-2-deoxyuridine and 5-fluorouracil. Cancer Res 38: 3784–3792
5. Reed ML, Vaitkevicius VK, Al-Sarraf M, Vaughn CB, Singhakowinter A, Sexton-Porte M, Izbicki R, Baker L, Straatsm GW (1981) The practicality of chronic hepatic artery infusion therapy of primary and metastatic hepatic malignancies. Cancer 47: 402
6. Buchwald H, Grage TB, Vassilopoulos PP (1980) Intraarterial infusion chemotherapy for hepatic carcinoma using a totally implantable infusion pump. Cancer 45: 866–869
7. Ensminger W, Niederhuber J, Dakhil S, Thrall J, Wheeler R (1981) Totally implanted drug delivery system for hepatic arterial chemotherapy. Cancer Treat Rep 65: 393
8. Kemeny N, Daly J. Oderman P, Shike M, Chun HG, Petroni GR, Geller NL (1984) Hepatic artery pump infusion toxicity and results in patients with metastatic colorectal carcinoma. J Clin Oncol 2: 595–600
9. Hohn DC, Stagg RJ, Price DC, Lewis BJ (1985) Avoidance of gastroduodenal toxicity in patients receiving hepatic arterial 5-fluoro-2′-deoxyuridine. J Clin Oncol 3: 1257–1260
10. Ensminger W, Niederhuber J, Gyves J, Thrall J, Cozzi E, Doan K (1982) Effective control of liver metastases from colon cancer with an implanted system for hepatic arterial chemotherapy. Proc ASCO 1: 94

11. Hohn DC, Melnick J, Stagg R (1985) Biliary sclerosis in patients receiving hepatic arterial infusions of floxuridine. J Clin Oncol 3: 98-102
12. Gluck WI, Akwari OE, Kelvin FM, Goodwin BJ (1985) A reversble enteropathy complicating continuous hepatic artery infusion chemotherapy with 5-fluoro 2-deoxyuridine. Cancer 56: 2424
13. Wood CB, Gillis CR, Blumgart LH (1976) A retrospective study on the natural history of patients with liver metastasis from colorectal cancer. Clin Oncol 2: 285-288
14. Gennari L, Doci R, Bozzetti F, Veronesi U (1982) Proposal for a clinical classification of liver metastases. Tumori 68: 443-448
15. Kemeny N, Daly J, Oderman P, Niedzwiecki D, Shurgot B (1985) Prognostic variables in patients with hepatic metastases from colorectal cancer: Importance of medical assessment of liver involvement. Proc ASCO 4: 88
16. Kemeny N, Braun DW (1983) Prognostic factors in advanced colorectal carcinoma: The importance of lactic dehydrogenase, performance status, and white blood cell count. Am J Med 74: 786-794
17. Kemeny N, Daly J, Reichman B, Geller N, Botet J, Oderman P (1987) Intrahepatic or systemic infusion of fluorodeoxyuridine in patients with liver metastases from colorectal carcinoma. Ann Int Med 107: 459-465
18. Hohn D, Stagg R, Friedman M (1987) The NCOG randomized trial of intravenous (IV) vs hepatic arterial (IA) FUDR for colorectal cancer metastatic to the liver. Proc ASCO 6: 85
19. Chang AE, Schneider PD, Sugerbaker PH, Simpson C, Culnane M, Steinberg SM (1987) A prospective randomized trial of regional versus systemic continuous 5-fluorodeoxyuridine chemotherapy in the treatment of colorectal liver metastases. Ann Surg 206: 685-693
20. Niederhuber JE (1985) Arterial chemotherapy for metastatic colorectal cancer in the liver. Conference Advances in Regional Cancer Therapy. Giessen, Federal Republic of Germany
21. Kemeny MM, Goldberg D, Beatty JD, Blayney D, Browning S, Doroshow J, Ganteaume L, Hill RL, Kokal WA, Riihimaki DU, Terz JJ (1986) Results of a prospective randomized trial of continuous regional chemotherapy and hepatic resection as treatment of hepatic metastases from colorectal primaries. Cancer 57: 492
22. Niederhuber JE, Ensminger W, Gyves, Thrall J, Walker S, Cozzi E (1984) Regional chemotherapy of colorectal cancer metastatic to the liver. Cancer 53: 1336
23. Balch CM, Urist MM (1986) Intraarterial chemotherapy for colorectal liver metastases and hepatomas using a totally implantable drug infusion pump. In: Herfarth C, Schlag P, Hohenberger P (eds) Therapeutic strategies in primary and metastatic liver cancer. Springer, Berlin Heidelberg New York Tokyo, pp 123-147 (Recent results in cancer research, vol 100)
24. Shepard KV, Levin B, Karl RC, Faintuch J, DuBrow RA, Hagle M, Cooper RM, Beschorner J, Stablein D (1985) Therapy for metastatic colorectal cancer with hepatic artery infusion chemotherapy using a subcutaneous implanted pump. J Clin Oncol 3: 161
25. Cohen AM, Kaufman SD, Wood WC, Greenfield AJ (1983) Regional hepatic chemotherapy using an implantable drug infusion pump. Am J Surg 145: 529-533
26. Weiss GR, Garnick MB, Osteen RT, Steele GD Jr, Wilson RE, Schode D, Kaplan WD, Boxt LM, Kandarpa K, Mayer RJ, Rei ET III (1983) Long-termp hepatic arterial infusion of 5-fluorodeoxyuridine for liver metastases using an implantable infusion pump. J Clin Oncol 1: 337-344
27. Schwartz SI, Jones LS, McCune CS (1985) Assessment of treatment of intrahepatic malignancies using chemotherapy via an implantable pump. Anal Surg 201: 560-567
28. Johnson LP, Wasserman PB, Rivkin SE (1983) FUDR hepatic arterial infusion via an implantable pump for treatment of hepatic tumors. Proc Am Soc Clin Oncol 2: 119

Regional Chemotherapy in Hepatic Metastases of Colorectal Carcinoma: Continuous Intra-arterial Versus Continuous Intra-arterial/Intravenous Therapy

F. SAFI,[1] R. BITTNER,[1] R. ROSCHER,[1] K. SCHUMACHER,[2] W. GAUS,[3] and H. G. BEGER[1]

Introduction

About 25% of patients have already liver metastases when the diagnosis of colorectal carcinoma is established. In another 30%-40% of the patients, metachronic metastases of a primary tumor settle in the liver, indicating that liver metastases are a significant factor for the prognosis of colorectal carcinoma [1]. The median survival time of the patients is approximately 6 months; only 7% live longer than 1 year [3]. Lymphogenous spread of metastases is not the decisive factor; rather, it is the invasion of the primary tumor into the vascular system [4].

The systemic treatment of hepatic metastases with cytostatic agents does not have a response rate greater than 25% [2]. Besides, survival time is not extended with this type of treatment.

The literature shows that response rates of liver metastases to regional intra-arterial perfusion of floxuridine (FUDR) can vary between 43% and 88% [5-7]. On the basis of these rates, the median survival time is said to range between 17 and 26 months [8, 9]. The therapeutic efficacy of a regionally applied cytostatic agent is directly dependent on an optimal concentration at the metastatic site. This again is directly influenced by the individual conditions of perfusion in the liver [10].

Different incidence rates for the appearance of extrahepatic metastases after the beginning of regional chemotherapy, ranging from 42% to 75%, have been reported. It is the formation of metastases that causes the death of patients, even in those patients responding to regional chemotherapy [6, 7].

The aim of the present study was to treat patients both regionally and systemically in order to delay or prevent the occurrence of extrahepatic metastases. In addition, we wanted to evaluate the survival time of patients with isolated hepatic metastases, the response rate of metastases, and the toxicity of regional therapy with FUDR.

To determine whether regional chemotherapy really prolongs patient survival, we divided our patient population into two groups:

- Group 1: Patients demonstrating remission (partial or total) of liver metastases in the computed tomographic (CT) scan
- Group 2: Patients with stable disease or progression of metastases

[1] Department of General Surgery, University of Ulm, Steinhövelstraße 9, 7900 Ulm, FRG.
[2] Department of Radiology, University of Ulm, Steinhövelstraße 9, 7900 Ulm, FRG.
[3] Department of Clinical Statistics and Documentation, University of Ulm, Steinhövelstraße 9, 7900 Ulm, FRG.

H. G. Beger et al. (Eds.), Cancer Therapy

The following questions were investigated:

1. Are the two groups comparable with respect to the spread of metastases and the primary tumor stage in the colorectal region?
2. If so, can a clear difference in survival time be found between responders and nonresponders?

Patients and Methods of Treatment

Pilot Study

From March 1983 to January 1985, we treated 20 patients with hepatic metastases of colorectal carcinomas by means of regional intra-arterial chemotherapy via the Infusaid pump.

Randomized Study

From February 1985 until December 1987, an additional 44 patients were randomized into two groups, depending on their primary tumor stage in the colorectal region and the metastatic spread in the liver. The intra-arterial (i.a.) group ($n=$ 23 patients) were treated only intra-arterially. In the intra-arterial/intravenous (i.a./i.v.) group ($n=21$), i.a./i.v. dual-catheter Infusaid pumps were implanted. The characteristics of the patients are summarized in Tables 1 and 2 a and b. The patients in the randomized study were comparable with respect to the stage of the primary tumor, metastatic spread in the liver, age, and sex ($p>0.1$) (Table 1, 2a). The serum concentration of carcinoembryonic antigen (CEA) and liver enzymes (median values) were also comparable in the two randomized groups (Table 2b).

Table 1. Regional chemotherapy of liver metastases of colorectal cancer – Patient characteristics

	Pilot study ($n=20$)	Randomized study		Total ($n=64$)
		i.a. ($n=23$)	i.a./i.v. ($n=21$)	
Sex ratio women/men	1/1	1/1.3	1/2	1/1.3
Average age (years)				
Women	51.9	52.5	55.14	52.96
Men	63.5	60.46	56.36	59.73
Location of primary tumor (n)				
Rectum	8	1	8	27 (42%)
Colon	8	2	8	18 (28%)
Sigma	4	10	5	19 (30%)
Primary tumor stage (n)				
$pT_{1-3}\ N_0$	6	10	11	27 (42%)
$pT_{1-3}\ N_1$	8	9	9	26 (41%)
$pT_{1-3}\ N_2$	6	4	1	11 (17%)

Table 2a. Regional chemotherapy of liver metastases of colorectal cancer – Metastatic spread in the liver

	Pilot study ($n=20$)	Randomized study		Total ($n=64$)
		i.a. ($n=23$)	i.a./i.v. ($n=21$)	
Volume of metastases (n)				
<50% of liver volume	13	20	16	49 (77%)
>50% of liver volume	7	3	5	15 (23%)
Synchronous metastases (n)	12	9	9	30 (47%)
Metachronous metastases (n)	8	14	12	34 (53%)

Table 2b. Regional chemotherapy of liver metastases of colorectal cancer – Initial values of liver enzymes and CEA serum level

	Pilot study		Randomized study				Total	
			i.a.		i.a./i.v.			
	Median	Min.–Max.	Median	Min.–Max.	Median	Min.–Max.	Median	Min.–Max.
CEA (ng/ml)	17.8	2.2–100.1	36.6	1.9–604	29.3	3.8–1600.1	23.2	1.9–1600.1
GOT (U/L)	14	8–50	12	6–59	16	7–76	14	6–76
GPT (U/L)	15	8–50	17	2–44	23	7–100	17.5	2–100
APH (U/L)	260	104–1047	180	101–1512	228	104–1990	209	101–1990
γ-GT (U/L)	61	12–325	52	12–516	34	15–750	59.5	12–750
LDH (U/L)	306	141–967	210	74–596	211	153–412	211	74–967

GOT, glutamic oxaloacetic transaminase; *APH*, alkaline phosphatase; *γ-GT*, γ-glutamyl transpeptidase; *LDH*, lactic dehydrogenase.

Surgical Technique

Blach and Urist [6] described the method of pump implantation and catheter placement into the arterial system. The arterial catheter was also implanted in the common hepatic artery in those patients in whom an i.a./i.v. pump had been placed. The venous catheter was inserted into the inferior vena cava via the testicular or ovarian vein following Kocher's maneuver and mobilization of the duodenum. The tip of the arterial or venous catheter was placed in the opening of the gastroduodenal/hepatic artery or the ovarian vein/inferior vena cava, respectively.

Complete perfusion was controlled during surgery by injection of a fluorescein solution and checked by ultraviolet light (Woods lamp). This control was performed again postoperatively and then every 3 months via the arterial angio-CT. The pump was placed subcutaneously into the lower abdominal region and secured to the fascia.

Chemotherapy

No patient had previously been treated with cytostatic drugs. The FUDR therapy was initiated from the 8th to the 14th day after pump implantation. FUDR was the basic chemotherapeutic agent (0.2 mg/kg daily) administered in 2-week cycles, alternating with double distilled water.
All patients with i.a. pumps received this dose. Patients with i.a./i.v. pumps were administered FUDR at a dose of 0.3 mg/kg daily, during the course of which 0.21 mg/kg was perfused intra-arterially (regionally) and 0.09 mg/kg intravenously (systemically). Thus, the regional dose was the same in both the i.a. and i.a./i.v. groups.
An additional administration of mitomycin C at a dose of 10 mg/m^2 during a ½-h infusion via the sideport of the pump was carried out for the following reasons:

1. Owing to chemically induced hepatitis or sclerosing cholangitis, the dose of FUDR had to be reduced by half.
2. Progression of hepatic metastases could be detected in spite of FUDR therapy.

If extrahepatic metastases occurred during therapy, an additional treatment of systemic intravenous 5-fluorouracil (5-FU) at a dose of 12.5 mg/kg daily for 5 days was added.

Monitoring of Regional Chemotherapy

The following parameters were investigated preoperatively and at 2-week intervals postoperatively: blood count, liver parameters [gamma-glutamyl transpeptidase (γGT), glutamic pyruvic transaminase (GPT), alkaline phosphatase (APH), lactic dehydrogenase (LDH), bilirubin] and CEA. An arterial angio-CT of the liver, sonography of the abdomen, and a chest X-ray film were performed preoperatively and every 3 months during treatment. If the bilirubin value increased, an endoscopic retrograde cholangiopancreatographic (ERCP) examination was carried out for the differential diagnosis "chemical hepatitis/mechanical obstruction of the biliary tracts." Persistent epigastric symptoms during the course of treatment represented an indication for duodenoscopy.
The patient's follow-up was supervised regularly in the outpatient department and sometimes by the patient's general practitioner.

Definition of Response

1. A complete response denotes the disappearance of liver metastases in the CT scan.
2. A partial response indicates a reduction greater than 25% in metastatic volume.
3. Stable disease indicates unchanged metastatic size.

The above criteria had to be fulfilled for at least two subsequent investigations, equivalent to a minimum of 3 months. Progression was defined as an increase in

metastatic volume in spite of FUDR therapy. The response to regional chemotherapy was determined after the first 3 months of FUDR therapy and every 3 months thereafter.
To determine the metastatic volume prior to and after treatment, metastases were demarcated in all CT layers with the help of "regions of interest" and compared with the healthy liver tissue. The region was established by a calculation program integrated into the system. Since the layer thickness of 10 mm was known, we determined the volume as the product of region multiplied by layer thickness. The whole-liver volume was determined in the same way. The quotient of metastatic and liver volume reveals the proportional metastatic volume.

Statistics

Patient survival time from the time of pump implantation was calculated in accordance with the Kaplan-Meier method [11]. The test devised by Mantel and Haenzel was used for comparison of survival rates [12]. For categorical variables, the chi-squared test and Fisher exact test were used [13].

Results

Postoperative Complications

All patients survived the surgical implantation of the pump. Immediate complications, such as peritonitis or hemorrhage did not occur. An infection of the pump pocket occurred postoperatively in one patient. Seromas of the pump pocket were observed in 13 patients; these disappeared in 11 patients following transcutaneous tapping. In two patients, a recurrence of seroma was observed. After transcutaneous tapping, which was performed at least 20 times, infection of the pump pocket occurred. Transposition of the pump to another abdominal region was necessary in these two patients, as well as in three patients who developed skin necrosis in the region of the pump sideports. The reoperation rate was 9%.

Toxicity of FUDR

In 14 of 64 patients (21%), gastroduodenitis or duodenal ulcers occurred. In two patients (3%), a macroscopic diagnosis of malignant growth could not be excluded. Histologically, constant severe dysplasia of the mucus membrane was diagnosed; this was misinterpreted as carcinoma [14]. In one of the first patients of our group, a painful chemical cholecystitis occurred, which necessitated a cholecystectomy. The cholecystectomy was then carried out as a matter of routine during surgery.
In 37 patients (57%), a twofold elevation above the standard values of at least two of the following liver parameters, glutamic oxaloacetic transaminase (GOT), GPT, APH, and γGT, was observed owing to a chemical hepatitis resulting from the

Table 3. Regional chemotherapy of liver metastases of colorectal cancer - FUDR toxicity

	Pilot study ($n=20$)	Randomized study		Total	
		i.a. ($n=23$)	i.a./i.v. ($n=21$)	($n=64$)	(%)
Stomatitis	0	4	4	8	12.0
Diarrhea	0	1	2	3	4.0
Esophagitis	0	0	1	1	1.5
Ulcer/gastritis	3	6	5	14	21.0
Chemical hepatitis	13	15	9	37	57.0
Sclerosing cholangitis	5	6	5	16	25.0

FUDR medication. This risk increases proportionally with the duration of administration and dosage of FUDR. In 16 additional patients (25%), a sclerosing cholangitis was detected by ERPC or percutaneous transhepatic cholangiogram (PTC) after elevation of serum bilirubin. Sclerosing cholangitis was reversible in seven patients only after discontinuation of the FUDR therapy.
Three patients (one in the i.a. and two in the i.a./i.v. randomized groups) complained of diarrhea that was severe enough for them to be hospitalized for rehydration. Stomatitis was seen in four patients of each randomized group, which disappeased after reduction of the FUDR dosage. Myelosuppression, alopecia, and emesis did not occur with either treatment (i.a. and i.a./i.v.). Gastrointestinal tract and liver toxicities did not differ significantly between the i.a. and i.a./i.v. treated patients ($p>0.1$) (Table 3).

Response

Computed Tomographic Scan

With regard to the development of intrahepatic metastases, the control angio-CTs showed a complete response in 18 patients - there were no detectable metastases shown on the CT. Fourteen patients showed a reduction in metastatic volume by more than 25%. These results were obtained by means of volumetric measurements of metastases and liver volume in our department of radiology. In 14 other cases, no change in metastatic size was seen on the CT scan. Progression of metastases in spite of FUDR therapy was also observed in 18 patients (Table 4).

Clinical Relevance of the Tumor Marker CEA

A total of 88% of the patients ($n=56$) had increases in CEA levels of over 4 ng/ml compared with CEA levels before chemotherapy. Of these 75% of these patients ($n=42$) showed a reduction in CEA serum levels following therapy. A regression rate of more than 60% (compared with baseline values) was seen in 79% of the latter patients (52% of the entire group) (Table 5).

Table 4. Regional chemotherapy of liver metastases of colorectal cancer – Response according to computed tomography

	Pilot study ($n=20$)	Randomized study		Total	
		i.a. ($n=23$)	i.a./i.v. ($n=21$)	($n=64$)	(%)
Total response	6	6	6	18	28
Partial response	4	6	4	14	22
Stable disease	2	6	6	14	22
Progression	8	5	5	18	28
Follow-up period (months)	5–43	5–43	4–27	4–43	
Minimum–Maximum Median	20	16	16	18	

Table 5. Regional chemotherapy of liver metastases of colorectal cancer – The clinical relevance of the tumor marker

	Pilot study		Randomized study				Total	
	($n=20$)	(%)	i.a.		i.a./i.v.		($n=64$)	(%)
			($n=23$)	(%)	($n=21$)	(%)		
CEA before chemotherapy >4 ng/ml	$n=16$	80%	$n=20$	87%	$n=20$	95%	$n=56$	88%
Minimum–Maximum	7–100		4–720		4–1600		4.3–1600	
Median	23.4		58.4		24.2		27.9	
CEA serum concentration in comparison with the starting values								
Decrease 30%–60%	$n=5$	31%	$n=2$	10%	$n=2$	10%	$n=9$	16%
60%–90%	$n=5$	31%	$n=10$	50%	$n=8$	40%	$n=23$	41%
>90%	$n=0$	0%	$n=4$	20%	$n=6$	30%	$n=10$	18%
Increase of CEA serum level	$n=6$	38%	$n=4$	20%	$n=4$	20%	$n=14$	25%

In accordance with the identical intra-arterial dose of chemotherapy, the metastases in both groups (i.a. and i.a./i.v.) responded equally to regional chemotherapy. Remission of the metastases (partial or total) was evident in 52% ($n=12$) of the patients treated by i.a. and in 48% ($n=10$) of the patients treated by i.a./i.v. A decrease in the CEA serum level exceeding 60% during the course of treatment could be found in 14 patients from the i.a. group (60%) and in 14 patients from the i.a./i.v. group (67%) $p>0.1$ (Tables 4 and 5).

Extrahepatic Spread of Metastases During Therapy

The median observation time for the patients in our pilot study was 20 months (5–43 monts). During this period of time, 14 patients developed extrahepatic metastases (70%). During treatment, 61% ($n=14$) of the i.a. and 33% ($n=7$) of the i.a./i.v. group developed extrahepatic metastases, the locations of which are given in Table 6. This spreading of the carcinoma was found in a median observation

Table 6. Regional chemotherapy of liver metastases of colorectal cancer – Extrahepatic spread of metastases

	Pilot study ($n=20$)	Randomized study		Total ($n=64$)
		i.a. ($n=23$)	i.a./i.v. ($n=21$)	
Extrahepatic metastases	14 (70%)	14 (61%)	7 (33%)	35 (55%)
Lung	8	6	4	18
Bone	1		3	4
Lymph nodes	1			1
Peritoneum	3	3		6
Pelvic recurrence	1	3		4
Colonic recurrence	–	2		2
Follow-up period (months)				
Minimum–Maximum	5–43	5–34	4–27	4–43
Median	20	16	16	18

period of 16 months. The difference between the two randomized groups was not significant at that point in time ($p>0.1$). Eight of the 14 patients in the i.a. group and one of the seven patients in the i.a./i.v. group responded to therapy. Although the metastases responded in the i.a. group in 12 patients, extrahepatic metastases occurred in eight, while only one of the 10 responders in the i.a./i.v. treated group developed metastases outside the liver.

Additional Treatment with 5-Fluorouracil (5 FU) and Mitomycin C

One patient with a recurrence of carcinoma of the colon was treated surgically. Thirteen patients were treated with 5 FU because of extrahepatic tumor progression, but none showed a decrease in the CEA serum level. In 13 other patients, the tumor spread intra- as well as extrahepatically. These were treated with 5 FU and mitomycin C. A temporary reduction of the CEA serum level was found in only four of these patients. In 5 patients, there was progression of the intrahepatic metastases despite the FUDR therapy; a decrease in the CEA serum concentration due to the mitomycin C therapy was seen in only one of these patients. The additional systemic or regional chemotherapy in the 31 patients gave rise to a temporary regression of the pulmonary metastases in one patient and of the hepatic metastases in another patient, as documented by the imaging procedure. Three patients refused further therapy.

Survival

The 1-year survival rate of the entire group ($n=64$) was 80%; 2-year survival was 50%. The median survival time was 24 months (Fig. 1). No significant difference in survival was found between the i.a./i.v.-treated patients up to 3 years (1-year sur-

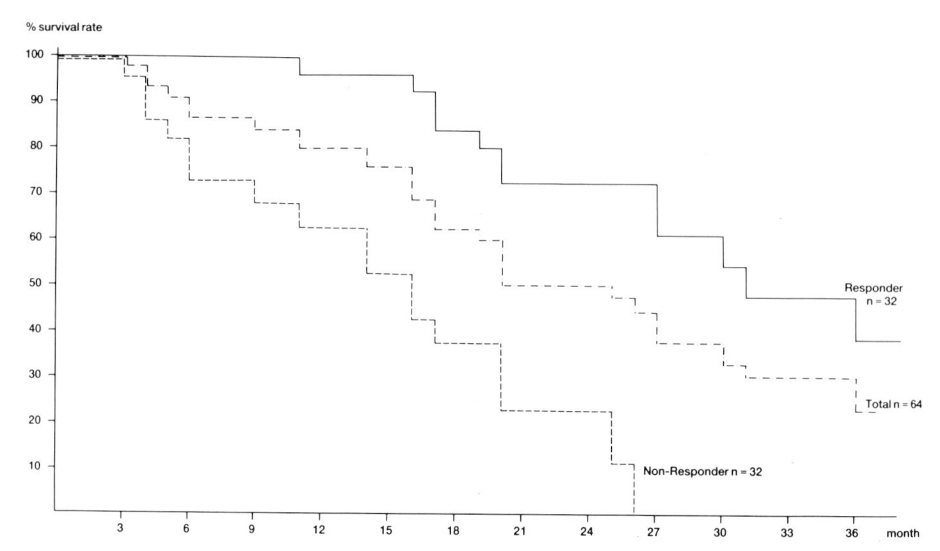

Fig. 1. Regional chemotherapy of liver metastases of colorectal cancer – Survival (responders vs non-responders)

vival: 89% and 86% respectively, 2 year survival: 55% and 43% respectively. Beyond 3 years, the survival rate was 0% and 43% respectively (Fig. 2).
Depending on our response criteria, we divided our patient population into two groups:

1. group 1 ($n=32$): Patients showing remission (partial or total) of the liver metastases in the CT scan
2. group 2 ($n=32$): Patients with stable disease or progression of metastases.

For the comparison of both groups, we used the chi-squared test. No significant difference resulted between the two groups with respect to primary tumor stage and spread of metastases ($p>0.1$) (Table 7a). The serum concentrations of CEA and liver enzymes were comparable for responders and nonresponders (Table 7b). The median survival time of group 1 was 31 months, for group 2, it was 16 months. This difference, calculated according to the logrank test, is statistically very significant ($p>0.0001$) (Fig. 1).

Discussion

The principle of intra-arterial chemotherapy has been increasingly employed. Transcutaneous intra-arterial dislocation of the catheter, thrombosis of the hepatic artery, and defective perfusion of the liver present major problems [7]. Technical advances as well as the introduction of a totally implantable, continuous infusion system have once again aroused interest in intra-arterial infusion of the liver [6, 9]. The advantage of this type of therapy has remained controversial, the main reason for this being the development of extrahepatic metastases, which are responsible

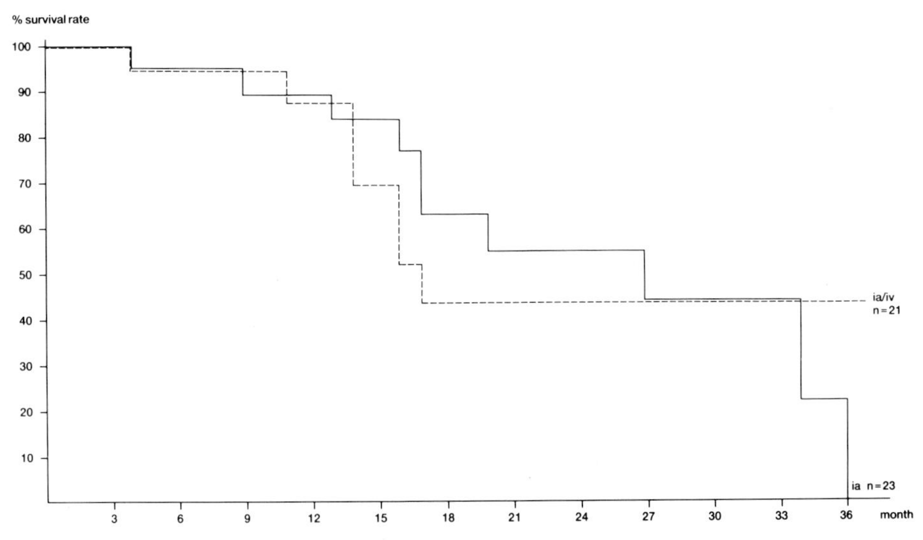

Fig. 2. Regional chemotherapy of liver metastases of colorectal cancer - Survival (randomized i.a. vs radomized i.a./i.v. group)

Table 7a. Regional chemotherapy of liver metastases of colorectal cancer - Survival (responders vs nonresponders)

Primary tumor stage of colorectal cancer	Responders (n=32)	Nonresponders (n=32)
T_{1-3} N_0	17	10
T_{1-3} N_1	10	16
T_{1-3} N_2	5	6
Metastatic spread in the liver		
<50% of liver volume	27	22
>50% of liver volume	5	10

Table 7b. Regional chemotherapy of liver metastases of colorectal cancer - Initial values of liver enzymes and CEA serum level

	Responders		Nonresponders	
	Min.-Max.	Median	Min.-Max.	Median
CEA (ng/ml)	1.9- 208	11.0	6-1600.1	44.0
APH (U/L)	101.0-1512	202.0	104-1990.0	218.0
γGT (U/L)	12.0- 750	46.0	12- 524.0	61.0
LDH (U/L)	74.0- 596	184.0	145- 967.0	280.0
GOT (U/L)	7.0- 59	14.0	4- 76.0	13.0
GPT (U/L)	7.0- 100	19.0	2- 88.0	16.0

APH, alkaline phosphatase; *γ-GT*, γ-glutamyl transpeptidase; *LDH*, lactic dehydrogenase; *GOT*, glutamic oxaloacetic transaminase.

for the patients' deaths [15]. Surgical implantation of the pump and insertion of the catheter do not cause mortality or any major morbidity. The pumps were accepted by the majority of the patients. Skin necrosis in the region of the pump sideports was treated sucessfully in three patients by transposition and subfascial placing of the pump to another abdominal region.

Side effects due to regional chemotherapy did occur during treatment. Gastritis or duodenal ulcers and induced cellular atypias following chemotherapy are probably due to the antimitotic effect of FUDR [16, 17]. The time of occurrence of epigastric pain was, according to our observations, independent of the duration and dosage of FUDR therapy [14]. The incidence of gastritis as quoted in the literature is variable; in our patient population, it was 21%. Balch and Urist found it to be 25% in their patients [6]; Kemeny et al., 15% [18]; and Niederhuber et al., 56% [7]. The reported difference in the incidence depend on whether a gastroscopy was carried out on all patients or whether this was performed only when symptoms appeared. Since these gastroduodenal changes occurred in spite of surgical ligation of the right gastric and duodenal arteries, it can be assumed that regional collateral arteries develop postoperatively from the proper hepatic artery that supply the duodenum or the antrum. The infused FUDR can then pass through these branches into the mucous membrane of the duodenum or antrum, thus affecting the cells of the mucous membrane.

Chemical cholecystitis, whose incidence was 25% [19], can be avoided by routine cholecystectomy during implantation of the pump.

According to the literature, chemical hepatitis occurs in 13%–83% of the patients [6, 19]. In our group of patients, it was 57%. This hepatitis subsides when the FUDR dose is reduced or when the therapy is discontinued.

The difference in the reported frequency stems from the fact that no uniform definition for chemical hepatitis yet exists. We speak of chemical hepatitis when a twofold increase over the normal values in two liver parameters (GOT, GPT, APH, and γGT), is present. Bilirubinemia must be excluded since it is caused only by progression of the intrahepatic metastases, by malignant occlusion of the bile duct, or by sclerosing cholangitis.

As a result of FUDR infusion, segmental stenosis (sclerosing cholangitis) of the intra- and extrahepatic bile ducts developed. This occurred independently of duration and dosage of the FUDR therapy. The incidence rate varies between 17% and 25% [20]. Our incidence was 25%. The pathogenesis of this complication is not yet known. The best marker for early detection of sclerosing cholangitis is a short-term determination of bilirubin in serum, since the other liver parameters were elevated in more than 50% of the patients who did not have any signs of sclerosing cholangitis. Therapy with FUDR must be discontinued even if the increase in bilirubin is minimal. If, after restarting the FUDR therapy, the bilirubin level again increases of if there is morphological evidence of sclerosing cholangitis, the chemotherapeutic agent (FUDR) must definitely be discontinued. Regional treatment can be continued with other cytostatic agents.

The additional intravenous administration of FUDR at a dose of 0.09 mg/kg daily in the i.a./i.v. group did not cause further significant systemic side effects when compared with the i.a. group. The FUDR toxicity, both regional and systemic, was the same in both groups.

Chemical hepatitis as a clinical picture without symptoms could be treated by reducing the FUDR dose. Gastritis or ulcers were revealed by epigastric pain, which subsided after a temporary discontinuation of FUDR therapy and treatment with cemitidine. There was a decrease in obstructive jaundice due to sclerosing cholangitis in seven patients after discontinuation of the FUDR therapy, reducing the incidence of sclerosing cholangitis from 25% to 13%. Three other patients had to undergo drainage (in two patients the jaundice subsided; one patient died of myocarditis). While, suffering from sclerosing cholangitis, five other patients developed extrahepatic tumor progression, which caused their deaths. Only one patient died, 2 years after the onset of therapy, of liver cirrhosis (there had been no evidence of intra- or extrahepatic metastases in any imaging procedure).

Evaluation of response of hepatic metastases to this type of therapy was carried out by examining several parameters. Our experience has shown that the best assessment criteria are the patient's survival time, arterial angio-CT, and follow-up of CEA. In 59% of the patients with prechemotherapeutic pathological CEA concentrations (52% of the overall collective group), a decrease in the CEA serum levels of over 60% took place during treatment. Of the entire collective group, 50% had a proven reduction of metastatic spread, as seen in the CT.

The i.a. and i.a./i.v. groups responded similarly to chemotherapy (52% vs 48% for CT and 60% vs 66% for tumor marker criteria, respectively). This observation is not surprising since, prior to initiation of therapy, the metastatic spread in the two groups has been identical and the FUDR intra-arterial dose amounted to 0.21 mg/kg daily in the i.a.- and the i.a./i.v.-treated patients. The literature documents different response rates: Balch et al. report 80% [6]; Niederhuber et al., 83% [7]; and Cohen et al., 51% [9]. This discrepancy is the result of response criteria that are not yet uniform.

The i.v. therapy prevented the growth of micrometastases that had not been detected at the time of pump implantation, as well as of cancer cells that had passed from the hepatic metastases into the blood stream. Extrahepatic metastases occurred during therapy in 70% of the patients in the pilot study, in 61% in the randomized i.a. group; and in 33% in the randomized i.a./i.v. group. This difference is not statistically significant ($p < 0.1$). The literature shows a discrepancy concerning the frequency of extrahepatic metastases after the onset of regional chemotherapy. Balch et al. report an incidence of 42% [6]; Niederhuber et al., 42% [7]; Rothmund et al., 77% [21]; and Kemeny et al., 56% [22]. Ultimately, the death of most patients, especially the ones who responded to regional chemotherapy, resulted from extrahepatic metastases. Owing to the high incidence of patients with extrahepatic carcinoma spread (42%-77%), both regional and systemic chemotherapy are indicated. The success of this additional therapeutic principle can be expected particularly in patients responding to regional chemotherapy.

Based on our experience with patients who underwent an additional 5 FU and/or mitomycin C therapy (only five patients showed a temporary reduction in their CEA serum levels), we believe that this therapy does not affect survival time in any way. Median survival time without therapy in patients with hepatic metastases that originate from colorectal carcinoma is 6-9 months [23]. Systemic chemotherapy with various antimetabolites such as 5-FU or FUDR, with a response rate of 15-24%, does not offer a therapeutic alternative [2]. In applying the pump catheter system and treatment with FUDR, Balch and Urist [6] achieved a median survival time of 26 months, and Ensminger et al. reported 21 months [24]. The response rate in these studies was above 80%.

In all of our patients ($n=64$), the response rate was 50% and 52% for CT and tumor marker criteria, respectively. Median survival time of these patients was 25 months. We noticed no improvement of survival in the two groups during the 36-month period. Later, however, no patient in the i.a. group survived beyond this period; in the i.a./i.v. group, 43% of the patients survived beyond 36 months (Fig. 2).

A highly significant difference in survival time was found among those patients who responded to regional chemotherapy and those having progressive or stable disease of the hepatic metastases (median survival time: 31 months vs 16 months respectively). This indicates that a clear prolongation of survival time can be expected in the presence a of detectable response by CT or tumor markers. The life expectancy of nonresponders can be compared to that of patients whose liver metastases are not treated (natural course of disease). The prolongation of survival among responders supports the efficacy of regional chemotherapy.

References

1. Kemeny N, Golbey R (1980) A chemotherapeutic approach to colorectal carcinoma. In: Stearns MR Jr (ed) Neoplasms of the colon, rectum and anus. Wiley, New York, pp 155-168
2. Kemeny N (1983) The systemic chemotherapy of hepatic metastases. Sem Oncol 10 (2): 148-158
3. Jaffe B, Donegan W, Watson F, Spratt I (1968) Factors influencing survival in patients with untreated hepatic metastases. Surg Gyn Obstet 127: 1-11
4. Brown CE, Warren S (1938) Visceral metastases from rectal carcinoma. Surg Gyn Obstet 66: 611-621
5. Sigurdson ER, Ridge JA, Kemeny N, Daly J (1987) Tumor and liver drug uptake following hepatic artery and portal vein infusion. J Clin Oncol 5 (11): 1836-1840
6. Balch CM, Urist MM (1984) Intraarterielle Chemotherapie mit einer implantierbaren Infusionspumpe bei Lebermetastasen, colorektaler Tumoren und Hepatomen. Chirurg 55: 485-493
7. Niederhuber JE, Ensminger W, Gyves J, Thrall J, Walker S, Cozzi E (1984) Regional chemotherapy of colorectal cancer metastatic to the liver. Cancer 53: 1336-1343
8. Reed ML, Vaitkevicius VK, Al-Sarraf M, Vaughn CB, Singhakowinta A, Sexon-Porte M, Izbicki R, Baker L, Straatsma GW (1981) The practicality of metastatic hepatic malignancies: Ten-year results of 124 patients in a prospective protocol. Cancer 47: 402-409
9. Cohen AM, Greenfield A, Wood WC, Waltman A, Novelline R, Athanasoulis Ch, Schaeffer NJ (1983) Treatment of hepatic metastases by transaxillary hepatic artery chemotherapy using an implanted drug pump. Cancer 51: 2013-2019
10. Safi F, Roscher R, Stahl S, Schuhmacher K, Pralle U, Bittner R, Beger HG (1987) Erfolgskontrolle der regionalen Chemotherapie der Metastasenleber durch arterielle Angio-Computertomographie. Tumor Diagn Ther 5: 181-186
11. Kaplan E, Meier P (1958) Nonparametric estimation from incomplete observations. J Am Stat Ass 53: 457-481
12. Mantel N (1966) Evaluation of survival data and two new rank order statistics arising in its consideration. Cancer Chemother Rep 50: 163-170
13. Conover WJ (1980) Practical nonparametric statistics, 2nd edn. Wiley, New York, pp 143-212
14. Safi F, Roscher R, Heymer B, Bittner R, Beger HG (1988) Erosive Gastroduodenitis mit schweren Epotheldysplasien als Komplikation der locoregionalen intraarteriellen Chemotherapie bei Lebermetastasen. Aktuel Chir 2 (23): 43-88

15. Ensminger WD, Rosowsky V, Raso DC, Glode M, Come S, Steele G, Frey E (1978) A clinical-pharmacological evaluation of hepatic arterial infusions of 5-fluoro-2-deoxyuridine and 5-fluorouracil. Cancer 38: 3784
16. Chuang VP, Wallace S, Stroehlein J, Xap HG, Patt YZ (1981) Hepatic artery infusion chemotherapy: Gastroduodenal complications. Am J Radiol 137: 347
17. Hall DA, Clouse ME, Gramm HF (1981) Gastroduodenal ulceration after hepatic arterial infusion chemotheraphy. J Radiol 136: 1216
18. Kemeny MM, Goldberg DA, Browning S, Metter GE, Miner PA, Terz JJ (1985) Experience with continuous regional chemotherapy and hepatic resection as treatment of hepatic metastases. Cancer 55: 1265
19. Kemeny N, Daly J, Oderman P, Shiku M, Chun H, Petroni G, Geller N (1984) Hepatic artery pump infusion: Toxicity and results in patients with metastatic colorectal carcinoma. J Clin Oncol 2 (6): 595
20. Kemeny MM, Battifora H, Douglas W, Blayney GC, David AG, Lucille AL, Kim AM, Jose JT (1985) Sclerosing cholangitis after continuous hepatic artery infusion of FUDR. Ann Surg 202: 176
21. Rothmund M, Brückner R, Keller E, Quint B, Knuth A, Schicketanz KH (1986) Regionale Chemotherapie bei Lebermetastasen kolorektaler Karzinome mit implantierbaren Druckpumpen. Dtsch Med Wochenschr 17: 652-658
22. Kemeny N, Daly J, Reichmann B, Geller N, Botet J, Oderman P (1987) Intrahepatic or systemic infusion of fluorodeoxuridine in patients with liver metastases from colorectal carcinoma. Ann Int Med 107: 459-465
23. Pestana C, Reitermeyer RJ, Moertel CG, Judd ES, Dockerty MB (1964) The natural history of carcinoma of the colon and rectum. Am J Surg 108: 826
24. Ensminger W, Niederhuber J, Dakhil S, Thrall J, Wheeler R (1981) Totally implanted drug delivery system for hepatic arterial chemotherapy. Cancer 65: 393

Isolated Regional Hyperthermal Liver Perfusion: Indications, Technique and Results

K. H. MUHRER[1] and H. GRIMM[1]

Introduction

In the treatment of liver metastases, surgical intervention has gained importance in the last few years [8]. Refined resection techniques and the development of various regional therapeutic procedures for nonresectable or disseminated metastases [2, 9] have led to an increase in therapeutic possibilities and defined new indications for surgery.

Regional chemotherapy offers a convincing therapeutic approach. Since liver metastases are supplied arterially, intra-arterial application of cytostatic agents provides the tumor with much higher drug concentrations. Isolated liver perfusion (ILP) [3] increases the advantages of regional chemotherapy by combining high drug concentrations to the tumor with low systemic side effects, thereby improving the therapeutic results.

Angioarchitecture of Liver Tumors as a Basis of Intra-arterial Chemotherapy

The liver is the first organ to filter hematogenous metastases of gastrointestinal carcinomas. Tumor cells are transported into the liver via the portal vein but soon gain access to the intrahepatic arterial system [1,5]. The metastases are then supplied by the hepatic artery making the intra-arterial infusion of cytotoxic drugs effective because it is founded on a pathophysiologic basis. Only the periphery of the metastases is supplied by the portal system, or there exist anastomoses between the arterial and the portal system [14].

Surgical Technique

Preparation of Liver Vessels

We prefer a median epigastric and mesogastric laparotomy. After snaring the hepatoduodenal ligament, the gastroduodenal, common, and proper hepatic arteries are exposed and snared. It is important to be aware of anatomic variations, e.g.,

[1] Department of General and Thoracic Surgery, Justus Liebig University, Gießen, Klinikstraße 29, 6300 Gießen, FRG.

H. G. Beger et al. (Eds.), Cancer Therapy

the right hepatic artery branching off from the superior mesenteric artery. The portal vein is then exposed in the hepatoduodenal ligament over a distance of 2 cm and doubly snared (Fig. 1).

Preparation and Cannulation of the Inferior Vena Cava

After division of the falciform ligament, the liver is displaced caudally, its anterior portion is detached from the diaphragm, and the point of passage through the diaphragm of the inferior vena cava is identified. At a distance of 2 cm from the inferior vena cava, the diaphragm and the pericardium are incised transversely. Inside the pericardial cavity, the inferior vena cava is snared (Fig. 2).

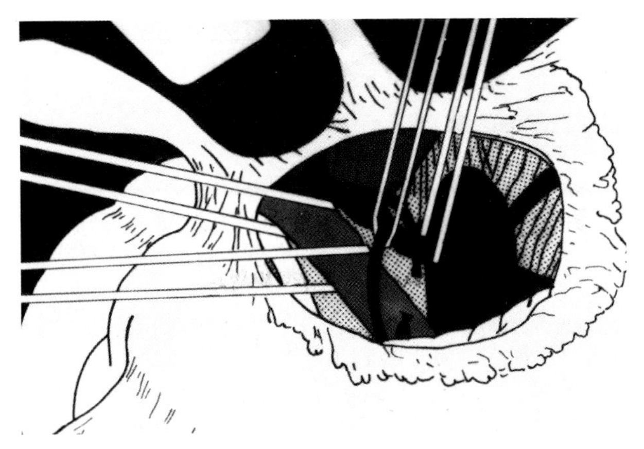

Fig. 1. Snared vessels in the hepatoduodenal ligament: *(from left to right)* portal vein, hepatic artery, gastroduodenal artery

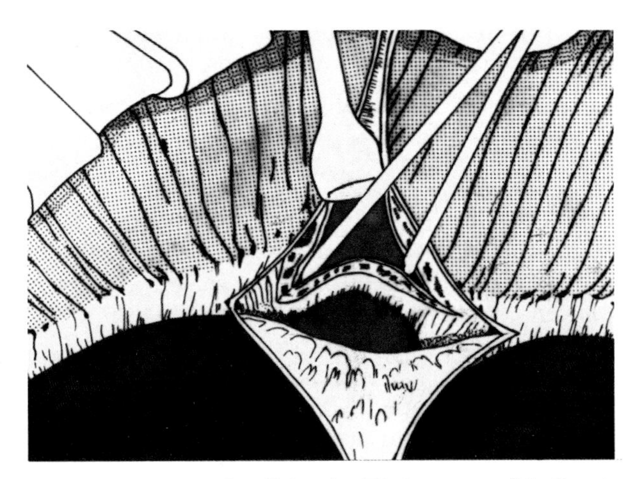

Fig. 2. Snaring of the inferior vena cava inside the pericardial cavity. The bare part of the liver is mobilized, and the diaphragm and the pericardium are incised transversely

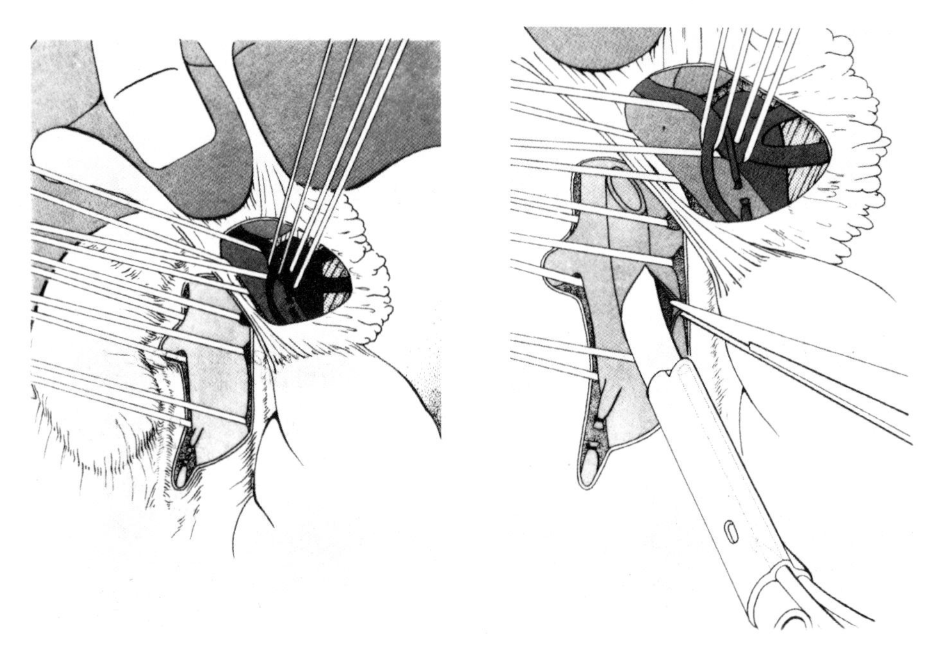

Fig. 3 *(left)*. Exposed and snared inferior vena cava. Spermatic/ovaric vein is ligated and divided

Fig. 4 *(right)*. Insertion of the liver perfusion catheter into the inferior vena cava via a longitudinal incision over 3 cm

To expose the infrahepatic part of the inferior vena cava, the duodenum is mobilized according to Kocher's maneuver. The inferior vena cava is then exposed over a distance of 8–10 cm, including the junction of the renal veins. Some lumbar veins and the right spermatic or ovaric vein are ligated and divided. Three tourniquets are put around the mobilized vein, one cranial and two caudal to the renal vein junction (Fig. 3). After heparinization, the inferior vena cava is incised longitudinally over a distance of 3 cm, the perfusion catheter is inserted, and the tourniquets are fixed (Fig. 4).

Arterial Cannulation

Following transverse incision of the portal vein, one catheter is inserted in the direction of the liver and the other, in the opposite direction. Both are fixed with rubber strings. The portocaval shunt is established by connecting the peripheral portal catheter to the corresponding nozzle of the perfusion catheter (Fig. 5). Next, the central portal catheter and the venous backflow tube from the perfusion catheter are connected to the heart-lung machine. After closure of the intrapericardial torniquet, the venous backflow from the liver is interrupted. The liver is then perfused only via the portal vein in a "partial bypass".

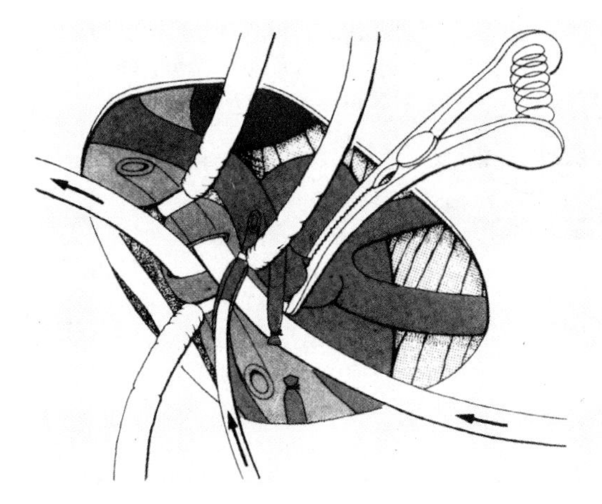

Fig. 5. Cannulated vessels of the hepatoduodenal ligament. The transversely incised portal vein is cannulated centrally and peripherally; the tubes are fixed with tourniquets. The hepatic artery is cannulated via the gastroduodenal artery

Principle and Aims of Isolated Regional Liver Perfusion

The principle of ILP is to disconnect the liver "in situ" from the systemic circulation by catheterizing the liver's efferent and afferent blood vessels and connecting them to an extracorporeal circulation. During ILP, high doses of cytostatic drugs may be injected in this extracorporeal circuit without provoking systemic side effects. High local drug concentrations and additional hyperthermia make a tumor toxic effect probable [3, 12, 13].

Quantitative extracorporeal drainage of hepatic venous blood is more difficult than limb perfusion anatomical reasons. The decisive step was brought about by the introduction of a special, double-luminal catheter, which is inserted into the inferior vena cava. This catheter separates the venous blood of the liver from the venous blood flowing from the kidneys and the lower half of the body [3]. The arterial supply of the liver is established by cannulation of both the hepatic artery and the portal vein. Thus, two separate circulations are provided to maintain physiologic flow rates. The perfusion of the intrahepatic portal system is the therapeutic attempt to reach micrometastases and the tumor periphery which is supplied by blood from the portal vein.

The gastroduodenal artery is ligated peripherally and incised transversely about 1 cm from its origin. Through this arteriotomy, a special catheter is inserted into the proper hepatic artery. The central part of the hepatic artery is blocked by a bulldog clamp (Fig. 5). This arterial catheter is also connected to the extracorporeal circulation. Thus, a total bypass - isolated liver perfusion - is started. After 10 min, a temperature of 39° -39.5 °C is established. The cytostatics are injected into the arterial inflow of the perfusion circuit. After a 60-min perfusion, the liver is flushed with 1 l of Ringer's solution, and the liver circulation is filled with erythrocyte concentrates and plasma. After the removal of the tubes, the incisions in the vessels are sutured. Finally, a catheter is implanted in the gastroduodenal artery for additional therapy cycles. On principle, we remove the gallbladder in order to prevent wall necrosis due to therapy.

Cytostatic Drugs and Pharmacokinetics

In nearly all perfusions, 5-fluorouracil (5-FU) was applied as a cytostatic agent. We increased the initial dose of 300 mg to a maximum of 1250 mg 5-FU. The drug concentration in the perfusion circuit peaked to 500 µg/ml after an injection of 1000 mg 5-FU, dropping slowly to 300 µg/ml. Even the minimum concentration was distinctly above the level that can be achieved by an intravenous bolus injection (Fig. 6).
Later, we additionally administered mitomycin C, starting with a dose of 5 mg, which we increased to up to 50 mg. After administrating 20 mg mitomycin C, a concentration peak of 100 µg/ml was obtained, which decreased to 0.2 µg/ml after perfusion. Table 1 shows a list of the cytostatic drugs administered in a total of 49 liver perfusions.

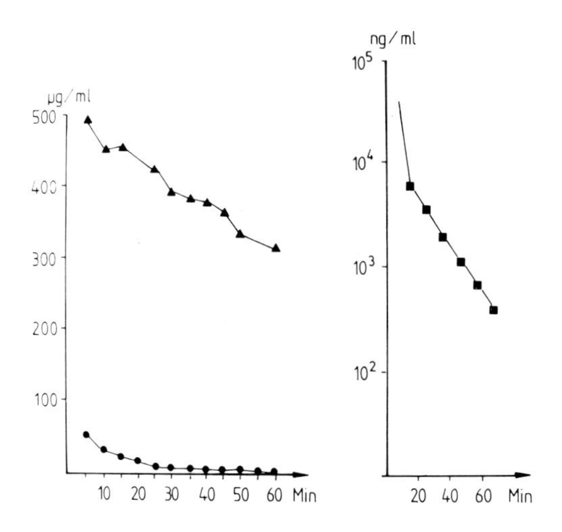

Fig. 6. Drug concentrations in the isolated liver circuit after injection of 1000 mg 5-FU (▲–▲–▲) or 20 mg MMC (■–■–■). At the end of the 60-min perfusion, 5-FU levels are higher than after intravenous bolus administration (●–●–●)

Table 1. Cytostatic drugs-used in isolated liver perfusion

Drug	Patients (*n*)
5-FU	31
5-FU + Mitomycin C	13
Mitomycin C	1
DDP	1
DDP + Mitomycin C	1
DDP + Mitomycin C + 5-FU	2

5-FU, 5-fluorouracil; *DDP*, cisplatinum.

Indications

We considered ILP to be indicated for liver tumors that could not be resected surgically or in disseminated metastases. Inoperability of the primary tumor, local tumor recurrence, and extrahepatic metastases were rated as contraindications for isolated liver perfusion. Main indications were liver metastases of colorectal carcinomas or carcinoids.

Patients

ILP was applied to a total of 49 patients - 28 men and 21 women. The youngest patient was 28 and the eldest, 65 years of age. Most of these patients suffered from nonresectable liver metastases of colorectal carcinomas (Table 2). Almost two-thirds of the patients were evaluated as stage II of the Lausanne Classification (hepatomegally or increased alkaline phosphatase), one-third as stage III (hepatomegally and increased alkaline phosphatase), and only a few patients as stage I (normal liver size and alkaline phosphatase levels) [13].
Of the 49 patients, 15 were treated with isolated liver perfusion applying 5-FU only. Another 34 patients received additional cycles of regional chemotherapy as maintenance therapy. Of these 34 patients, 19 were treated with 5-FU perfusions only, while the remaining 15 received combinations of cytostatic drugs (Fig. 7) [4].

Results

In August 1987, we updated the evaluation of our results. Of the 49 patients, 4 (8%) died after ILP. One of them died of uncontrollable hemorrhage due to simultaneous right hemihepatectomy and the other, of diffuse hemorrhage due to disseminated intravascular coagulation. Another died of generalized sepsis after simultaneous colonic resection and the fourth, of heart and kidney failure. No other life-threatening complications occurred (Table 3).

Table 2. Type of liver tumors treated by isolated liver perfusion

	Patients (*n*)
Liver metastases	
- Colorectal cancer	45
- Carcinoid tumors	2
Primary liver-cell Carcinoma	2
	49

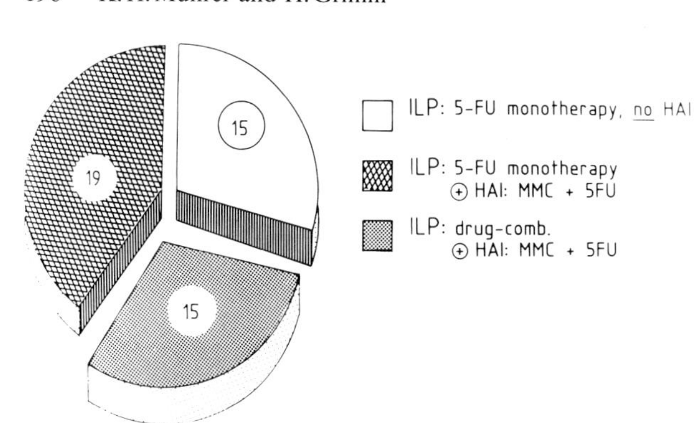

Fig. 7. Therapy schemes in 49 patients treated with ILP. *5-FU*, 5-fluorouracil; *HAI*, hepatic artery infusion; *MMC*, mitomycin C

Table 3. Postoperative complications after isolated liver perfusion

	Patients (*n*)	Deaths (*n*)
Pleural effusion	9	0
Hemorrhage	3	2
Sepsis	2	1
Cardiac disturbances	3	1
Subphrenic abscess	1	0

Table 4. Response rates after isolated liver perfusion

Complete remission	22%
Partial remission	68%
Nonresponder	10%

Remission Rates

An important criterionto judge the therapeutic effect is the definition of remission rates by means of diagnostic imaging procedures and laboratory findings. The disappearance of all evidence of tumor in computerized tomography or evident calcification of tumor areas, normalization of increased carcinoembryonic antigen (CEA) levels, and clinical well-being were defined as "complete remission." A "partial remission" was thought to be present if the tumor marker dropped to 50% of previously elevated levels and if the metastases decreased to 50% of their previous sizes in computerized tomography [13]. On the basis of these criteria, the initial remission rate of liver tumors after ILP was relatively high: 9 out of 41 patients had a complete remission (22%), and 28 had a partial remission (68%) (Table 4).

Survival Times

Of the 49 patients treated with liver perfusion, 4 died during the postoperative period (8% mortality). The median survival time of all 45 surviving patients was 15.5 months. As for survival times, decisive differences are revealed if both therapy groups are compared: the median survival time was 7 months in patients per-

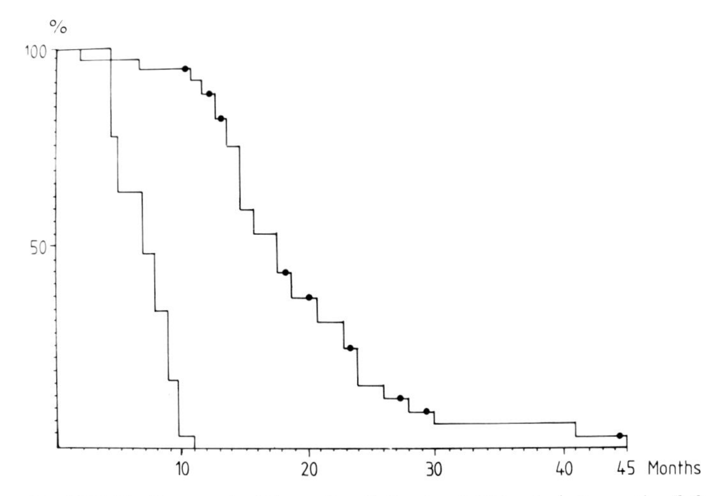

Fig. 8. Survival curves after ILP. Median survival time after ILP using 5-FU only is 7 months *(left curve)*. Using a combination of 5-FU and MMC and additional regional chemotherapy, median survival time is 18 months *(right curve)*

Table 5. Occurrence of extrahepatic metastases

	Median times of occurrence (months)
After isolated liver perfusion (5-FU)	4
After isolated liver perfusion (5-FU + MMC) *and* hepatic artery infusion (MMC + 5-FU)	11.6

5-FU, 5-fluorouracil; *MMC*, mitomycin C.

fused with 5-FU only, but 18 months in patients who were perfused with a combination of 5-FU and mitomycin and who additionally received maintenance therapy after operation (Fig. 8) [4].

All the 36 patients who passed away had extrahepatic metastases at the time of death. Extrahepatic metastases are also present in four out of nine patients still alive. That means that a total of 40 patients (88%) developed extrahepatic metastases after ILP [4]. After an average of 4 months, extrahepatic tumor progression was seen if only 5-FU was applied in liver perfusion. In combination with mitomycin C and additional regional chemotherapy, extrahepatic tumor progression appeared after an average of 11.6 months (Table 5).

A summary of the therapeutic procedures implemented to stop extrahepatic tumor progression is provided in Table 6. Chemoembolization served as a final therapeutic attempt if liver metastases showed progression in spite of ILP and regional chemotherapy [11]. After isolated liver perfusion, three of the five patients still

Table 6. Procedures used in conjunction with isolated liver perfusion

	Case (*n*)
Liver resection (segments)	6
Hemihepatectomy	4
Chemoembolization	5
Intra-arterial infusion of lung metastases	2
Resection of lung metastases	2
Whole-body hyperthermia	1

alive and free of metastases have lived without tumor recurrence for 45, 30, and 28 months, respectively, and two of them have survived for 14 and 7 months respectively.

Discussion

The aim of ILP is to increase toxicity to the tumor by means of high-dose therapy and to minimize side effects. This aim is realized by sophisticated surgical techniques and technical equipment. Through ILP, the tumor can be confronted with cytostatic concentrations that other regional methods cannot achieve. Hyperthermia employed in ILP provides the liver parenchyma with a temperature of 39°-39.5 °C. Although this temperature does not have a toxic effect on the tumor cells, it increases the blood flow through the tumor by dilating its blood vessels [15]. However, higher temperatures would reduce tumor perfusion and damage liver cells.

Systemic side effects are brought to a minimum by separating the liver from the systemic circulation. The previously described surgical technique reduces the leakage rate to less than 6% [13]. Arterialization of the portal vein guarantees the perfusion of the tumor periphery supplied by the portal system. During the 1-h perfusion, we diverted the portal blood flow from the gastrointestinal tract into the inferior vena cava, interposing a hemofilter to eliminate toxic substances (especially ammonia). By gradually reducing the filtration rates, we found that the ammonia concentrations registered during the anhepatic phase were well tolerated [4]. Thus, we were able to simplify the perfusion system and the technical devices establishing a simple portacaval shunt.

ILP has only a short-term, slightly toxic effect on liver parenchyma. The serum concentrations of serum glutamic oxaloacetic transaminase (SGOT) and serum glutamic pyruvic transaminase (SGPT) increased to an average of 80-100 U/l but dropped back to normal within 2 weeks. Cholinesterase concentrations fell to 600-1200 U/l, rising to normal values within 3-4 weeks [3, 4, 13]. After the deaths of two patients, we avoided combining major surgical procedures, especially large-bowel resections, with ILP.

The indication for ILP is mainly limited to nonresectable metastases disseminated in both liver lobes evaluated as stages II or III of the Lausanne Classification [10]. In stage III, however, we have become extremely restrictive because of the poor results and technical problems imposed by hepatomegaly [13].

Some patients were reoperated about 4 weeks after ILP for other indications, providing the chance to take biopsies from the metastases. Up to 90% of the tumor masses were found to be necrotic - with vital tumor formations still present [6, 7]. Tumor necroses are difficult to evaluate. Spontaneous tumor necroses are known to result from an impaired ratio of tumor growth to nutritive blood supply without being differentiable from therapy-induced necroses. The demonstration of vital tumor formations gives evidence that perfusion alone - even if carried out with very high cytostatic drug concentrations - is not sufficient to damage the tumor decisively. Since ILP cannot be repeated, the oncologic principle of repeated therapy had to be realized by combining ILP with additional cycles of intra-arterial chemotherapy. An increase of cytostatic doses in the perfusion circuit and especially the administration of mitomycin C seemed to increase the remission rates.

As far as the interpretation of CEA levels is concerned, one has to be aware that immediately after perfusion a considerable increase in CEA may be observed. In responders, these peaks dropped below the pretherapeutic levels within a few days.

Post-therapeutic results of computerized tomography have to be interpreted with caution. Slight differences in size and density should not be interpreted as tumor response. Only disappearance or evident elimination of metastases, an unmistakable decrease in density, or a manifest calcification should be regarded as tumor response.

Remission rates effected by ILP are much superior to those of systemic chemotherapy and other regional procedures, but ILP requires a relatively high standard of surgical technique. Finally, ILP has yet to stand its hardest test - the increase in survival time. ILP is difficult to evaluate from this point of view: patients treated with ILP only had an obviously shorter survival time (median, 7 months) than patients treated with additional intra-arterial chemotherapy (median, 18 months). We have to admit that our previous expectation of stopping tumor growth for a long-term period by a single, high-dose therapy has not been realized. A prolongation of survival times was effected only if various therapeutic means were implemented, starting with ILP. However, a comparison of both therapy groups (ILP vs. multimodal therapy) is problematic, since both groups differed in tumor stages, cytostatic agents, and drug doses.

Extrahepatic metastases represent the main problem confronting regional chemotherapy. Lung metastases and local tumor recurrence seem to appear more often than after systemic chemotherapy [9]. The incidence of extrahepatic metastases and/or local tumor recurrence after ILP is extremely high, averaging 88%. How are these findings to be interpreted? Committed supporters of regional chemotherapy claim that patients live through this stage of generalized metastases only because tumor growth in the liver is brought "under control" by regional chemotherapy. Liver metastases, they argue, are "surpassed" by other tumor manifestations [4].

One has to assume that, at the time of perfusion, the disease was much more extensive than was detectable by clinical and diagnostic methods [15]. This makes the indication for isolated liver therapy questionable. As long as these conflicting results cannot be resolved, we must maintain a skeptical attitude towards isolated regional liver perfusion.

References

1. Ackerman NB (1972) Experimental studies on the circulatory dynamics of intrahepatic tumor blood supply. Cancer 29: 435
2. Aigner KR, Link KH, Helling HJ, Stemmler S (1985) Intraarterielle Infusion, experimentelle und pharmakokinetische Grundlagen – Klinik In: Aigner KR (ed) Regionale Chemotherapie der Leber. Isolierte Perfusion, intraarterielle Infusion und Resektion. Karger, Basel (Beiträge zur Onkologie, vol 21)
3. Aigner KR, Walther H, Helling HJ, Link KH (1985) Die isolierte Leberperfusion. In: Aigner KR (ed) Regionale Chemotherapie der Leber. Isolierte Perfusion, intraarterielle Infusion und Resektion. Karger, Basel (Beiträge zur Onkologie, vol 21)
4. Aigner KR (1987) Regionale Leberperfusion. In: Schumpelick V, Pichlmayr R (eds) Springer-Verlag Berlin Heidelberg New York Tokyo
5. Breedis C, Young G (1954) Blood supply of neoplasmas in the liver. Am I Pathol 30: 969
6. Fischer HP (1985) Histomorphometry of spherical tumors using holoptical cross-sections. Virchows Arch [A] 405: 277
7. Fischer HP, Schulz A, Kracht J, Aigner K (1984) Perfusionstherapie von Lebermetastasen – Morphometrische Auswertung der spontanen und therapiebedingten Tumorregression. Verh Dtsch Ges Pathol 68: 230
8. Häring R, Bauknecht KJ, Boese-Landgraf J (1987) Chirurgie der Lebermetastasen. In: Schumpelick V, Pichlmayr R (eds) Chirurgie der Leber. Springer-Verlag, Berlin Heidelberg New York Tokyo
9. Hottenrott C, Lorenz M (1987) Stellenwert der regionalen Chemotherapie der Leber. Z Gastroenterol 25: 364
10. Pettavel J, Morgenthaler F (1976) Dix ans d'expérience de chimiothérapie artérielle des tumeurs primaires et secondaires du foie. Ann Gastroenterol Hepatol 12: 349
11. Schultheis KH (1985) Embolisation – Chemoembolisation. Zur Behandlung maligner primärer und sekundärer Lebertumoren. In: Aigner KR (ed) Regionale Chemotherapie der Leber. Isolierte Perfusion, intraarterielle Infusion und Resektion. Karger, Basel (Beiträge zur Onkologie, vol 21)
12. Schwemmle K, Aigner KR (1987) Regionale Chemotherapie. In: Heberer G, van Dongen RJAM (eds) Kirschnersche allgemeine und spezielle Operationslehre: Gefäßchirurgie, vol XI. Spinger-Verlag, Berlin Heidelberg New York
13. Schwemmle K, Link KH, Rieck B (1987) Rationale and Indications for Perfusion in Liver Tumors: Current Data World J Surg 11: 534
14. Strohmeyer T, Hangeberg G, Lierse W, Farthmann EM (1986) Die Blutversorgung und Angioarchitektur von Lebermetastasen. Z Gastroenterol 24: 47
15. Vaupel P, Thwes R, Wendling P (1976) Kritische Sauerstoff- und Glukoseversorgung maligner Tumoren. Dt med Wochenschr 101: 1810

Chemoembolization of Liver Tumors

K.-H. SCHULTHEIS,[1] M. PLIESS,[1] H.-H. GENTSCH,[1] H. BÖDEKER,[1]
C. GEBHARDT,[1] and K. SCHWEMMLE[2]

Introduction

In malignant primary and secondary liver tumors, surgical therapy should be considered first because of superior long-term results if a curative resection can be performed. For inoperable tumors, the choice of therapy is not clear, and a variety of palliative forms of treatment are available.

One of these is chemotherapy with various cytostatics, which can be administered systematically or locoregionally. The advantage of regional over systemic therapy is that higher local concentrations of cytostatics can be achieved with less severe systemic effects. In general, higher remission rates are observed with regional application. However, it has not been possible to achieve a significant improvement in survival times so far [32]. Obviously, there is an urgent need for new therapeutic concepts with higher efficiency.

Another form of palliative treatment is dearterialization of the liver. Ligation of the hepatic artery is only rarely performed today; instead, occlusion of the arterial system is effected by some form of embolization [11, 16, 45].

Physiologic Considerations

The normal liver is supplied by a dual vascular system in which 70% of the blood supply is provided by the portal vein and 30% by the hepatic artery. Oxygenation of hepatocytes is derived in equal parts from the artery and the portal vein. The ability to achieve high extraction rates of oxygen allows the hepatocytes to adapt to a reduced oxygen supply. Hepatotrophic factors reach the liver cell by way of the portal vein [4, 19, 43]. Therefore, the portal vein has special significance in the supply of the normal liver [43]. Primary and secondary liver tumors are much more dependent on oxygen supply from the hepatic artery [1, 2, 5, 19, 41]. These physiologic facts are the basis for regional therapy and explain why the arterial blood supply can be interrupted without ill effects if there is normal supply by the portal vein.

[1] Department of General and Thoracic Surgery, Clinic of Nuremberg, Flurstraße 17, 8500 Nuremberg, FRG.
[2] Department of General and Thoracic Surgery, Justus Liebig University Gießen, Klinikstraße 29, 6300 Gießen, FRG.

H. G. Beger et al. (Eds.), Cancer Therapy

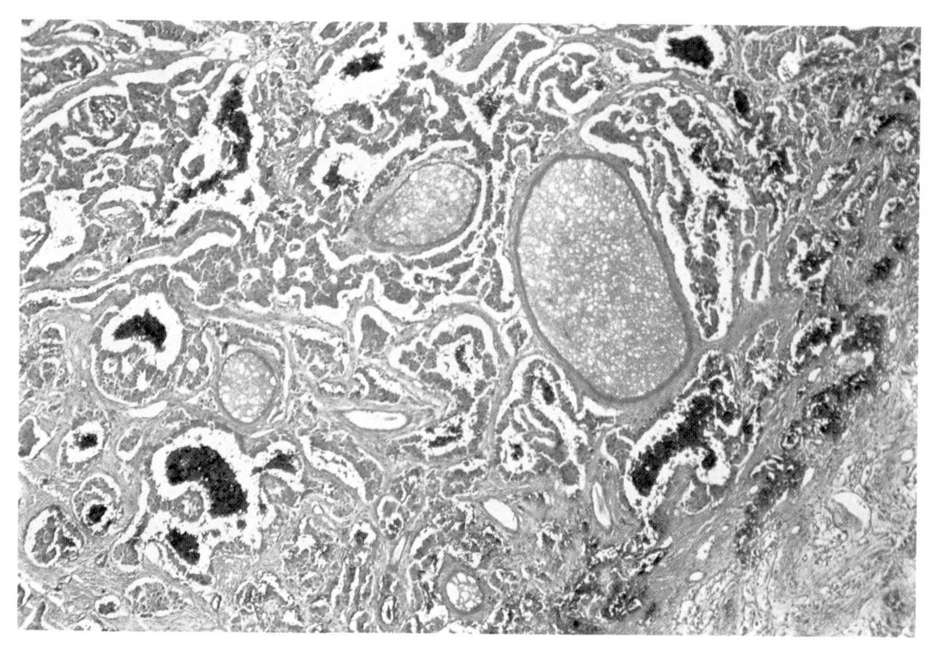

Fig. 1. Histologic picture of a metastasis after chemoembolization (Ethibloc can be seen in tumor vessels)

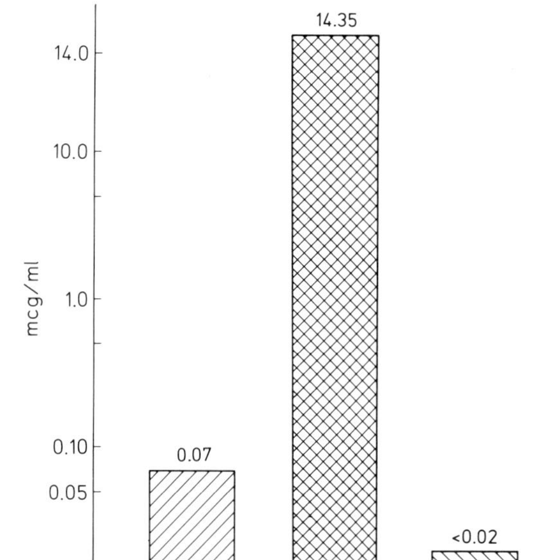

Fig. 2. Tissue and serum concentrations after chemoembolization (patient P. M.)

Substances Used in Embolization

In performing tumor embolization, one has to differentiate between materials achieving central or peripheral occlusion, as well as between those having a short-term or a long-term effect [21]. Embolization effecting the very peripheral branches of the artery is the only alternative to vascular ligation and has the advantage of preventing the early formation of collateral vessels [11, 12]. This formation of an effective collateral circulation is one of the main reasons for the limited therapeutic effect of a central embolization, in addition to a possible revascularization of the artery. For these reasons, when embolization is indicated, we use a solution of prolamine in alcohol (Ethibloc, Ethicon, Hamburg-Norderstedt), which, after the preliminary injection of 40% glucose solution, effects a long-term occlusion of the very peripheral (50 µm) arterial branches. Under favorable conditions occlusion of the vascular system of the tumor itself occurs (Fig. 1) [30].

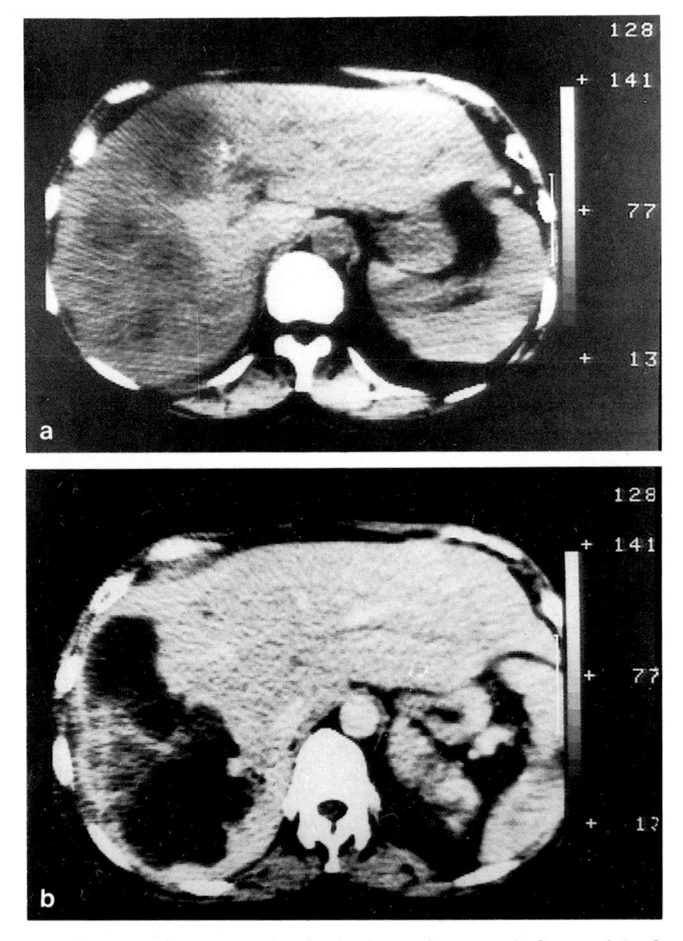

Fig. 3a, b. Computed tomographic scan of a metastasis of colonic carcinoma **a** before and **b** after chemoembolization

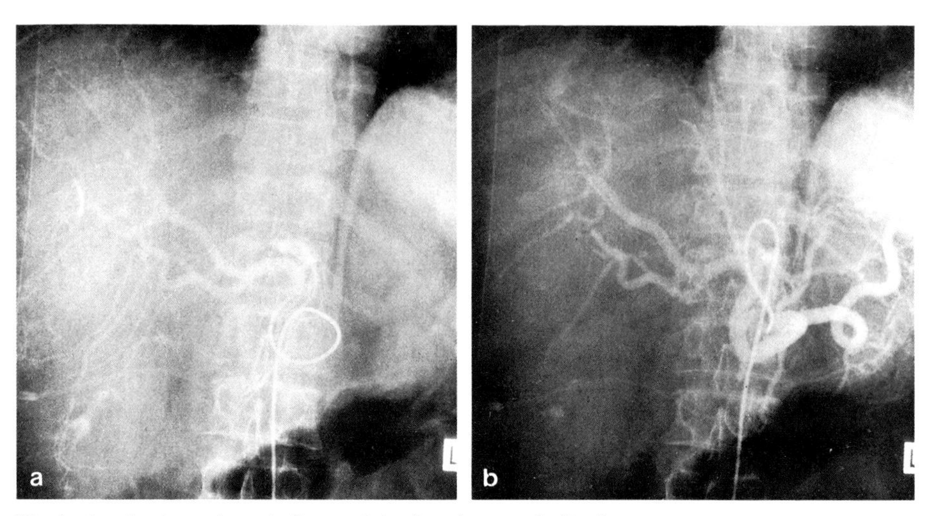

Fig. 4 a, b. Angiography **a** before and **b** after chemoembolization

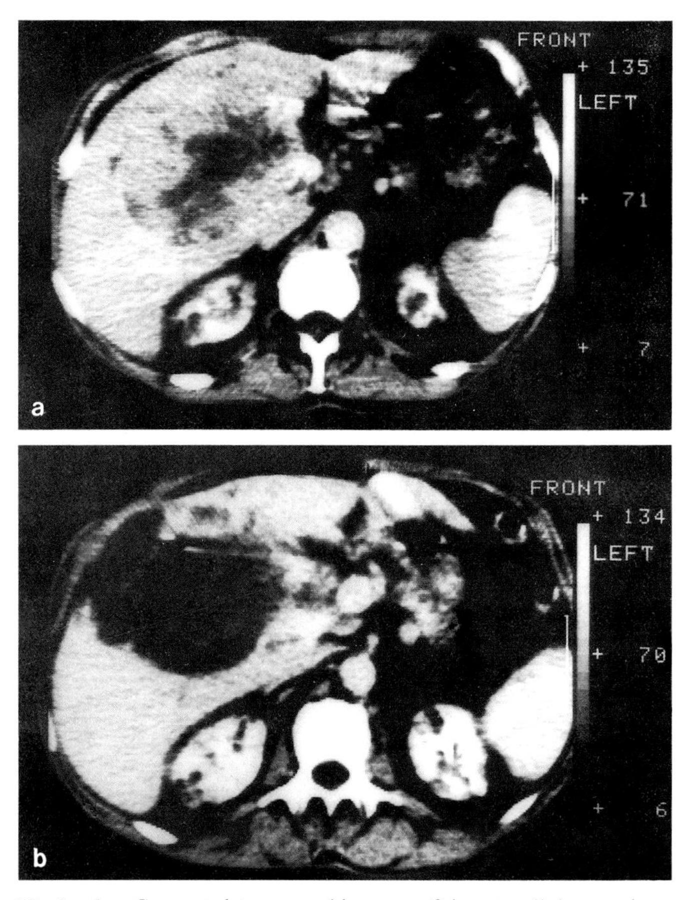

Fig. 5 a, b. Computed tomographic scan of hepatocellular carcinoma **a** before and **b** after chemoembolization

One of the advantages of this substance is that various pulverized of lyophilized cytostatics can easily be admixed and there is a gradual release of these substances [33-35]. This leads to high concentrations of cytostatics in the tumor with minimal systemic effects (Fig. 2). This form of embolization is called chemoembolization. The combination of hypoxia, cutting off of energy supplies, and concomitant liberation of high doses of cytostatics leads to an increased effectiveness and results in a rather quick destruction of tumor mass (Figs. 3, 5-7, 9, and 10).

The concentration of cytostatic drugs within the tumor can also be increased by a short-term interruption of blood supply (15-20 min) by using microspheres [40] or intermittent occlusion of the hepatic artery with the aid of balloon catheters or external occlusion [3, 46]. In our opinion, because of the very short duration of the occlusion, the additional therapeutic advantage of this method over simple intra-arterial infusion of cytostatics comes about solely through the increase in the regional concentration of cytostatics.

The application of this method seems to be indicated in adjuvant chemotherapy, since micrometastases of the liver are mainly supplied by diffusion [1, 2]. A mix-

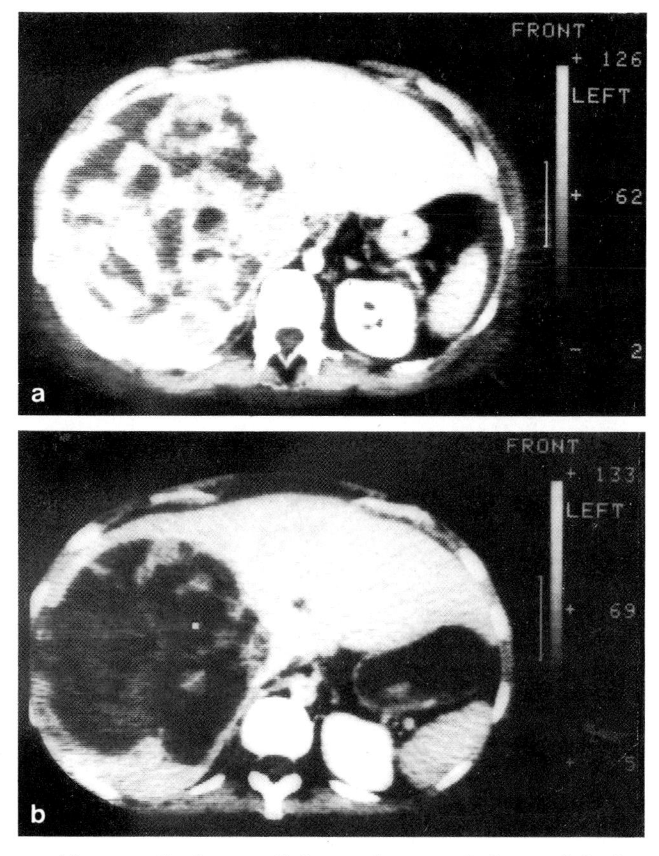

Fig. 6 a, b. Computed tomographic scan of a hepatocellular carcinoma **a** before and **b** after chemoembolization

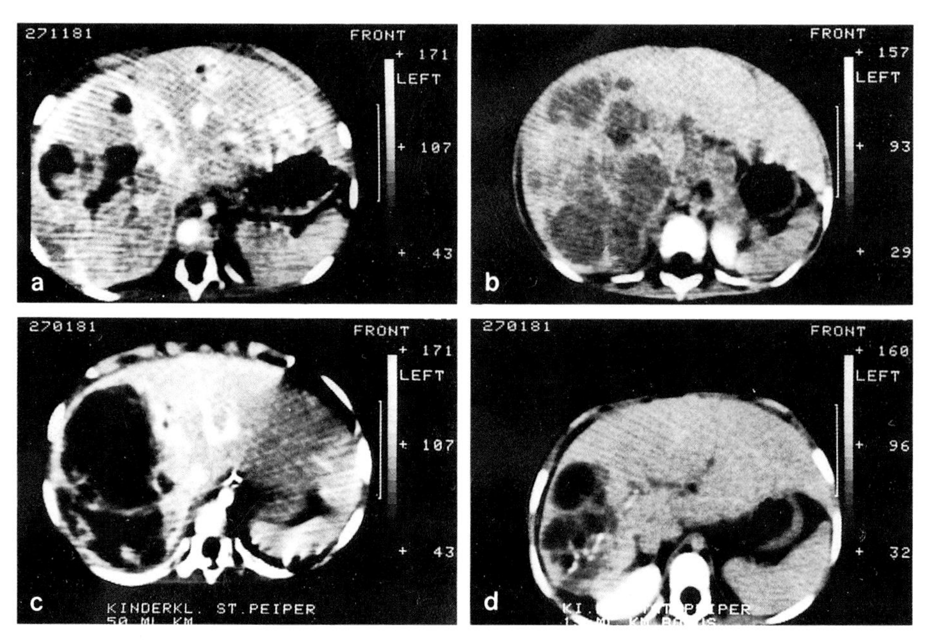

Fig. 7a–d. Computed tomographic scan of hepatoblastoma. **a** Before treatment; **b** after systemic chemotherapy; **c** after chemoembolization; **d** before resection

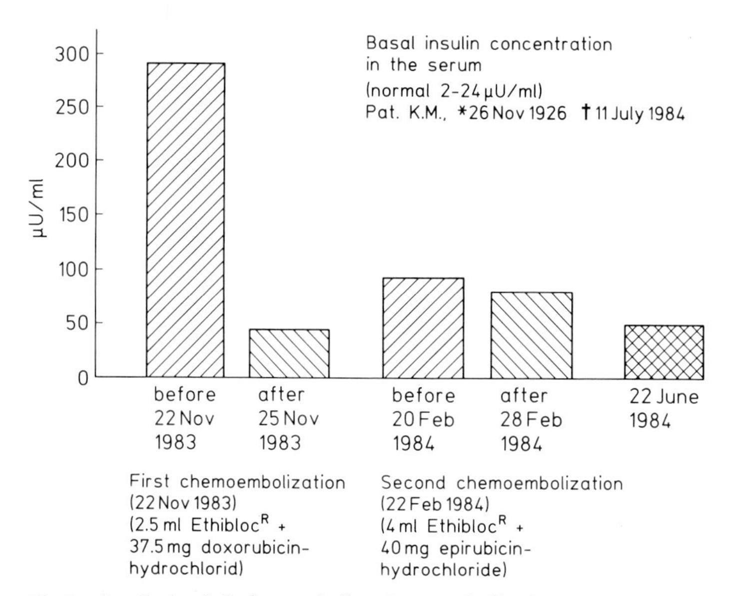

Fig. 8. Insulin levels before and after chemoembolization

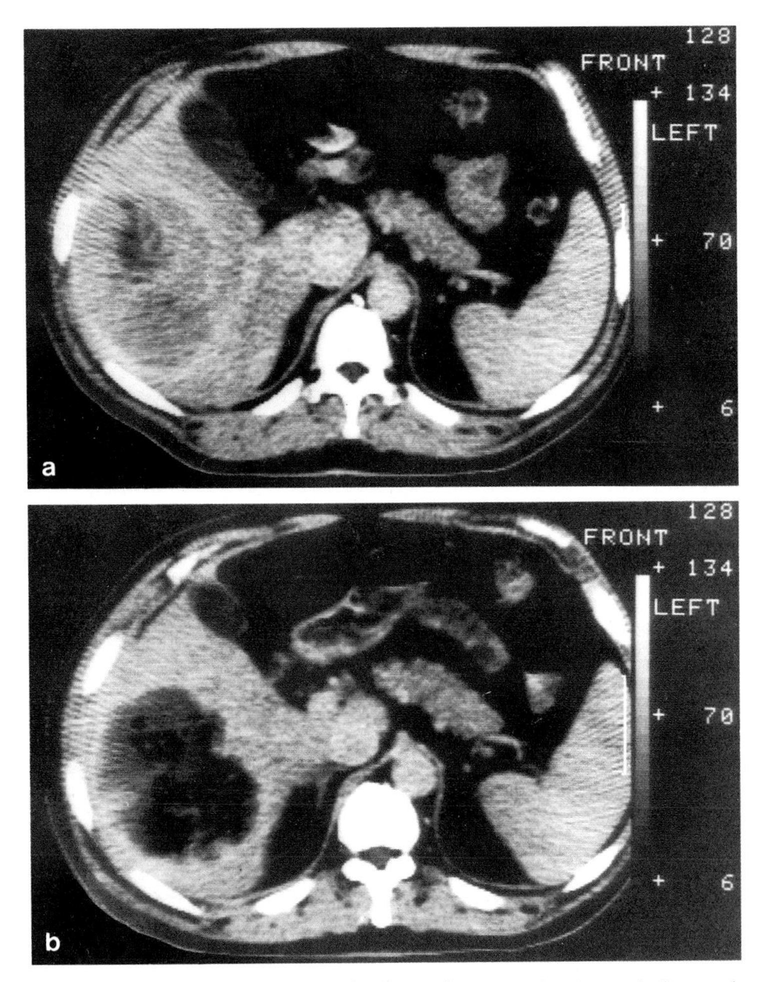

Fig. 9 a, b. Computed tomographic scan of a metastasis of a malignant melanoma **a** before and **b** after chemoembolization

ture of microspheres and cytostatic agents would lead to prolongation of contact time and thereby of diffusion time of the cytostatic agent with the micrometastasis. Confirmation of this hypothesis by experimental results is still pending.

Mode of Application

Chemoembolization of the hepatic artery is usually performed angiographically after selective visualization of the common hepatic artery. A preliminary evaluation has to be made of the type of vascular supply of the liver. In about 40% of the cases, variations in the anatomy of the arterial vascular supply of the liver are present [9, 25]. In rare cases, a selective visualization of the hepatic artery distal to the

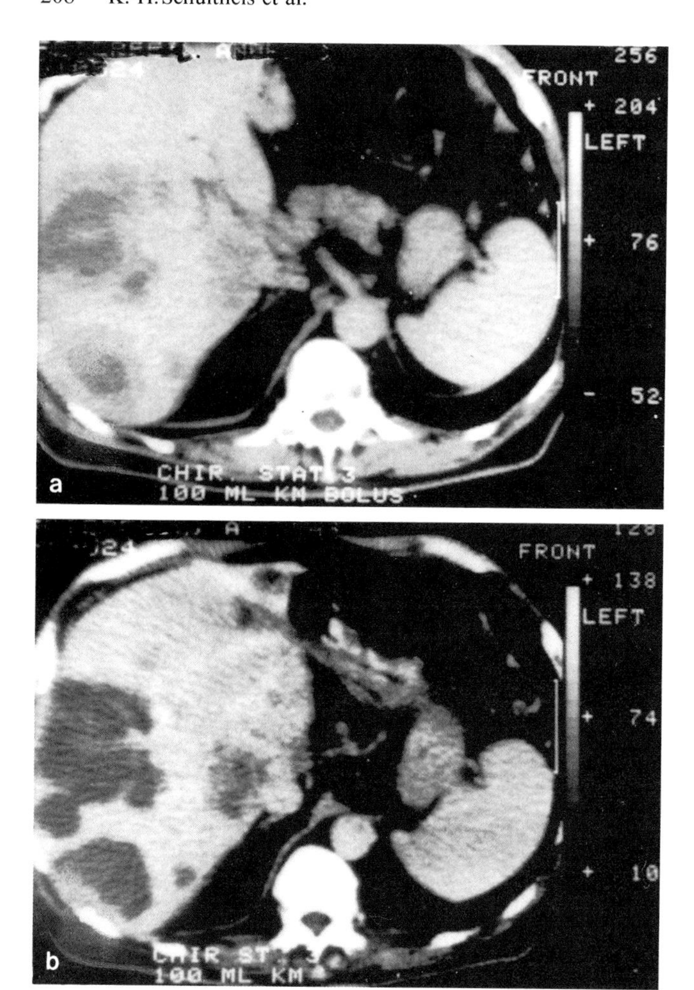

Fig. 10 a, b. Computed tomographic scan of a metastasis of a colorectal carcinoma **a** before and **b** after chemoembolization

origin of the gastroduodenal artery is not possible, and, in these cases, laparotomy and operative exposure of the artery are necessary.

Although we have initially performed chemoembolization of both branches of the hepatic artery simultaneously, at the present time we prefer a sequential procedure, whereby selective chemoembolization of the right or left hepatic artery is performed initially. One month later, the other side is chemoembolized, aiming at a total occlusion of the hepatic arterial supply. One has to make sure that only the peripheral branches of the artery are occluded in order to be able to repeat the procedure of chemoembolization if necessary (Fig. 4).

As mentioned above, our preferred agent for chemoembolization at the present time is a solution of prolamine with an admixture of cytostatics. Our choice of a combination of 10 mg mitomycin C, 25 mg adriamycin, and 25 mg cisplatin is

based on the results of studies in cell cultures performed by K.-H. Link [22]. Systemic levels of cytostatics that can be expected by the application of this method are minimal compared with those concentrations achieved in the tumor and can be neglected. In the 91 chemoembolizations performed so far, there was not a single incidence of systemic side effects due to the cytostatics.
A concomitant regional or systemic chemotherapy with the aim of destroying the tumor margins with mainly portal-venous supply is possible and seems to be a logical choice of therapy after chemoembolization. So far, this has not been performed on our patients. However, we have startet a prospective, randomized study comparing chemoembolization and intraportal infusion of cytostatics with intra-arterial infusion plus intraportal infusion and no therapy.
The mixture of prolamine and cytostatics is injected via a catheter into the hepatic artery after a preliminary injection of 40% glucose solution. The injection of this highly concentrated glucose solution is necessary to postpone precipitation of the embolisate within the blood, ideally leading to a capillary chemoembolization [21].

Complications

After chemoembolization, a so-called postembolization syndrome can be expected [13, 45]. Temporary nausea, fever, subileus, or intestinal paralysis und upper abdominal pain may occur and should be treated symptomatically. High peridural anesthesia seems to be most effective for pain relief. In addition, we carry out prophylactic antibiotic therapy to prevent infection of the necroses that result from the embolization. An incipient hepatorenal syndrome can be recognized early by close check-ups of the urine output. This complication can usually be prevented by increasing diuresis and administering cortisone (1 g) at the time of chemoembolization.
Laboratory parameters can be expected to show a temporary increase of transaminases and leukocytes and a reduction of cholinesterase [35]. These parameters return to normal quickly if the course is uncomplicated.

Indications

The experience of other authors cited in the literature and our own results suggest the following indications for chemoembolization at the present time:

Emergency Indications

Bleeding in ruptured tumors and complications in paraneoplastic syndromes constitute emergency indications for chemoembolization [27].

Clear Indications

Chemoembolization is definitely indicated in the case of primary liver-cell tumors of the nodular type (Figs. 5–7) [38], metastases of hormonally active tumors if other forms of treatment are ineffective (Fig. 8), and painful hepatomegaly caused by tumor bulk (Figs. 6, 7) [7, 16, 36].
After chemoembolization, there is a rapid decrease in tumor bulk, which can be demonstrated by computed tomography. Under favorable circumstances, this can make an initially inoperable tumor resectable (5 out of 33 primary liver tumors). If the tumor is hormonally active, chemoembolization leads to almost immediate cessation of symptoms. This results in a pronounced improvement in the quality of life. Only after the artery is recanalized can renewed hormone production be expected, which can be treated again by chemoembolization. The reduction in tumor bulk leads to a decrease in the size of the tumorous portion of the liver and, thereby, to pain reduction. In favorable cases, a side effect can be the prolongation of life.

Relative Indications

Hepatic metastases appearing or remaining after unsuccessful regional or systemic chemotherapy (Figs. 3 and 10), and primary liver tumors (diffus type) constitute relative indications for chemoembolization. In these cases, it has to be decided whether a renewed attempt at therapy is feasible in the individual patient. In both our own experience and that of other authors [11], chemoembolization resulted in pronounced tumor cell necrosis, even in those cases where other forms of chemotherapy had been ineffective. Prolongation of life, however, was observed only under exceptional circumstances. It would be worthwhile investigating whether chemoembolization, as the most effective method with regard to initial reduction in tumor cell mass, should not be the primary form of treatment. Since the rate of complications is low (30-day mortality: 5%), it would be possible to combine this method with other modes of treatment that are only effective with a small tumor cell mass.

No Indication

Operable primary and secondary liver tumors are no indication for chemoembolization at the present time. However, based on the results of Okamura [28] and Yamasaki [47], it should be discussed whether it would be possible to achieve an improvement in long-term survival rates by preoperative chemoembolization. These authors showed that this is possible in primary liver tumors. Yamasaki improved the 5-year survival rate from 27.2% to 50.6% with a combination of preoperative chemoembolization followed by resection.

Contraindications

An absolute contraindication is portal hypertension. In these cases, the portal-venous supply of the liver is considerably impaired, and after arterial occlusion, a satisfactory blood supply to the remaining liver tissue is not guaranteed. The best way to diagnose such a portal-venous insufficiency is by means of dynamic angio-computed tomography. After intravenous injection of contrast medium, there is an early phase with collection of dye mainly in the metastases while, at a later portal phase, the remaining part of the liver is opacified. If there is decreased perfusion of the healthy part of the liver, which is documented by delayed portal filling, chemoembolization is contraindicated.

Discussion

The only mode of treatment in malignant primary and secondary liver tumors to guarantee long-term survival in at least some patients is surgical resection. However, curative resection can only be performed in a few cases, and in all the other inoperable patients, some kind of palliative treatment should be employed. Methods used in this kind of palliative therapy should fulfill the criteria for minimal burdening of the patient, together with simplicity of application and improvement in the quality of life for these patients.
Chemoembolization of the hepatic artery is gaining importance because it is highly effective and has little influence on the general condition of the patient. Therefore, it is a valid alternative to arterial ligation. The latter loses its therapeutic effectiveness rather quickly because collateral vessels can form even after such short periods as 10 h [23]. Such collaterals can be prevented by a very peripheral embolization [11, 12]. However, Burgner [6] and Doppmann and coworkers [15] warn against such a peripheral embolization. They observed hepatic necroses in healthy livers of rabbits and rhesus monkeys after vessels below a diameter of 175 μm had been embolized. We have observed such necroses as well in the healthy livers of Goettingen mini-pigs [35].
Our method in clinical practice consists of preliminary injection of glucose into the hepatic artery followed by embolization or chemoembolization with prolamine solution. This leads to vascular occlusion of branches down to a diameter of 50 μm. It is of special interest that in diseased livers with widespread metastases or in primary liver tumors, chemoembolization of these small branches can be performed without ill effects [11, 12]. This is documented by the results of our own clinical experience, which have shown a very low complication rate ($n=91$, hospital mortality: 5%).
An explanation for this may be that the arterial bed of the tumor or metastases has some kind of steal effect in the arterial supply. In animal experiments, Maede and coworkers [24] showed that only with 30--50-μm particles is the embolization rate of the metastases higher than that of the healthy liver tissue (tumor/liver ratio 3:1). With microspheres of 50 μm, the amount of embolized tissues was equal in the tumor and the healthy liver tissue (tumor/liver ratio 1:1). This report indicates that different embolization materials might produce more effective chemoembolization.

It should be noted that chemoembolization can be performed with a low rate of complications only if portal vein function is intact. Portal hypertension or right cardiac failure are always contraindications.
What is the relative merit of chemoembolization as compared with the wide variety of other palliative modes of treatment? In 1987, Itoh [20] compared chemoembolization, embolization without cytostatics, and regional chemotherapy in animal experiments. He demonstrated that only chemoembolization resulted in significant reduction in tumor weight. With the other two modes of treatment, there was no difference in comparison to a control group.
Clinically, Monna and coworkers [26] and Charnsangavej [10] were the first authors to show the superiority of chemoembolization as compared to regional therapy. When comparing the results of chemoembolization with those of resectional therapy, it is apparent that the 1-year survival rates are comparable [29]. These good results were achieved only if adriamycin was part or the combination of cytostatics used. Whether the cytostatics or the embolizing substance is more important in bringing about the effect can only be clarified in prospective studies. Since there is no conclusive information on what would be the best cytostatic for chemoembolization, we adhere to a protocol - according to the recommendations of Link (1985, personal communication) - and use a combination of cisplatin, adriamycin, and mitomycin C. In cell cultures, it was possible to show that this triple combination has the highest effectiveness.
Long-term survival of 5 years or more has so far only been achieved by resectional therapy. Therefore, it seems to be desirable to reduce inoperable tumors to a size that makes resection possible. This final goal of any therapy could be reached in five of our patients with primary liver tumors ($n=33$). The good treatment results of the resectional therapy of liver metastases could not be approached by chemoembolization, either by us or by other authors. Only Chuang and Wallace [11] report a median survival time of 11.5 months in a very heterogeneous group of patients.
It should be mentioned, however, that this method is used in liver metastases usually after other treatment has failed or in tumors resistant to chemotherapy. The sequence in which the different modes of treatment should preferably be implemented should be clarified in prospective studies. Chemoembolization, in any case, results in the destruction of a large tumor cell mass, which creates favorable conditions for other forms of therapy.
The elimination of the blood supply to the tumor, which is the main principle of chemoembolization, achieves the desired effect in two ways: firstly, by causing hypoxia, and secondly by bringing about a long-lasting interruption of the delivery of important substrates, such as glucose. This leads to growth retardation and necroses, a process which can be observed in any growing tumor if lack of vascularization in a certain region results in underperfusion [44]. The concomitant release of cytostatics enhances the effectiveness of the treatment.
Several authors have offered explanations of this fact. However, they are not usually backed by experimental data. The following hypotheses exist:

1. Higher doses of cytostatics lead to higher remission rates [14, 22].
2. In vitro studies [31, 42] have shown that hypoxia increases the effectiveness of the cytostatics mitomycin C and adriamycin. The action of 5-Fluorouracil is im-

paired, however, which indicates that this cytostatic agent is not suited for chemoembolization.

3. Chemoembolization leads to early devitalization of large parts of the tumor, which makes locally active cytostatics more effective (because of the reduced mass of active tumor cells) [8].
4. Cytostatics of the anthracyclin type as well as vincaalkaloids seem to induce mechanisms of cell resistance that function by an energy-dependent pump system [17, 37, 39, 42]. The cytostatic agent is eliminated from the cell against a concentration gradient. This mechanism is obviously abolished by embolization, which leads to an interruption of oxygen and energy supply for an extended period of time. Cytostatics that are released at the same time will have full effect, since the mechanism of cell resistance is interrupted.

In general, chemoembolization seems to have many merits in the palliative treatment of liver tumors.

An optimal therapy, however, would probably include some other form of supportive chemotherapy. Chemoembolization can only reach the parts of the tumor with mainly arterial vascular supply. The marginal areas of the tumor, which have mainly portal-venous supply, as well as micrometastases can only be influenced by some additional type of treatment. Chemoembolization with its high local effectiveness but minimal systemic side effects permits other forms of supportive chemotherapy. Therefore, it has a good chance of becoming the primary and most important step in an optimal therapeutic concept for malignant primary and secondary liver tumors. This concept would allow a combined treatment by the arterial as well as the portal-venous route, which, in our opinion, is the most important prerequisite for maximal effect.

It has to be kept in mind, however, that all forms of treatment described above are only palliative, with the exception of those cases in which a "curative" resection can be performed. But even in these patients, tumor recurrence in the remaining part of the liver or in extrahepatic sites is frequent (in our own patients [Nürnberg, 1985–87], 19 out of 32 resected tumors within an average observation period of 16 months). Whether preoperative chemoembolization can lead to better long-term results will have to be determined by a prospective study. There are a few indications pointing in that direction.

Acknowledgement. We are grateful to Professor Bayindir (Gießen) for providing us with some of the roentgenograms.

References

1. Ackerman NB (1974) The blood supply of experimental liver metastases. Changes in vascularity with increasing tumor growth. Surgery 75: 589–596
2. Bassermann R (1984) Angiogenese und Vaskularisation in Metastasen. Verh Dtsch Ges Path 67: 1–16
3. Bengmark S, Fredlund P, Hafström LO, Vang I (1974) Present experience with hepatic dearterialization in liver neoplasm. Progr Surg 13: 141–166
4. Biersack HJ (1980) Die quantitative Leberperfusions-Szintigraphie. Langenbecks Arch Chir 351: 23–27

5. Breedis C, Young G (1954) The blood supply of neoplasms in the liver. Am J Pathol 30: 969-985
6. Burgener FA (1980) Peripheral hepatic artery embolization in rabbits with VX2 carcinoma of the liver. Cancer 46: 56-63
7. Carrasco H, Pichmang V, Wallace S (1983) Apudomas metastatic to the liver: Treatment by hepatic artery embolization. Radiologie 149: 79-83
8. Carter SK (1984) Einige Gedanken zur Resistenz bei der Chemotherapie maligner Erkrankungen. In: Seeber S, Osieka R, Sack H, Schönenberger H (eds) Das Resistenzproblem bei der Chemo- und Radiotherapie maligner Tumoren. Karger, Basel, pp 93-100
9. Charnsangavej C, Chuang VP, Wallace S, Soo CS, Bowers T (1982) Angiographic classification of hepatic artery collaterals. Radiology 144: 485-494
10. Charnsangavej C, Chuang VP, Wallace S, Soo CS, Bowers T, Obe W (1983) Work in progress: transcatheter management of primary carcinoma of the liver. Radiology 147: 51-55
11. Chuang VP, Wallace S (1981) Heaptic artery embolization in the treatment of hepatic neoplasms. Radiology 140: 51-58
12. Clouse ME, Lee RG, Duszlank EJ, Lokich JJ, Trey C, Alday M (1983) Peripheral hepatic artery embolization of primary and secondary hepatic neoplasms. Radiology 147: 407-411
13. Clouse ME, Lee RG (1984) Management of the posthepatic artery embolization syndrome. Radiology 152: 238
14. Collins JM (1984) Pharmacokinetic rationale for intra-arterial therapy. Proceedings Interarterial and intracavitary chemotherapy, American Society for Clinical Oncology, San Diego, 24-25 Feb 1984, pp 9-13
15. Doppman JL, Girton M, Kahn ER (1978) Proximal versus peripheral hepatic artery embolization: experimental study in monkeys. Radiology 128: 577-588
16. Doyon D, Mouzon A, Jourde AM, Regensberg C, Frileux C (1974) L'embolisation artérielle hépatique dans les tumeurs malignes du foie. Ann Radiol 17: 593-603
17. Friche E, Skovsgaard T, Nissen NI (1987) Effect of verapamil on daunorubicin in Ehrlich ascites tumor cells. Cancer Chemother Pharmacol 19: 35-39
18. Frei E, Cannellos GP (1980) Dose: a critical factor in cancer chemotherapy. Am J Med 69: 585-594
19. Gelin LE, Lewis DH, Nilsson L (1968) Liver blood flow in man during abdominal surgery. Acta Hepatosplenologica 15: 13-21
20. Itho J (1985) Gan-To-Kagaku-Ryoho 12: 258-264
21. Kaufmann GW, Wenz W, Rohrbach R, Richter R, Rassweiler J, Strecker EP (1981) Renal embolization: Indications and material. Ann Radiol 24: 386-389
22. Link KH, Aigner KR, Kühn W, Roetering N, Schwemmle K (1985) Chemosensitivitätsbestimmung in vitro bei regionaler Chemotherapie von Lebertumoren. Tumor Diagn Ther 6: 238-243
23. Mays ET, Wheeler CS (1979) Demonstration of collateral arterial flow after interruption of hepatic arteries in man. New Engl J Med 290: 993-996
24. Maede VM, Burton MA, Gray BN, Self GW (1987) Distribution of differenz sized microspheres in experimental hepatic tumors. Eur J Cancer Clin Oncol 23: 37-41
25. Michels NA (1960) Newer anatomy of the liver-variant blood supply and collateral circulation. J Am med Ass 172: 125-132
26. Monna T, Kanno T, Marumo T, Harihara S, Kuroki T, Yamamoto S (1982) A comparison of transcatheter arterial embolization with one-shot therapy for the patients with hepatic cell carcinoma. Gastroenterol Jpn 17: 542-549
27. Nouchi T, Nishimura M, Maeda M, Funatsu T, Hasumura Y, Takeuchi J (1984) Transcatheter arterial embolization of rupture hepatocellular carcinoma associated mit liver cirrhosis. Dig Dis Sci 29: 1137-1141
28. Okamura J, Monden M, Kabayashi J, Gothoh M, Sakurai M, Wakasa K (1984) Experience of the multidisciplinary treatment of hepatocellular carcinoma: Follow-up studies on chemoembolization with surgical excision. In: Ogawa M, Muggia FM, Rozencweig M (eds) Adriamycin. Excerpta Medica, Amsterdam
29. Okuda K, Ohtsuki T, Obata H, Tomimatsu M, Okazaki I, Hasegawa H, Nakajima Y, Ohnishi K (1985) Natural history of hepatocellular carcinoma and prognosis in relation to treatment. Cancer 56: 918-928

30. Richter G, Rohrbach R, Kauffmann GW, Rassweiler J (1981) Verschluß des gesamten arteriellen Gefäßsystems experimentell erzeugter Nierentumoren. Fortschr Röntgenstr 135: 85-97
31. Rockwell S (1982) Cytotoxicities of mitomycin C and X-rays to aerobic and hypoxic cells in vitro. Int Radiat Oncol Biol Phys 8: 1035-1039
32. Schlag P, Hohenberger P (1988) Regionale Chemotherapie von Lebertumoren - Eine Situationsanalyse. Chirurg 59: 218-224
33. Schultheis K-H, Schulz A, Schiefer HG (1981) Schnellhärtende Aminosäurelösung als mögliche Chemotherapeuticaträgersubstanz. Unfallchirurgie 7: 324-333
34. Schultheis K-H, Henneking K, Rehm KE, Ecke H, Schiefer HG, Breithaupt H (1982) Untersuchungen über die Freisetzungskinetik verschiedener Chemotherapeutika aus einer viskösen, im feuchten Milieu schnell aushärtenden Aminosäurenlösung und ihre klinische Bedeutung. Langenbecks Arch Chir [Suppl]: 200-205
35. Schultheis K-H (1985) Neue Möglichkeiten der lokalen chemotherapeutischen Behandlung von Lebertumoren und -metastasen mit Hilfe einer Prolaminlösung als Chemotherapeutikaträgersubstanz. Habilitationsschrift, University of Giessen
36. Schuster R, v Romatowski HJ, Kreutzfeld W, Stöckmann F (1983) Transluminale Occlusionsbehandlung von Lebermetastasen hormonbildender Geschwülste. Röntgenpraxis 36: 386-373
37. Seeber S (1980) Sensitivität und Resistenz bei der Tumortherapie. Verh Dtsch Ges Inn Med 86: 367-377
38. Shichijo Y, Inoue Y (1985) Embolisierung der A. hepatica beim primären hepatozelulären Carcinom. Fortschr Röntgenstr 143: 63-68
39. Skovsgard T, Dano K, Niessen NJ (1984) Die Wirkung von Chemosensitizern bei erworbener Antracyclin- und Vinca Akaloid-Resistenz in vivo. Beitr Onkol 18: 124-138
40. Starkhammer H (1987) On the effect of degradable starch microspheres in intraarterial chemotherapy. Linköping University Medical Dissertations No. 243, Linköping, Sweden
41. Taylor J, Bennett R, Sheriff S (1979) The blood supply of colorectal liver metastases. Br J Cancer 39: 749-756
42. Teicher BA, Lazo JS, Sartorelli AC (1981) Classification of antineoplastic agents by their selective toxicities toward oxygenated and hypoxic tumor cells. Cancer Res 41: 73-81
43. Tittor W, Schwalbach S (1981) Leberdurchblutung und Kreislauf. Thieme, Stuttgart
44. Vaupel P, Thews R, Wendling P (1976) Kritische Sauerstoff- und Glucoseversorgung maligner Tumoren. Dtsch Med Wschr 101: 1810-1816
45. Wallace S, Charnsangavej C, Carrasco H, Bechtel W (1984) Infusion - Embolization. Canver 54: 2751-2765
46. Wopfner F (1981) Therapie inoperabler Lebermetastasen. Erste Erfahrungen mit der intrahepatischen Chemotherapie unter Verwendung eines neuen Verweilkatheters. Dtsch Med Wschr 106: 1099-1102
47. Yamasaki S (1986) Surgical treatment of hepatocellular carcinoma. Gan No Rinsho 32: 1267-72

New Cancer Treatment with Lasers - Photodynamic Therapy and Interstitial Hyperthermia

S. G. BOWN[1]

Lasers are sophisticated light sources that can deliver energy to living tissue with a great deal of precision. However, many of their current clinical applications, although more accurate than the available alternatives, are still relatively crude, and the effects are judged largely on the immediate visual changes alone. The real future of lasers in medicine lies in harnessing the precision available and applying it to biological systems. Inevitably, it is far more difficult to control all the factors that influence the nature and extent of laser effects in living tissue than it is in inanimate materials, but one can do considerably better than with other energy sources, such as diathermy. High-power lasers have an established role in clinical practice as, for example, the carbon dioxide laser in gynaecology and the neodymium yttrium aluminium garnet (YAG) laser for the endoscopic palliation of advanced obstructing tumours of the gastrointestinal tract and major airways [1].

This paper will look at much lower-power applications of lasers with wavelengths that penetrate well into living tissue. Relatively little work has yet been done in this field, but tissue effects can be produced with greater accuracy than with high-power instruments, both by thermal and non-thermal mechanisms. Conventionally, the term therapeutic hyperthermia has been used to mean relatively uniform heating of tissues to temperatures in the range of 42.5°-50° C for extended periods of time (often over 1 h) [2]. Local hyperthermia with lasers is normally less uniform, as the light energy is usually delivered via flexible fibres either held above the target tissue (external therapy) or inserted into it (interstitial therapy), and the light intensity drops exponentially with increasing distance from the fibre, seldom producing biological effects through more than 7-10 mm of tissue from each treatment point. With the laser, the highest temperatures may exceed 100° C, but at the margins of the tissue influenced by the heat, the temperatures are comparable to those found with conventional hyperthermia. The non-thermal techniques currently under most intensive study are the photochemical effects produced by administering exogenous photosensitising agents, which are activated by light to produce a local cytotoxic effect (photodynamic therapy).

[1] National Medical Laser Centre, The Rayne Institute, 5, University Street, London WC1E 6JJ, UK.

H. G. Beger et al. (Eds.), Cancer Therapy

Hyperthermia

The range of biological responses to local heat from a high-power laser with a deeply penetrating wavelength, like the infrared beam of the neodymium: YAG laser at 1064 nm, can be summarised as:

1. Total destruction	Instant vaporisation Necrosis with later sloughing
2. Destruction with reconstruction	Necrosis with healing by scarring or regeneration
3. Reversible effects	Oedema and inflammation Local warming only

Under appropriate circumstances, all these effects can be seen in the same organ. For example, a neodymium:YAG shot of 3 s at 70 W onto a 3-mm spot on the normal stomach wall will instantly vaporise a small area of mucosa, necrose the muscularis mucosae and submucosa, which slough during the next few days, and cause partial necrosis in the external muscle layer, which heals with fibrosis, while there is a regeneration of the mucosa and submucosa. This same range of effects can be observed in neoplastic tissue [3]. This has major therapeutic implications, as it means that there is the potential for destroying localised tumours, particularly in thin-walled organs, and replacing the diseased tissue either with a scar or by regeneration of the normal tissue. For therapeutic purposes, one must be sure that a scar rather than perforation results. There exist few experimental data so far concerning this problem. The extent of lesions produced with particular laser parameters is reasonably predictable with the high-power laser. With the low-power laser (1–2 W), no vaporisation is seen, and there is a more gradual and more prolonged tissue hyperthermia, which is easier to control and can be applied with much greater precision. This approach will be explored in this paper.

Photodynamic Therapy

Photodynamic therapy (PDT) has attracted a lot of interest in the last few years as a new technique with the potential for localisation (by fluorescence) and selective destruction of malignant tumours (particularly small, multi-focal lesions) [4]. It is based on the systemic administration of certain sensitising drugs, which are retained with some selectivity in tumours and can be activated by light to produce a local cytotoxic effect. Undoubtedly, local tumour destruction by this method is possible although, for comparable light doses, the extent of tissue damage in tumours is often very little more than in adjacent normal tissue. The real value of PDT will probably lie more in the nature of the biological effects produced, as these differ from thermal damage.

Most experimental work to date has used haematoporphyrin derivative (HpD) as the sensitising drug. However, HpD and dihaematoporphyrin ether/ester (DHE) thought to contain a higher percentage of the active ingredients or ingredients of HpD, are both incompletely defined mixtures of porphyrins [5]. New groups of drugs with similar biological properties, but which are much easier to handle chemically, are now being studied, particularly the phthalocyanines [6]. Tissue damage by photodynamic therapy is thought to involve the production of singlet oxygen [7]. Following its systemic (usually intravenous) administration, the sensitising agent can be activated by light of a wavelength matched to one of its absorption peaks. This activated form can elevate oxygen from its ground state (triplet oxygen) to the much more reactive singlet state. Singlet oxygen is short lived and can produce a toxic effect (most likely on the cell membrane, though probably also on other cellular organelles) in the cell region where it is formed. The phthalocyanines have the major advantage that they absorb strongly in the red part of the spectrum, where light penetrates most living tissue well compared with HpD, which only has a weak absorption peak in the red spectral portion [8]. It is often thought that the key to tumour destruction with PDT is the selective retention of the sensitising agent in malignant neoplasms. It is now clear that, with the exception of intracranial tumours [9], this is a relatively minor factor. The final biological effect may depend more on the distribution of the applied therapeutic light and the local response of the target area (normal or neoplastic) to a particular level of absorbed light energy and singlet oxygen production. However, selective retention is the factor that has been used to characterise the technique in the scientific literature so far published.

Although PDT has been studied in many different centres worldwide for over 10 years, it is remarkable how little data are available on which factors control the extent of PDT necrosis, what the nature of the tissue damage produced is, and how it heals. It is even more remarkable how few studies have been carried out comparing its effects on tumours and on the normal tissue in which those tumours arose. Chaudhuri et al. [10] have shown that PDT can produce extensive sloughing of the jejunal mucosa and submucosa in rats while sparing the muscular and serosal layers. Okuda et al. [11] found that extensive necrosis of normal mucosa can occur when treating gastric tumours. In recent work at the National Medical Laser Centre in London, we have tried to tackle this type of problem both for low-power hyperthermia and for PDT, comparing the effects of each type of tissue damage on the normal liver and the colon and on chemically induced colon tumours in rats.

Experimental Studies on the Liver

The liver was chosen for the first studies on both hyperthermia and PDT, as it is large enough in rats to be able to measure the extent of tissue necrosis produced by laser treatment in a relatively homogeneous organ. In addition, it is easily accessible, and the liver is known to take up more of the sensitising agents used for PDT than any other organ [12]. For the studies of hyperthermia, Matthewson et al. [13] chose a simple experimental model in which a 0.4-mm diameter fibre from a low-power neodymium:YAG laser was inserted directly into the centre of a liver lobe exposed at laparotomy in Wistar rats. They originally used a pulsed laser (0.1-ms pulses at 40 Hz) but subsequently showed that the results were identical to those with a continuous wave laser [14].

A similar experimental arrangement was explored for the PDT studies on liver parenchyma [8]. A slightly thinner fibre was used (0.2 mm in dameter), and the light

source was an argon ion pumped dye laser tuned to emit at 675 nm, the best absorption peak for the photosensitising agent, aluminium sulphonated phthalocyanine (AISPc). Control experiments showed that when the laser power at the tip of the fibre was raised above 100 mW, significant thermal effects were seen in unsensitised animals. Therefore, all quantitative studies of PDT were performed at 100 mW. The width of necrosis in the liver was correlated with the total laser energy, the dose of AISPc used, and the time from photosensitisation to phototherapy. Maximum necrosis was seen 2–4 days after treatment, and lesions were examined at other times to assess healing.
The results for PDT and hyperthermia can be summarised as follows:

1. Well-defined areas of necrosis, roughly spherical in shape, were produced around each treatment point.
2. The diameter of the necrotic zone increased with the logarithm of the applied light energy.
3. The best power of hyperthermia was 1–1.5 W (higher power caused charring; lower power reduced the effect for the same energy), whereas the best of PDT was 100 mW (higher power caused thermal effects). Thus, for the same energy, the exposure time was ten times as long with PDT.
4. Following sensitisation with 5 mg/kg AISPc 3 h prior to phototherapy, the width of necrosis was about the same for PDT and for hyperthermia when the same total light energy was applied.
5. Further studies on PDT showed that the width of necrosis correlated with the concentration of AISPc in the tissue (measured by alkali extraction) and also that the PDT effect (but not the hyperthermal one) could be completely prevented by occluding the blood supply to the liver prior light exposure, thereby making the tissue hypoxic during phototherapy.

The histological studies provided some interesting contrasts [15]. Vascular damage occurred after both types of treatment but was much more obvious after PDT. The inflammatory response was more florid and occurred earlier after PDT. Lesions produced by PDT and by hyperthermia healed mostly by regeneration of normal liver tissue, but the thermal lesion healed more slowly and left a small fibrous scar, whereas scarring in the healed PDT lesions was barely detectable. Thus, both hyperthermia and PDT produce areas of necrosis of a predictable extent in normal liver parenchyma, which heal safely.

Experimental Studies on the Colon

Our first experiments focused on the liver, as it is a solid organ in which the extent of laser lesions can be measured easily in three dimensions. The next series of experiments focused on the colon, partly to assess the risks of full-thickness damage and perforation on a hollow organ, and partly because there is a convenient animal model of an autochthonous tumour (colon cancer induced by dimethyl hydrazine in Wistar rats).
The laser sources used were the same as for the liver experiments, as was the photosensitising agent for the PDT. In the studies on normal rats [16, 17], the colon

was exposed at laparotomy and the laser fibre pushed through the wall of the colon into the lumen and held gently against the mucosa of the opposite site. In addition to the parameters varied and measurements made as in the experiments on the liver, the mechanical strength of the colon was tested immediately after the animals were killed by isolating the treated section of colon, slowly distending it with air, and measuring the bursting pressure.
The results of studies on normal colon can be summarized as follows:

1. Well-defined areas of necrosis, roughly circular in shape, were produced by both hyperthermia and PDT. The size of the necrosis depended on the total light energy delivered and for PDT, on the tissue concentration of the photosensitiser.
2. At light energies that produced full-thickness damage to the colonic wall of the rat, (this was the case for most specimens, as the wall is less than 1 mm thick), thermal lesions showed a marked reduction in bursting pressure for the first 7 days after treatment, whereas there was no reduction in bursting pressure at any time in lesions of comparable extent produced by PDT.

Histological studies [18] suggested that submucosal collagen was preserved in PDT-induced lesions but not in thermal ones, which could explain the difference in bursting pressure results. There was also a marked difference in the healing. Lesions produced by PDT healed in about 2 weeks with essentially complete regeneration of all layers of the colonic wall, whereas thermal lesions healed more slowly with some residual fibrosis.
Results with a transplantable fibrosarcoma [19] show that the extent of necrosis varies with the treatment parameters in the same way in this malignant tissue as it does in normal liver parenchyma. Fewer experimental data are available so far on the response of the chemically induced colonic cancers, but with both techniques [17], tumour necrosis followed by sloughing was observed, and if the extent of necrosis matched the size of the tumour, only a shallow ulcer was left behind. Overtreatment with hyperthermia could lead to perforation, whereas PDT-induced necrosis of larger tumours was sometimes followed by secondary haemorrhage, which was not seen after thermal treatment.

Conclusions

The experiments reviewed in this paper were designed to compare low-power neodymium: YAG laser hyperthermia with photodynamic therapy. It is clear that, although local necrosis of a predictable extent can be produced in both normal and neoplastic tissue by both mechanisms, the nature of the tissue damage and the form of healing may differ. If the submucosal collagen is intact, there is little risk of perforating the colon with PDT. Since lesions in normal bowel wall heal by regeneration, PDT would seem suitable for treating small and multiple colonic lesions. However, secondary haemorrhage may occur after treating larger tumours with PDT, and for these, hyperthermia seems more appropriate. However, care must be taken not to cause deep damage that could lead to perforation, and it should be kept in mind that local scarring is likely on healing. No studies are available on the response of intrahepatic tumours, but from the data reviewed here, it would seem that hyperthermia would be more appropriate for treating these, as the time required to produce an area of necrosis of any particular size is much less than with PDT, and the healing is fairly similar. These are very early results, and it may not be valid to extrapolate from results in rats to the treatment of human disease. Also, only two types of tissue have been studied. This type of experiment should facilitate evaluation of whether both or of which technique is likely to be relevant to clinical practice. In addition, each technique must be fully understood on its own before one can assess whether there could be any synergy between them, as has been suggested [20], or between any of the laser techniques and other approaches, such as radiotherapy or chemotherapy.

References

1. Bown SG (1986) Laser endoscopy. Br Med Bulletin 42 (3): 307-313
2. Hahn GM (1982) Hyperthermia and cancer. Plenum, New York
3. Bown SG (1983) Phototherapy of Tumors. World J Surg 7: 700-707
4. Doiron D, Gomer C (eds) (1984) Porphyrin localisation and treatment of tumours. Plenum, New York
5. Dougherty TJ, Potter WR, Weishaupt R (1984) The structure of the active component of HpD. In Doiron D, Gomer C (eds) Porphyrin Localisation and Treatment of Tumours, Alan R. Liss, New York, pp 301-314
6. Spikes JD (1986) Phthalocyanines as photosensitizers in biochemical systems and for the photodynamic therapy of tumours. Photochem Photobiol 43 (6): 691
7. Weishaupt KR, Gomer CJ, Dougherty TJ (1976) Identification of singlet oxygen as the cytotoxic agent in photoactivation of a murine tumour. Cancer Res 36: 2326-2329
8. Bown SG, Tralau CJ, Coleridge-Smith PD, Akdemir D, Wieman TJ (1986) Photodynamic therapy with porphyrin and phthalocyanine sensitization: quantitative studies in normal rat liver. Br J Cancer 54: 43-52
9. Wharen RE, Anderson BAS, Laws ER (1983) Quantitation in HpD of human gliomas, experimental central nervous system tumours and normal tissues. Neurosurg 12 (4): 446
10. Chaudhuri K, Goldblatt PJ, Kreimer-Birnbaum M, Keck RW, Selman SH (1986) Histological study of the effect of HpD photodynamic therapy on the rat jejunum. Cancer Res 46: 2950-2953
11. Okuda S, Mimura S, Otani T, Ichii M, Tatsuta M (1984) Experimental and clinical studies on HpD photodynamic therapy for upper gastrointestinal cancers. In: Andreoni A, Cubeddu R (eds) Porphyrins in tumour phototherapy, Elsevier, Amsterdam, pp 413-422
12. Gomer CJ and Dougherty TJ (1979) Determination of ^{3}H and ^{14}C HpD distribution in malignant and normal tissue. Cancer Res 39: 146-51
13. Matthewson K, Coleridge-Smith PD, O'Sullivan JP, Northfield TC, Bown SG (1987) Biological effects of intrahepatic NdYAG laser photocoagulation in rats. Gastroenterology 93: 550-557
14. Matthewson K, Coleridge-Smith P, Northfield TC, Bown SG (1986) Comparison of continuous wave and pulsed excitation for interstitial NdYAG laser induced hyperthermia. Laser Med Sci 1: 197-201
15. Collins CM, Tralau CJ, Wieman TJ, Bown SG (1986) Histological comparison of photodynamic therapy with phthalocyanine sensitisation and thermal injury in normal rat liver. British Medical Laser Association, 4th annual congress, London
16. Barr H, Tralau CJ, MacRobert AJ, Krasner N, Boulos PB, Bown SG (1987) Photodynamic therapy in the normal rat colon with phthalocyanine sensitization. Br J Cancer 56: 111-118
17. Matthewson K, Barton T, Lewin MR, O'Sullivan JP, Northfield TC, Bown SG, Low power interstitial NdYAG laser photocoagulation in normal and neoplastic rat colon. GUT 29: 27-34

18. Barr H, Tralau CJ, Boulos PB, MacRobert AJ, Tilly R, Bown SG (1988) Contrasting mechanisms of colonic collagen damage between photodynamic therapy and thermal injury. Photochem Photobiol 46: 795–800
19. Tralau CJ, MacRobert AJ, Coleridge-Smith PD, Barr H, Bown SG, Photodynamic therapy with phthalocyanine sensitisation: quantitative studies in a transplantable fibrosarcoma of rats. Br J Cancer 55: 389–395
20. Henderson BW, Waldow SM, Dougherty TJ (1985) Interaction of photodynamic therapy and hyperthermia, tumour control and tumour cell survival after treatment in vivo. Lasers Surg Med 5: 139

Specificity, Kinetics, and Distribution of Monoclonal Antibodies to Carcinoembryonic Antigen in Human Colorectal Carcinoma by Ex Vivo Human Tumor Perfusion

E. KRAAS,[1] E. LÖHDE,[1] O. ABRI,[1] H. SCHLICKER,[2] S. MATZKU,[3] H. KALTHOFF,[4] and W. H. SCHMIEGEL[4]

Introduction

The use of monoclonal antibodies (MAB) for diagnostic and therapeutic purposes depends on their accumulation and retention in solid tumor tissue [1, 2, 4, 5, 8, 13, 14]. The accuracy of presently available methods is subject to inherent limitations with respect to scintigraphic localization. Furthermore, the therapeutic application appears only rarely succussful [3, 11, 12]. This situation demands a systemic investigation of factors determining the biodistribution of MAB in both tumor and normal tissue.

Scope of the Problem

In detail, the following problems have to be recognized:

1. Prerequisite is the presence of specific, tumor-associated antigens. Serum carcinoembryonic antigen (CEA) levels, however, have little descriptive value, since not all antigens may have been secreted.
2. To achieve an antibody enrichment in the tumor that can be demonstrated scintigraphically, the MAB must be specific to the tumor-associated antigen and show only a slight tendency toward nonspecific binding [7].
3. The MAB must reach the tumor antigen via the vascular system, i.e., the antibody must be able to pass through the basal membrane and the vascular endothelium.
4. Binding sites can be extracellular and intracellular, as well as on the cell membrane [10, 11, 16, 18].
5. The binding kinetics of the MAB important, i.e., how rapidly and tightly the antibody binds to the antigen [15].

[1] Department of Surgery I, Moabit Hospital, Turmstraße 21, 1000 Berlin 21, FRG.
[2] Department of Nuclear Medicine, Moabit Hospital, Turmstraße 21, 1000 Berlin 21, FRG.
[3] German Cancer Research Center, Im Neuenheimer Feld 280, 6900 Heidelberg, FRG.
[4] Department of Clinical Immunology, University Clinic Eppendorf, 2000 Hamburg, FRG.

H. G. Beger et al. (Eds.), Cancer Therapy

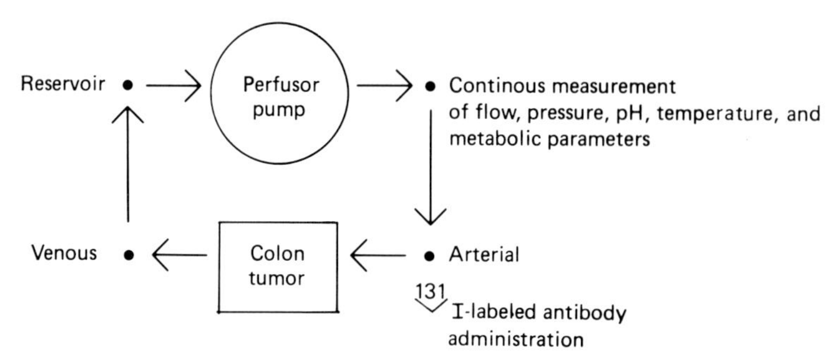

Fig. 1. Model of the ex vivo tumor perfusion system

Methods

A model for ex vivo perfusion of colonic tumors was developed (Fig. 1) [17]. For this purpose, the artery supplying the tumor segment of the colon is exposed intraoperatively. After cannulization of the main artery, the tumor-bearing segment is perfused with Eurocollins solution at 4 °C. The warm ischemic period due to this procedure is less than a few minutes. Afterwards, the colon segment is removed, and pulsative perfusion with fresh-frozen, heparinized plasma is administered at room temperature with continuous monitoring of pressure, flow, temperature, and pH. Methylene blue is injected to prove the tumor lay within the perfused area.

While controlling various metabolic parameters, such as pH, glucose, lactate, and CKMB, the ^{131}I-labeled, 180-kD CEA antibody C1 P83 are added (0.4–0.8 mg; 300–400 μCi). Simultaneously, the MABs' accumulation and clearance are measured immunoscintigraphically. After 45 min perfusion (approximate time interval for maximal uptake), the preparation is rinsed with fresh-frozen plasma and Ringer's solution in a ratio of 1:3 for another 45 min. The ratios of maximal uptake in tumor tissue to accumulation in the intestine are computed. Finally, tissue samples are taken from the center of the tumor, from the tumor periphery, from the (nontumorous) intestinal wall, fat, mucosal lymph nodes, and vascular tissue. Activity profiles are then performed (Fig. 2).

The distribution of the MAB in the tumor is detected by autoradiography. The immunohistologic examination of the perfused tumor should provide information about the antibody/antigen distribution and the accessibility of the antigen for the antibody.

Results

Eleven human colonic tumors (from 8 female and 3 male patients; 6 located in the colon ascendens, 1 in the colon transversum, and 4 in the sigmoid colon) were perfused as described. Three examples will be discussed to illustrate the process of ex vivo tumor perfusion.

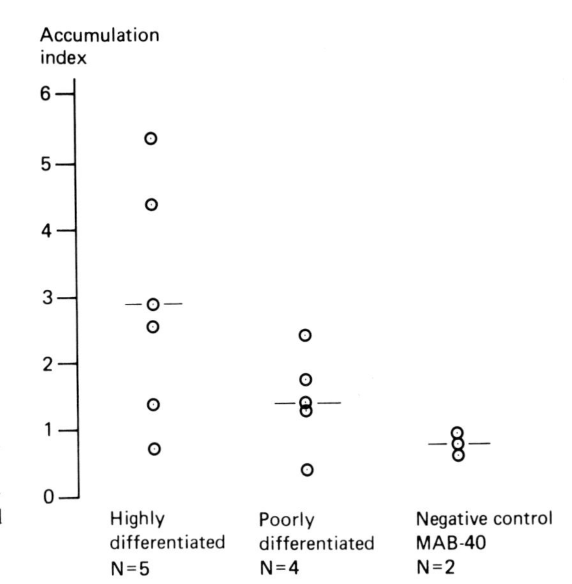

Fig. 2. Activity profile of ^{131}I-labeled MAB C1 P83. Antibody binding ratios of highly differentiated and poorly differentiated tumors are compared with negative controls. – ⊙ –, standard mean

Example 1. Initially, the ^{131}I-labeled MAB is diffusely distributed in the vascular system (Fig. 3 A–D; the circle indicated macroscopically the center of the tumor). Thereafter, an accumulation in the tumor takes place. The maximal uptake is reached after approximately 45 min. Subsequently, the colon segment is rinsed via the arterial line for another 45 min.
The vascular system and the surrounding intestinal tissue loses its scintigraphic activity almost completely. In the tumor, a marked residual activity can be observed even following the 45-min rinsing phase. The ratio of uptake activity in the tumor to the surrounding intestinal tissue is determined scintigraphically. In this experiment, a ratio of approximately 2:1 was achieved (Fig. 3 d).

Example 2. Similar continuous accumulation and clear retainment by the tumor, even after the rinsing procedure, are demonstrated in Fig. 4 a–d. In this second example, the distribution ratio of tumor to intestinal tissue is about 2.5:1.

Example 3. A nonretaining tumor with stenotic growth is shown in Fig. 5. The intestinal tissue surrounding the tumor shows a distinctly higher accumulation of radiolabeled MAB than the tumor itself. This occurred despite the fact that the patient showed clearly elevated serum CEA values.
Table 1 contains the data of the nine completed tumor perfusions and shows that an immunohistological differentiation between the types of adenocarcinomas might be possible. It is interesting to note that differentiated tumors (three from the ascending colon and two from the sigma), three of which had been found preoperatively to have elevated CEA levels, showed much higher antibody binding than poorly differentiated tumors. The tumor/mucosa binding ratio ranges between 0.89 and 5.4 (average, 2.9) for highly differentiated tumors and 0.18 and 2.3 (average, 1.3) for poorly differentiated tumors.

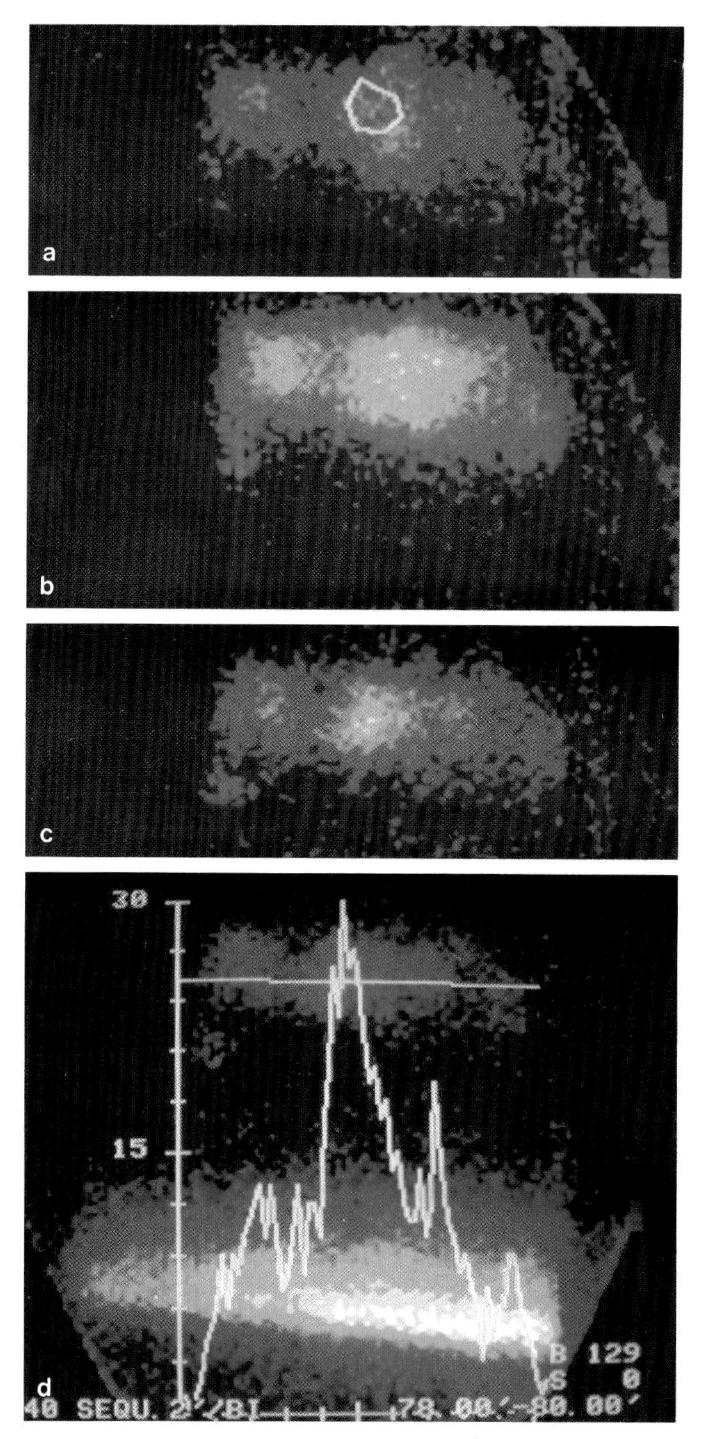

Fig. 3a–d. Immunoscintigram of ex vivo perfusion of a tumor of the sigmoid colon. **a** Diffuse distribution of ratiolabeled MAB; **b** accumulation in the tumor; **c** rinsing (wash out); **d** scintigraphic analysis of the activity accumulation in the tissue (*abscissa*, pixels; *ordinate*, counts)

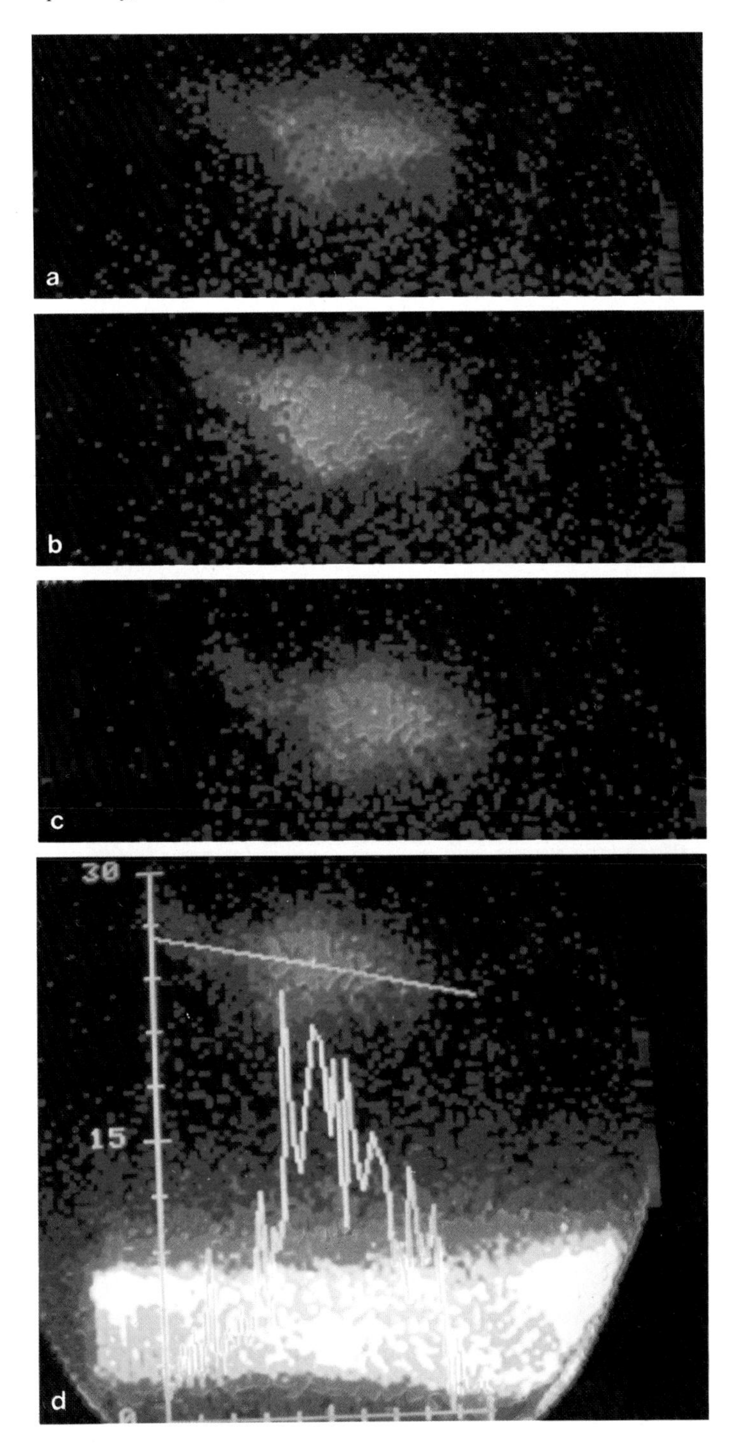

Fig. 4 a–d. Immunoscintigram of ex vivo perfusion of a tumor in the colon ascendens. Continuous accumulation, washout, and scintigraphic analysis of the activity enrichment in the tissue (*abscissa,* pixels; *ordinate,* counts)

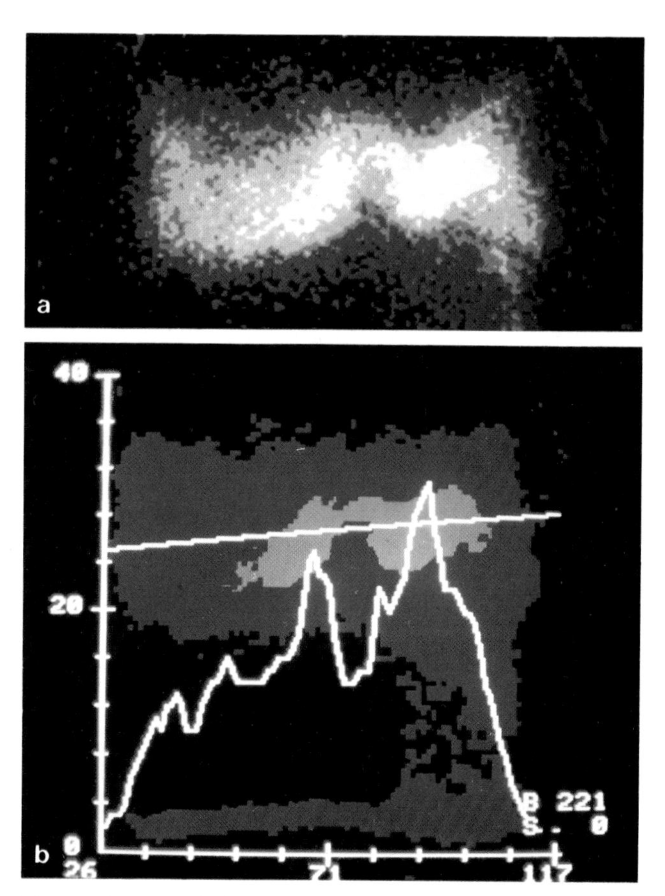

Fig. 5. a Immunoscintigram of a poorly differentiated colon tumor. **b** Between two peaks of low mucosal activity, there is no MAB enrichment in the central occluding tumor mass

The ratio is significantly lower in poorly differentiated tumors. Attempts to verify this tendency by immunohistology were somewhat disappointing: it was possible to demonstrate antibody binding immunohistologically in only two out of five of the differentiated carcinomas, although all tumors were highly positive for MAB C1 P83 by direct tissue staining. The same results are seen in nondifferentiated tumors.

Of the five well-differentiated, cylinder-cell carcinomas, three tumors showed good accumulation, while two tumors showed little accumulation. The accumulation quotient of tumor to normal intestinal tissue varies from nonaccumulation to 5.6:1. Figure 6 shows activity ratios in tumor, lymph nodes, mucosa, fat, and vascular tissue. This illustrates the general differences in antibody binding between highly differentiated tumors and their adjacent tissues.

The absolute amount of ^{131}I-labeled C1 P83 antibodies retained in the whole tumor tissue reaches 6% of the total injected activity. In Fig. 2, the binding ratios between the highly and the poorly tumors are contrasted to a negative control in

Table 1. Human colon adenocarcinoma - ex vivo perfusion with ^{131}I-labeled MAB C1 P83

n	Histology	Location	TNM	Elevated serum CEA levels (preoperative) (*n* tumors)	Tissue activity ratio (tumor/mucosa)	Scintigraphic accumulation index (range)	Immunohistologic cross-section	
							C1 P83 rediscovered in tissue (*n* tumors)	Binding specificity of C1 P83 (positive control) (*n* tumors)
5	High degree of differentiation	Colon ascendens *n*=3 Sigmoid colon *n*=2	$T_3N_0M_0$ *n*=4	3 of 5	2.9 (0.89-5.4)	2.3 (0.5-3.8)	2 of 5	positive 5 of 5
4	Low degree of differentiation	Colon ascendens *n*=2 colon transversum *n*=1 sigmoid colon *n*=1	$T_3N_0M_0$ *n*=2 $T_3N_0M_0$ *n*=2	1 of 4	1.3 (0.18-2.3)	0.84 (0.52-1.63)	2 of 4	positive 4 of 4

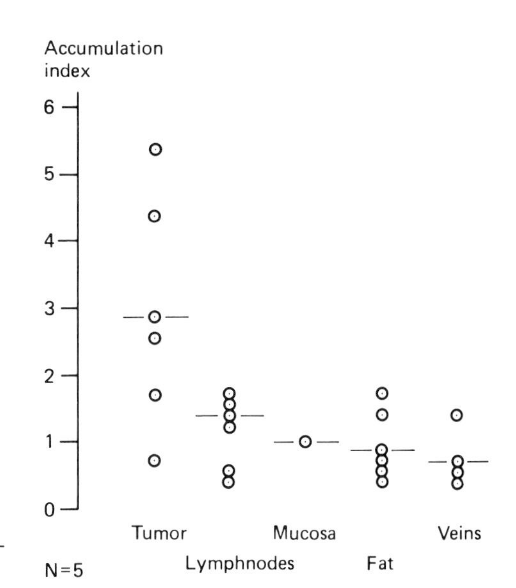

Fig. 6. Activity profile of ^{131}I-labeled MAB C1 P83 in highly differentiated carcinomas and in adjacent tissues. – ⊙ –, standard mean

which a nonspecific antibody was employed. The vascular supply system in the area of the tumor, which is shown by methylene blue staining or identification with technetium-marked erythrocytes, does not permit a correlation with the accumulation of MAB C1 P83-CEA in tumor tissue. The autoradiographic analysis of the tumor tissue (Fig. 7) does not show a homogeneous binding of the MAB in the

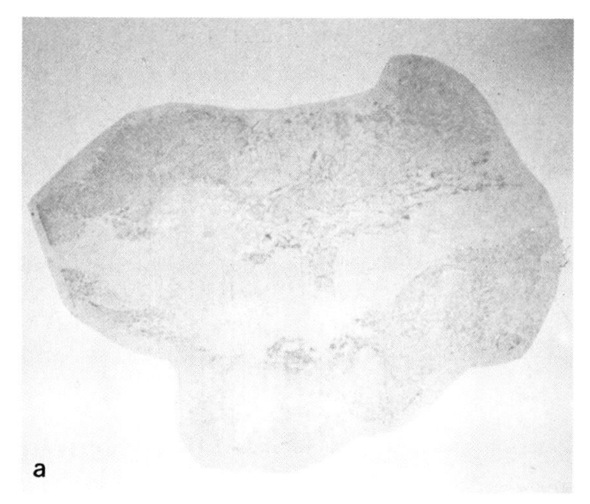

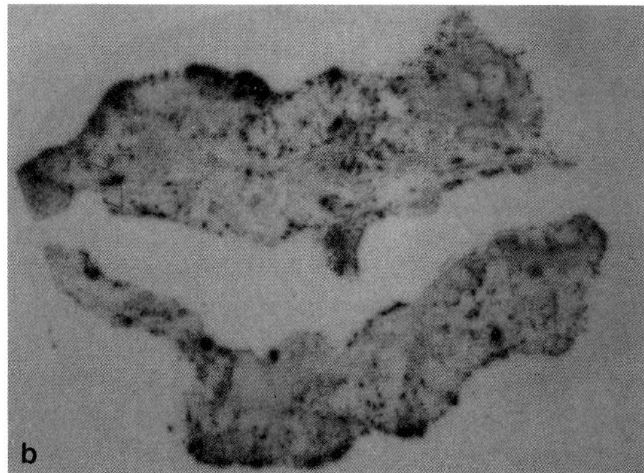

Fig. 7 a, b. Cross-section of an occluding colon carcinoma. **a** Morphological aspect of the probe. **b** Autoradiogram shows heterogenic MAB distribution. Regions of intense enrichment are localized on the tumor surface

tumor tissue. Centers of extremely strong accumulation (spots) versus areas of modest binding are observed.

Discussion

The ex vivo perfusion of human colonic with antibody-containing media tumors as described here allows both scintigraphic determination of the process of accumulation within human tumor tissue and autoradiographic examination of the biodistribution of retained antibodies. On the basis of this method, it is possible to investigate factors crucial to the transport of antibodies, the accessibility of antigen-positive tumor cells, and the permeation of the solid tissue with intact antibodies.

The differential adherence of the antibodies to the tumor tissue is striking; some of the tumors initially showed good scintigraphic accumulation during perfusion, which was later retained during the rinsing phase. Other tumors also showed accumulation; the antibody, however, could be rinsed away. A third group of tumors showed no specific accumulation.

Tumor targeting with MAB can however be successful only if relatively large quantities of antibodies accumulate in the solid tumor tissue [3, 6, 8, 9, 11]. The few published cases in which it was possible to measure the actual accumulation quotients of human tumors and normal tissue report suprisingly low values of less than 0.01% of the amount of MAB administered per gram of tumor [5, 6]. Without a doubt, the present technological possibilities allow accurate scintigraphic localization, even at quite low levels of antibody accumulation. Considering therapeutic concepts, at least a tenfold increase in the presently obtainable antibody targeting would be needed [11]. Therefore, it is very remarkable that in the ex vivo model described here up to 6% (500-fold higher uptake!) of the applied antibody is retained in the tumor tissue. A reason for the high uptake in the model may be the absence of the reticuloendothelial system, including liver and spleen.

Here, progress can be achieved only if the relevant mechanism of tissue-antibody binding can be explained and if, with respect to tumor type and tumor antigen, it is possible to elucidate the binding sites (extracellular or intracellular) of the MAB and the accessibility of the respective target antigens [5, 11, 15]. This problem has two basic aspects: first, antibody transport by the circulation into the tissue; second, the amount and distribution of the target antigen in the tumor itself [16, 18]. Both aspects are of major importance, in particular with respect to the deliberate manipulation of the targeting process. At present, only an incomplete study is possible. However, the ex vivo perfusion system seems to be an important link between animal models and implementation in humans.

Animal models, by their very nature, are artificial, since human tumors typically implanted in nude mice are (mono-)clonal. The antigen expression is generally homogeneous, and the intratumoral connective tissue - in particular, the vascular system of the tumor - is derived from the mouse. The clinical accessibility is restricted to the interpretation of the immunoscintigraphy, which in terms of time and space is relatively crude.

The perfusion of operatively acquired human tumor tissue can bridge this gap. The main advantages of the ex vivo perfusion technique are illustrated by the following facts:

1. The kinetics of binding and clearance in tumor tissue can be measured by direct scintigraphy after resection.
2. The final result, i.e., the local distribution of the antibody, can be documented with high-resolution equipment, quantitated, and determined by autoradiography.

Comparing the immunohistologic and autoradiographic measurements according to the tissue distribution of the antigen, conclusions about the accessibility of the target antigen can be reached. Of course, some limitations will have to be accepted with the ex vivo perfusion technique and must be considered in the interpretation of data. Most notable and in contrast to scintigraphy is the substantially shortened interval allowed for examination of the tumor patient, which is directly limited by the development of ischemic edema in the preparation. Another disadvantage of this method is based on the nature of the experiment, in which each variable will have to be tested in a number of individual experiments using different tumor preparations.

References

1. Beatty JD, Duda RB, Williams LE, Sheibani K, Paxtron RJ, Beatty BG, Philben VJ, Werner JL, Shively JE, Vlahos WG, Kokal WA, Riihimaki DU, Terz JJ, Wagman LD (1986) Preoperative imaging of colorectal carcinoma with ^{111}In-labeled anti-carcinoembryotic antigen antibody. Cancer Res 46: 6494-6502
2. Biersack HJ, Bockisch A, Vogel J, Oehr P, Hansen HH, Hartlapp J, Biltz H, Jaeger N, Bellmann O (1987) Szintigraphischer Malignomnachweis mit radioaktiv markierten Tumorantikörpern. Dtsch Med Wochenschr 112: 341-344
3. Bradwell AR, Vaughan ATM, Dykes PW (1986) Limitations in localising and killing tumours using radiolabelled antibodies. Nuklearmedizin 25: 245-248
4. Chatal JF, Saccavini JC, Fumoleau P, Douillard JY, Curtet C, Kremer M, Le Mevel B, Koprowsky H (1984) Immunoscintigraphy of colon carcinoma. J Nucl Med 25: 307-314
5. Epenetos AA, Snook D, Durbin H, Johnson PM, Taylor-Papadimitriou J (1986) Limitations of radiolabelled monoclonal antibodies for localization of human neoplasms. Cancer Res 46: 3183-3191
6. Esteban JM, Colcher D, Sugarbaker C, Carrasquillo JA, Bryant G, Thor A, Reynold JC, Larson SM, Schlom J (1987) Quantitative and qualitative aspects of radiolocalization in colon cancer patients of intravenously administered MAB B72.3. Int J Cancer 39: 50-59
7. Gold P, Freedman SO (1965) Specific carcinoembryonic antigens of the human digestive system. J Exp Med 122: 467-481
8. Goldenberg DM, LeLand F, Kim E, Bennett S, Primus FJ, van Nagell JR, Estes N, DeSimone P, Rayburn P (1978) Use of radiolabelled antibodies to carcinoembryonic antigen for the detection and localization of diverse tumours by external photoscanning. N Engl J Med 298: 1384-1388
9. Goldenberg DM, Kim EE, Bennett SJ, Owens-Nelson M, Deland FH (1983) Carcinoembryonic antigen radioimmunodetection in the evaluation of colorectal cancer and in the detection of occult neoplasms. Gastroenterology 84: 524-532
10. Griffiths AB, Burchel J, Gendler S, Lewis A, Blight K, Tilly R, Taylor-Papadimitriou J (1987) Immunological analysis of mucin molecules expressed by normal and malignant epithelial cells. Int J Cancer 40: 319-327
11. Halpern SE, Dillman RO (1987) Problems associated with radioimmunodetection and possibilities for future solutions. J Biol Response Mod 6: 235-262
12. Larson SM, Carrasquillo JA, Reynolds JC (1984) Radioimmunodetection and radioimmunotherapy. Can Invest 2 (5): 363-381
13. Mach JP, Buchegger F, Forni M, Ritschard J, Carrel S, Egley R, Donath A, Rohner A (1980) Tumour localization of radiolabeled antibodies against carcinoembryonic antigen in patients with carcinoma. N Engl J Med 303: 5-10
14. Mach JP, Bischof-Delaloye A, Curchod S (1987) L'immunoscintigraphie par les anticorps monoclonaux radiomarqués. Schweiz Med Wochenschr 117: 1076-1086
15. Moshakis V, Omerod MG, Westgood JH, Imrie S, Neville AM (1982) The site of binding of anti-CEA antibodies to tumour CEA in vivo: An immunochemical and autoradiographic approach. Br J Cancer 46: 18-21
16. Readin CL, Hutchins JT (1985) Carbohydrate structure in tumour immunity. Cancer Metastasis Rev 4: 221-260
17. Sears HF, Herlyn M, Grotzinger PJ, Steplewski Z, Gerhard W, Koprowski H (1981) Ex vivo perfusion of a tumour-containing colon with monoclonal antibody. J Surg Res 31: 145-150
18. Taylor-Papadimitriou J, Peterson JA, Arklie J, Burchell J, Ceriani RL, Wedmer WF (1981) Monoclonal antibodies to epithelium-specific components of the human milk fat globule membrane: Production and reaction with cells in culture. Int J Cancer 28: 17-21

CHEMOTHERAPY AND HORMONAL THERAPY

Chemotherapy: Benefits and Limits*

G. FALKSON[1]

Introduction

It is fortunate that the three treatment modalities for cancer, surgery, radiotherapy and chemotherapy (as given by a medical oncologist), are complementary and seldom compete with one another.

Significant advances have been made in the field of medical oncology, and these are attributed not only to the continued availability of better chemotherapy, but also to the better understanding of the biology of cancer that has resulted from clinical trials. The benefits and limits of chemotherapy, both on its own and in combination with other modalities, are currently being better delineated by prospective, randomised clinical trials. Increased input by statisticians has improved understanding in both planning and executing trials.

The ultimate benefit for the patient is cure. Control of the disease, especially when complete or good partial remission is obtained, is of definite benefit and is increasingly being achieved. The most accurate measure of the effects of control, even in the absence of cure, is survival time. Benefit also is obtained when the disease is partially controlled, even in the absence of survival gain. In all the above categories, there is no doubt that it is possible to improve the quality of life with chemotherapy.

Benefits Versus Limits

Knowing the limits of chemotherapy enables the informed doctor to withhold those agents when they would do more harm than good. There is, unfortunately, no panacea. The therapeutic index of treatment with chemotherapy is the all-important factor. There are no chemotherapeutic agents that do not have toxic side effects. The relationship between the effective dose and the toxic dose determines the therapeutic index for a particular drug in each disease. For example, a curative dose of cyclophosphamide can be given for Burkitt's disease but not for breast cancer; a curative dose of methotrexate can be given for choriocarcinoma but not for cancer of the head and neck.

---

* Supported in part by grants from the National Cancer Association of South Africa and the David and Freda Becker Trust.

[1] Department of Medical Oncology, University of Pretoria, Private Bag X169, Pretoria 0001, Republic of South Africa.

H. G. Beger et al. (Eds.), Cancer Therapy

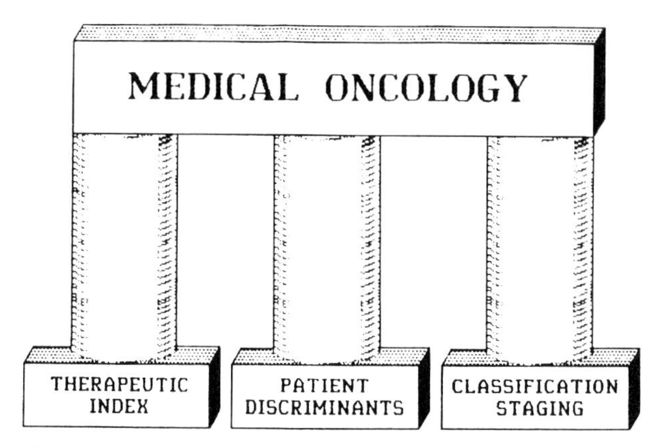

Fig. 1. Benefits and limitations of chemotherapy

The major indications for chemotherapy in the treatment of cancer are in the presence of advanced disease. The results that can be obtained are dominated by patient characteristics, the most important being age, sex, performance status, concurrent disease and site of metastases. These factors are the definition of the patient as an individual.

The benefits and limits of chemotherapy for patients with cancer in 1988 are determined by: (a) the therapeutic index of the agents currently available, (b) the relative importance of patient discriminants and (c) the classification and stage of a particular type of malignant neoplasm (Fig. 1). When the therapeutic index of an agent is good, the effect of patient characteristics becomes less important. At the present time, however, patient discriminants tend to have greater prognostic significance for most patients with solid tumors than the effect of the drugs available. For example, platinum-containing drug combinations give an expected cure rate for patients with testicular cancer, but if the patient has concomitant kidney disease, a therapeutic dose of platinum cannot be given. Similarly, in diffuse, large-cell non-Hodgkin's lymphoma, a good cure rate is expected when anthracycline combination chemotherapy is administered, but if the patient has concomitant heart disease, a therapeutic dose of anthracycline is contraindicated.

It is considered important to start chemotherapy at an optimal dose. A low dose has less chance of producing a response, and increasing the dose later is almost never of value in the clinic. It is important to attempt to administer an adequate dose to cross the therapeutic threshold.

Combination chemotherapy is usually so designed that different agents with different side effects are given together to gain a therapeutic effect without compounding the toxic side effects. Of increasing interest is the use of drug combinations in which one agent blocks at least some of the toxic effects of the others, e.g., nephrotoxicity and urothelial toxicity induced by ifosfamide can be prevented by giving mesna. In 1972, we concluded that a high dose of ifosfamide could not be administered because of nephrotoxicity [2], whereas by 1982 we could give a high dose by administering mesna concomitantly [3].

The schedule of chemotherapy and of the chemotherapy combinations used can sometimes increase the benefit obtained enormously, as in Hodgkin's disease. In diseases such as breast cancer [10, 13, 15], however, many of the theoretical models that predict much better results with different scheduling have not been validated by clinical trial data.

Limits

In limits of chemotherapy are the toxic effects on normal organ systems. The limiting toxic effects are predictable in time, and the type of toxicity is predictable for particular chemotherapy, be it a single drug or a drug combination. The organs that can be affected include the haemopoietic system, the mucous membranes, the gastrointestinal system including the liver, the genitourinary system including the kidneys and bladder, the heart and the central and peripheral nervous systems. Local toxicity can also be of importance.

Haematologic Toxicity

Haematologic toxicity is the most common limiting toxic effect of chemotherapy. The effects of different agents on white cells, platelets and haemoglobin all differ. In most treatment regimens, there is a tendency toward cumulative toxicity, which can be observed by comparing the values at the beginning of each treatment cycle. If, however, the nadir counts are plotted, by the third cycle of treatment, the nadir is lower. Some agents have a more cumulative toxic effect on the white blood cells and others, on platelets. An example is 4′epi-doxorubicin (given to patients with advanced colonic cancer), where the nadir white-cell count by the third cycle is significantly lower than after the first cycle, whereas these patients showed no difference in nadir platelet counts by the third cycle [5].

An illustration of the importance of haematologic toxicity can be seen in a series of more than 600 patients with advanced breast cancer (prospectively studied by the Eastern Cooperative Oncology Group [ECOG]), who were treated with 135 mg/m^2 dibromodulcitol orally days 2–11, 45 mg/m^2 doxorubicin (Adriamycin) IV on day 1 (maximum cumulative dose, 500 mg/m^2), 2.0 mg vincristine IV on day 1, 20 mg tamoxifen per os daily and 20 mg fluoxymesterone per os daily. Ten percent of the patients developed life-threatening leukopenia, 5% life-threatening thrombocytopenia, 37% severe leukopenia and 13% severe thrombocytopenia. An additional 4% of the patients developed mild to moderate leukopenia, and 3% developed mild to moderate thrombocytopenia. It is obvious that the dose could not be increased; the highest tolerated dose was used, and the good response rate could not have been improved by increasing the dose because only increased toxicity would have occurred. Investigations showed that most cases of life-threatening toxicity occurred during the first three cycles of chemotherapy. This shows that an optimal dose was given and that further toxicity was limited by correct dose modification [7].

Mucosal Toxicity

Mucosal toxicity can be minimized by prophylactic hygienic measures, especially in the oral cavity.

Urologic Toxicity

Toxicity to the kidneys and bladder can be decreased by prophylactic diuretic procedures.

Cardiotoxicity

Cardiotoxicity can be predicted and is usually related to the high total dose of the drug administered. Radionuclide angiography can be used to measure baseline ventricular ejection function, and changes in the cardiac ejection fraction can be monitored. In studies conducted in Pretoria for example, the median dose administered before a $>10\%$ reduction in left ventricular ejection fraction (LVEF) in patients treated with 4′epi-doxorubicin was 753 mg/m^2. The median cumulative dose administered before clinical indications of cardiotoxicity were observed was 1030 mg/m^2. The median dose given before a $\geq 10\%$ reduction in LVEF in patients treated with mitoxantrone was 51.4 mg/m^2. None of the patients treated with mitoxantrone developed clinical indication of cardiotoxicity. This shows that, although there was a significant decrease in LVEF in 30% of our patients who were treated for longer than 3 months with both 4′epi-doxorubicin and mitoxantrone, there is a definite difference in the degree of cardiotoxicity between those treated with 4′epi-doxorubicin and those treated with mitoxantrone. The cardiotoxicity documented with mitoxantrone occurred mainly in patients previously treated with doxorubicin, and non of the patients treated with mitoxantrone alone developed clinical manifestations of heart disease [16].

Alopecia and Local Toxicity

Some side effects, while only of cosmetic importance (e.g., alopecia), cannot be ignored, while other side effects (e.g., local toxicity) can be avoided by taking greater care with drug-administering techniques.

Benefits

Chemotherapy is absolutely indicated because of its definite predictive value in most forms of haemopoietic neoplasia, in pediatric cancer and in some types of urologic cancer. It is of value for breast cancer, ovarian cancer and small-cell lung cancer. It is of limited value for gastrointestinal cancer, malignant melanoma and sarcoma. It is of doubtful value for non-small-cell lung cancer, head and neck and other squamous-cell carcinomas (Fig. 2).

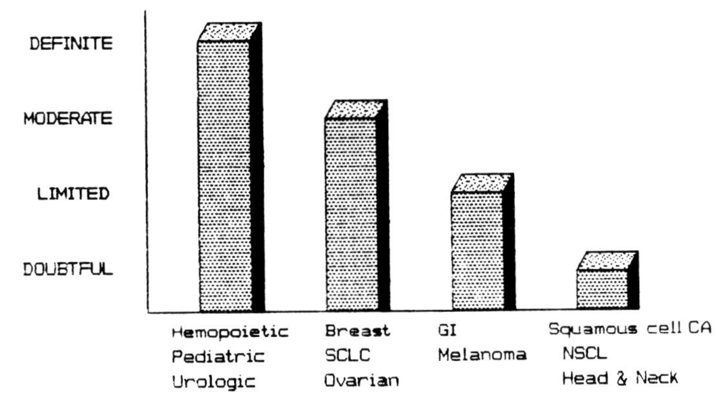

Fig. 2. Chemotherapy: benefit relative to limitations

The results being achieved in childhood cancer, especially acute lymphatic leukemia, are well known and, like the results in Hodgkin's disease and lymphoma, are reproducible with high cure rates throughout the world. The dramatic change in the prognosis of patients with testicular cancer illustrates how even a very toxic chemotherapy treatment can be accepted when it results in cure. Short-term toxic chemotherapy has changed non-seminomatous testicular cancer from a usually incurable, short-prognosis disease to a usually curable disease.

The limited but sometimes visually dramatic results in symptomatic chemotherapy are illustrated by the use of mitotane in functional adrenal cancer and somatostatin in amine precursor uptake and decarboxylation cell (APUD) tumors. The gonadotropin-releasing hormone analogs (GnRhA) not only give response on their own in prostate [9] and breast cancer, but combinations with chemotherapy are producing interesting preliminary results. The benefits and limitations of chemotherapy are illustrated in two diseases based on our own experience, namely metastatic breast cancer and hepatocellular carcinoma.

Metastatic Breast Cancer as an Example of Benefits Versus Limits

In metastatic breast cancer, the ±20%-response rate on LPAM clearly differs from the 65%-79%-response rate on cyclophosphamide, doxorubicin and fluorouracil (CAF) [1, 4, 8] and the 79%-response rate obtained in premenopausal women (with estrogen receptor (ER)-unknown disease). The best response rate (89%) is obtained with CAF in conjunction with oophorectomy for patients with ER-unknown disease.

The improved response rates in metastatic breast cancer are being translated into survival times. In our experience, the median survival time for patients treated with single agents, such as melphalan, was 7 months and improved to 13 months on cyclophosphamide, methotrexate and fluorouracil (CMF) and to 19 months on CMF plus prednisone. The median survival time with CAF is more than

20 months and for premenopausal women, 29 months, rising to 41 and 43 months respectively if they have ER-positive or ER-unknown disease.

While this clearly shows increasing benefits for treatment with chemotherapy, the limits of current chemotherapy are illustrated by the finding that patient discriminants continue to play a relatively important role. When patients are treated with CAF (the best of the currently used combination cytostatics), the median survival times obtained for patients with one metastatic site are 31 months, with two metastatic sites, 23 months and with three metastatic sites, 11 months. For patients with osseous metastases, the median survival is 30 months, whereas it is ± 19 months for those with visceral or soft-tissue metastases. While the number of organs afflicted with metastases affects the response rate and the survival time, the organ predominately afflicted with metastases does not affect the response rate but does affect the survival time [4].

We were able to show that a combination of dibromodulcitol (DBD) plus doxorubicin (Adriamycin) (ADM) was superior to either DBD or ADM alone [12] and that DBD + ADM in combination with tamoxifen (TMX) was superior to DBD + ADM [14]. Dibromodulcitol + ADM + vincristine + TMX + fluoxymesterone (DAVTH) proved slightly more effective in treating metastatic breast cancer than CAF [13] and was effective in treating patients with metastatic breast cancer [7].

Recent cumulative experience has shown that a small percentage of the patients treated with DBD develop myelodysplasia and/or acute non-lymphatic leukemia. As this occurs in the long-term survivors, it is important and illustrates one of the limits of chemotherapy. Dibromodulcitol could, therefore, not be considered for inclusion in an adjuvant regimen.

In a study in which 18 prognostic factors in 1168 patients undergoing treatment for metastatic breast cancer by ECOG were analyzed, it was clearly shown that younger patients, irrespective of menopausal status, had shorter survival times [6]. The predicted median survival times after the first recurrence of disease were 491 days for patients ≤ 35 years of age, 590 days for patients 36–45 years of age and 700 days for those > 45 years of age. The only age group in which menopausal differences relative to age was significant was the 46–55-year-old group, where premenopausal patients had a median survival time of 30 months compared with 20 months for postmenopausal patients.

A further important effect of age as a limitation for chemotherapy is seen in a study of elderly patients. Data from most cooperative group studies of breast cancer show few, if any, significant differences in chemotherapy tolerance between younger and older patients with breast cancer. It must, however, be borne in mind that there is a strong selection factor, and the number of patients over the age of 65 entered on trials is limited. In the ECOG study [11] comparing CMF to TMX as the first treatment for patients over 65 with metastatic breast cancer, it was shown that response rates were 38% for CMF and 45% for TMX with a median duration of response of 7.9 and 10.4 months, respectively. Furthermore, survival rates tended to favor TMX as the initial treatment, even in ER-negative patients [11].

Metastatic breast cancer serves as a good example of how the benefits of chemotherapy are slowly but steadily increasing owing to the availability of better chemotherapy and a better understanding of patient discriminants or the limits of chemotherapy.

Hepatocellular Carcinoma as an Example of the Limits Versus the Benefits of Chemotherapy

Hepatocellular carcinoma serves as a second illustration of the advances made in understanding the importance of patient factors, enabling future chemotherapy trials to be performed more scientifically. The ECOG studied 432 patients with hepatocellular carcinoma. As standard eligibility criteria were used in all the studies and as the same endpoints were defined for all the studies, valid statistical conclusions could be made (G. Falkson et al., 1988, Prognostic Factors for Survival in Hepatocellular Carcinoma, unpublished work). The 301 North American and 131 South African patients received similar treatment at the same time.
Bedridden patients, patients with other serious disease or inadequately functioning organs were not included in the studies. The overall median survival time was 14 weeks. Single factors associated with survival were age, sex, race, country of origin, performance status (PS), weight loss, disease symptoms and cirrhosis. A more complete analysis of multifactors showed important prognostic factors to be performance status (PS)[1], sex, country of origin, age, disease and disease symptoms, while race and cirrhosis were insignificant. Among 368 patients with a PS of 0–2, the median survival time was 16 weeks; among 64 patients with a PS of 3, the median survival time was only 7 weeks ($P = <0.01$). Patients with a PS of 4 were not included in the study. The importance of these findings in interpreting the results obtained with chemotherapy are apparent in the following examples: a) a North American female with a good PS without jaundice or loss of appetite who is less than 45 years of age has a 68% probability of surviving 6 months; b) a South African male with a good PS, jaundice and loss of appetite who is more than 45 years old has only a 5%-chance of surviving 6 months. In this analysis, only two of the chemotherapy regimens were associated with survival. Oral 5-fluorouracil, despite very little toxicity, was associated with a shorter survival time. This finding is of importance to those seeking non-toxic chemotherapy. The intravenous application of 5-fluorouracil plus methyl-Semustine appeared to result in a longer survival time. Studies of hepatocellular cancer show how the benefits and limitations of chemotherapy can be better understood by examining the individual patients. This may be helpful in planning future treatment with chemotherapy.
The benefits obtained with chemotherapy in the treatment of patients with cancer continue to expand as the limits of chemotherapy are better understood. The number of patients with different types of cancer being cured by chemotherapy is slowly but steadily increasing. In some types of cancer, better disease control and longer survival times are being achieved. For many of the major types of cancer, the benefits of chemotherapy remain limited, but both expanding knowledge of the biology of cancer and increasing experience with chemotherapy are enabling us to make advances in treating patients with malignant neoplasms. Despite toxicity, chemotherapy, when used judiciously, can improve the quality of the patient's life by helping control disease.

[1] Performance status key: 0, normal activity; 1, symptoms but ambulatory; 2, in bed less than 50% of time; 3, in bed more than 50% of time; 4, 100% bedridden; 9, unknown.

The medical doctor who hopes to enable all of his patients to live forever will quickly be disillusioned when dealing with cancer patients. Chemotherapy is, however, often effective if the doctor is informed about its possible benefits and limits.

References

Bull JM, Tormey DC, Li S-H, Carbone PP, Falkson G, Blom J, Perlin E, Simon R (1978) A randomized comparative trial of adriamycin versus methotrexate in combination drug therapy. Cancer 41: 1649-1657

van Dyk JJ, Falkson HC, van der Merwe AM, Falkson G (1972) Unexpected toxicity in patients treated with iphosphamide. Cancer Res 32: 921-924

Falkson G, van Dyk JJ, Stapelberg R, Falkson HC (1982) Mesnum as a protector against kidney and bladder toxicity with high-dose ifosfamide treatment. Cancer Chemother Pharmacol 9: 81-84

Falkson G, Gelman RS, Tormey DC, Cummings FJ, Carbone PP, Falkson HC (1985) The Eastern Cooperative Oncology Group experience with cyclophosphamide, adriamycin, and 5-fluorouracil (CAF) in patients with metastatic breast cancer. Cancer 56: 219-224

Falkson G, Klein B, Falkson H (1985) Hematological toxicity: experience with anthracyclines and anthracenes. Exp Hematol [Suppl 16] 13: 64-71

Falkson G, Gelman RS, Pretorius FJ (1986) Age as a prognostic factor in recurrent breast cancer. J Clin Oncol 4 (5): 663-671

Falkson G, Gelman RS, Glick JH (1987) The induction efficiency of dibromodulcitol, adriamycin, vincristine, tamoxifen and fluoxymesterone in the treatment of patients with metastatic breast cancer. Proc Am Soc Clin Oncol (abstr) 6: 49

Falkson G, Gelman RS, Tormey DC, Falkson CI, Wolter JM, Cummings FJ (1987) Treatment of metastatic breast cancer in premenopausal women using CAF with or without oophorectomy: An Eastern Cooperative Oncology Group study. J Clin Oncol 5 (6): 881-889

Falkson G, Vorobiof DA (1987) Intranasal buserelin in the treatment of advanced prostatic cancer: a phase II trial. J Clin Oncol 5 (9): 1419-1423

Loprinzi CL, Tormey DC, Rasmussen P, Falkson G, Davis TE, Falkson HC, Chang AYC (1986) Prospective evaluation of carcinoembryonic antigen levels and alternating chemotherapeutic regimens in metastatic breast cancer. J Clin Oncol 4 (1): 46-56

Taylor SG, Gelman RS, Falkson G, Cummings FJ (1986) Combination chemotherapy compared to tamoxifen as initial therapy for stage IV breast cancer in elderly women. Ann Intern Med 104: 455-461

Tormey DC, Simon R, Falkson G, Bull J, Band P, Perlin E, Blom J (1977) Evaluation of adriamycin and dibromodulcitol in metastatic breast carcinoma. Cancer Res 37: 529-534

Tormey DC, Falkson G, Simon RM, Blom J, Bull JM, Lippman ME, Li S-H, Cassidy JG, Falkson HC (1979) A randomized comparison of two sequentially administered combination regimens to a single regimen in metastatic breast cancer. Cancer Clin Trials 2: 247-256

Tormey DC, Falkson G, Crowley J, Falkson HC, Voelkel J, Davis TE (1982) Dibromodulcitol and adriamycin ± tamoxifen in advanced breast cancer. Am J Clin Oncol (CCT) 5: 33-39

Tormey D, Gelman R, Falkson G (1983) Prospective evaluation of rotating chemotherapy in advanced breast cancer: An Eastern Cooperative Oncology Group trial. Am J Clin Oncol (CCT) 6: 1-18

Vorobiof DA, Iturralde M, Falkson G (1985) Assessment of ventricular function by radionuclide angiography in patients receiving 4'epidoxorubicin and mitoxantrone. Cancer Chemother Pharmacol 15: 253-257

The Human Tumor Clonogenic Assay for the Prediction of Tumor Sensitivity

H. P. KRAEMER[1] and H. H. SEDLACEK[1]

It is well known that human tumors even of comparable histology are quite heterogeneous with respect to their sensitivity to cytotoxic drugs (Table 1). As a result, the response of individual patients to a standard treatment protocol with cytotoxic drugs is variable, and, for the majority of solid tumors, response rates of only 30%–40% are quite common. Those patients who do not respond will nevertheless be subjected to all the problems of drug toxicity in spite of the ineffectiveness of the treatment. Finally, new drugs with an interesting spectrum of activity can only be given to patients who do not respond to standard chemotherapy. These nonresponders, however, will have a decreased probability of response to new drugs as a consequence of their pretreatment with toxic but ineffective standard drugs.
Consequently, it is clear that any pretherapeutic test that could predict the sensitivity or resistance of an individual patient to a treatment regimen would help to overcome some of the above-mentioned problems. For example, the test would help to identify those patients with tumors resistant to the standard protocol, thus sparing them an ineffective but toxic standard treatment. If the pretherapeutic assay has sufficient selectivity and specificity, the treatment of the individual patient could even be directed by the test results, provided a sufficient number of potentially active drugs (standard drugs or new drugs under development) are included in such a pretherapeutic test. This individualization of chemotherapy would be comparable to the treatment of bacterial infections after having tested the sensitivity of the bacteria by an antibiogram (Table 2).
During the last 10 years, the human tumor clonogenic assay has been used as such a pretherapeutic chemosensitivity assay for cancer patients [1–4]. In this test sys-

Table 1. Chemotherapy today

- Low response rate to standard protocols
- Toxic but ineffective treatment
- New drugs available only for patients who have not responded to previous treatment

Table 2. Advantages of pretherapeutic chemosensitivity tests

- Selection of those patients who might benefit from standard treatment
- Avoidance of toxic side effects of ineffective treatment for patients with resistant tumors
- Early selection of new agents for individualized treatment of otherwise resistant tumors

[1] Department of Experimental Medicine, Behringwerke AG Marburg, P.O. Box 1140, 3550 Marburg 1, FRG.

H. G. Beger et al. (Eds.), Cancer Therapy

Table 3. Human tumor clonogenic assay as a pretherapeutic test[a]

– Sensitivity (true positives/true negatives + false negatives):	80%	
– Specificity (TN/TN + FP):	86%	n=2166 patients 45 clinical trials 31 institutions
– Predictive value:		
for sensitivity:	69%	
for resistance:	95%	
– Increased response rate (and survival) for patients treated according to test results		
– About 70% of all tumors grow in vitro		

[a] According to von Hoff [3].
TN, true negative responses; *FP*, false positive responses.

tem, human tumor material is enzymatically digested, and the resulting tumor cell suspension is incubated with each test drug in several concentrations (related to peak plasma levels). After extensive washes, the cells are plated in soft agar, and the reduction in formation of tumor colonies seen after 2–4 weeks is used as an indicator of drug activity. The clinical correlations obtained with this assay are summarized in a review published recently by von Hoff (Table 3) [3]. During the last 10 years, 45 clinical trials at 31 different institutions were performed, including a total of nearly 2200 patients. From these trials, the sensitivity and specificity of the assay was calculated to be 80% and 86% respectively. The predictive value of the assay for sensitivity of a tumor was 69%; the predictive value for resistance was 92%. In addition, it was possible to demonstrate that, after treatment (according to test results), patients showed increased response rates and, in one study, even increased survival when compared with patients treated with drugs of their clinician's choice. Owing to technical modifications, it was possible to increase the growth rate of tumor biopsies in this assay from an average of 25% in 1983 [5] to 70% in 1986 [3].

The potential influence of such a pretherapeutic assay on cancer chemotherapy can be demonstrated in the following example (Table 4). A hypothetical tumor disease should have a clinical response rate to a standard protocol of 30%. Accordingly, treatment with the standard protocol would result in 30 responders and 70 nonresponders, who would however have to be treated with the standard protocol to identify their resistance. Those 70 pretreated patients could subsequently be treated with other standard drugs or, if available, with new drugs under development.

Using the clonogenic assay, 70% of all tumor biopsies can be tested in vitro, and, assuming a sensitivity and specificity of the assay as discussed above, 24 of the patients tested would show sensitivity in the assay to the standard drugs. Of those 24 patients, 17 would also respond clinically (true positives), whereas 7 patients would not respond clinically (false positives). In addition, 30 patients whose tumors are not testable in vitro would be treated with a standard protocol, resulting in 9 responders and 21 nonresponders. Finally, 42 patients would be correctly identified as resistant (true negatives). Those resistant patients could be excluded from the standard protocol and treated with other standard drugs (especially if

Table 4. Use of clonogenic assay as a pretherapeutic test[a]

Treatment	Responders (*n*)	Nonresponders		Available for "non"-standard drugs
		treated (*n*)	untreated (*n*)	
Protocol	30	70	none	70 pretreated
70% tested	17 (TP) 4 (FN)	7 (FP)	42 (TN)	42 untreated
Test 30% not testable	9	21	none	28 pretreated

[a] Assumption: tumor with 30%-response rate to a standard protocol; pV(S)=69%; pV(R)=92%; 70% of all tumors testable in vitro.

TP, true positive; *TN*, true negative; *FP*, false positive; *FN*, false negative; *pV(S)*, predictive value for sensitivity; *pV(R)*, predictive value for resistance.

those drugs proved to be effective in the pretherapeutic test) or, if no drug proved effective, the patients could be spared a toxic but ineffective treatment.

Up to now, the specificity of the assay is only 92%. Thus, four patients who would respond clinically would not be identified by the test (false negatives). It is obvious that the possibility of a small number of false-negative test results will limit the broad clinical application of any chemosensitivity test. A potential reason for false-negative test results is related to the fact that most patients are treated clinically with combinations of drugs, whereas the in vitro tests are performed for each single drug separately. However, the possibility exists that a combination of three drugs, each being only marginally active, might produce a clinical response as a consequence of synergism among the individual drugs. Therefore, one can speculate that, by testing drug combinations in vitro, the possibility of false-negative test results could be decreased in the future. Several theoretical and technical problems must just be solved, however.

In summary, the calculation summarized in Table 4 demonstrates that the use of the clonogenic assay as a pretherapeutic test will have some benefit for the majority of tumor patients, either by preventing unnecessary toxicity or by selecting an active drug, which would not have been selected by the clinician.

Several fundamental problems accompanying any in vitro test system should be mentioned (Table 5). First of all, it is obvious that the growth of tumor cells in vitro is quite different from the in vivo growth with respect to microenvironment, cell-to-cell contact, diffusion of nutrients and drugs, etc. In addition, it is known that the pharmacokinetics of an antitumor drug varies among different patients, and the vascularization of individual tumors is heterogeneous. As a consequence, one must expect that different drug levels within individual tumors and patients are reached after an identical drug dose. Therefore, the sensitivity of a tumor at the cellular level as measured by any in vitro assay might not lead to a clinical response for all patients because the drug might not reach the tumor in sufficient amounts. In addition, tumor nodules in a single patient might even differ in their sensitivity to cytotoxic drugs, and thus a biopsy from a single nodule might not predict the sensitivity of another nodule in the same patient.

Table 5. Principal problems of in vitro chemosensitivity tests

- In vitro tumor growth quite different from in vivo growth
- Patient variation in tumor vascularization and drug pharmacokinetics
- Heterogeneity of different tumor lesions in a single patient
- Necessity of relating in vitro dosage (concentration, incubation time) to in vivo situation

Finally, for any predictive test, the drug concentration and incubation time in vitro must be related to the in vivo situation with respect to tumor concentration and tumor cell exposure time. Because of the heterogeneity of individual patients, only approximative procedures are used. However, irrespective of these fundamental problems, the predictive value of the clonogenic assay lies between 70% and 92%, which demonstrates that the approximations used today are neither perfect nor completely unrealistic.

For 6 years, our group has used the clonogenic assay with human tumor xenografts to identify drugs with a new spectrum of activity, especially against slowly growing, solid human tumors which are refractory to treatment. In addition to this, we have recently started using the clonogenic assay to predict the sensitivity or resistance of individual patients. The first aim of this study was to establish a procedure which allows the transportation of tumor biopsies from different tumor centers to our institution for testing. Therefore, technical conditions that maintain the viability and sterility of the tumor cells have to be established. A summary of the technical performance status of the first 209 tumors is summarized in Fig. 1.

With the exception of 26 tumors transported from Italy by plane, we had no problems with transport logistics. A total of 178 tumors could be tested; 135 of these had a tumor weight of ≥1 g. The assay could be performed successfully in 66% of all tumor samples and in 76% of all tumors with a tumor weight >1 g. Of these successful assays, in 25% (or 29% for tumors >1 g) at least one active drug could be identified in vitro, whereas in 41% (or 47% of tumors >1 g), no drug proved effective.

Thirty-four percent of all tumors (or 24% of those tumors >1 g) showed technical problems. The main problems were the lack of a sufficient number of tumor cells for broad testing in 18% of all tumors (12% of the tumors >1 g) and the lack of any tumor growth in vitro in 10% of all tumors (7% of the tumors >1 g). Contaminated samples were seen only in 5% of all biopsies.

Owing to the short duration of this study (1 year), no final results are available making it possible to correlate the prediction by this assay and the final clinical outcome. From the data summarized in Fig. 1, it is obvious that there are some technical problems, which have to be improved for the clonogenic assay (Table 6). First of all, it is necessary to decrease the cell number needed for a single drug test because 12%–18% of all tumor samples could not be tested sufficiently owing to the low number of cells isolated from these biopsies. Furthermore, the in vitro growth conditions for some tumors (leukemia, breast tumor) must be improved because those tumors do not grow sufficiently in a number of cases. In addition, technical modifications of the assay to test drug combinations in vitro are also urgently needed because this might be a possibility to decrease the number of false-

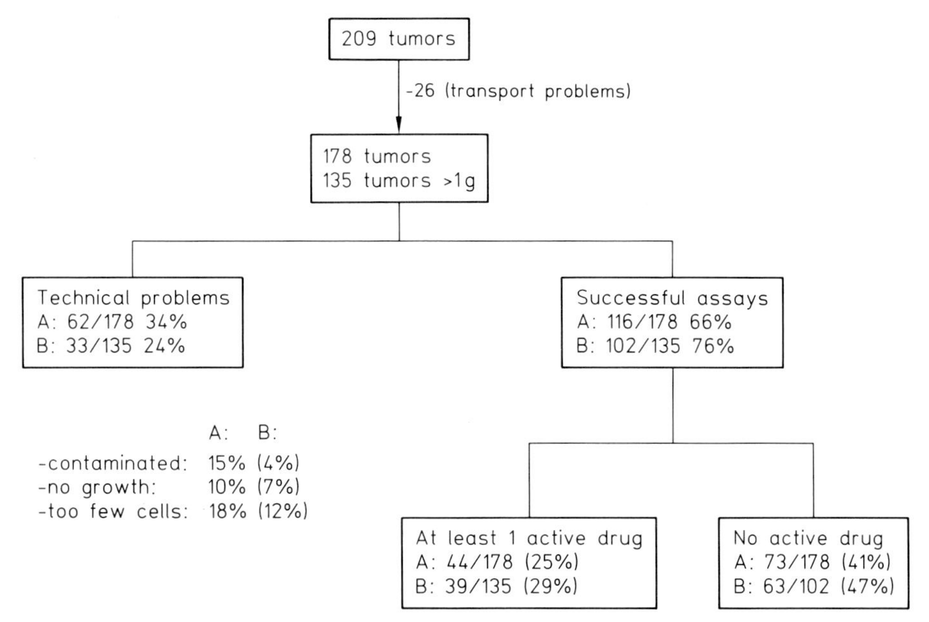

Fig. 1. Experience with the clonogenic assay at Behringwerke, Marburg, FRG. *A*, all tumors; *B*, tumors > 1 g

Table 6. How to improve the clonogenic assay

- Decrease the cell number per drug test (for 12%–18% of biopsies)
- Optimize growth conditions (for 7%–10% of biopsies)
- Test drug combinations in vitro
- Identify new drugs (for 40%–60% of all biopsies)

negative test results, as discussed above. Beside these technical problems, however, we feel that the real "rate-limiting step" of any tumor sensitivity assay today is the lack of active drugs for the majority of tumors. Therefore, we propose a combination of our human-tumor-based test systems, which would help to identify new active drugs by means of the patient-oriented pretherapeutic sensitivity assay. This could be used not only to identify new drugs for solid human tumors but also to improve the clinical results more individualized through treatment of patients with new drugs. A schematic standard treatment of tumors that prove to be resistant to the standard drug could be avoided by such a pretherapeutic assay.

We are optimistic that this combination of new preclinical selection criteria with an individualization of chemotherapy might help to identify new drugs, at least for some solid tumor types. Thus, the pessimistic argument that new antitumor drugs have not been detected because they do not exist might hopefully be refuted in the future.

References

1. Salmon SE, Trent JM (1984) (eds) Human tumor cloning. Grune and Stratton, Orlando
2. Hanauske AR, von Hoff DD (1985) Clinical correlations with the human tumor cloning assay. Cancer Invest 3: 541-551
3. von Hoff DD (1987) In vitro predictive testing: sulfonamide era. Int J Cell Cloning 5: 179-190
4. Kern DH, Bertelsen CA (1984) Present status of chemosensitivity assays. Int Adv Surg Oncol 7: 187-213
5. von Hoff DD, Clark GM, Stogdill BJ, Sarosdy MF, O'Brien MT, Casper JT, Mattox DE, Page CP, Cruz AB, Sandbach JF (1983) Prospective clinical trial of a human tumor cloning system. Cancer Res 43: 1926-1931

Chemosensitivity – Directed Regional Chemotherapy of Liver Metastases

K. H. LINK[1]

Introduction

Regional chemotherapeutic procedures like intra-arterial infusion, isolation perfusion, chemoembolization, and intracavitary drug instillation can effectively achieve locoregional tumor growth control in tumor resistant to systemic chemotherapy [1, 9, 15] by taking advantage of the dose-response behaviour of tumors to most cytotoxic drugs [3, 4]. Although response rates are higher in regional than in systemic chemotherapy [10], there are treatment failures with either no response or only short remission periods. A recent analysis of treatment results from various protocols concerning regional chemotherapy of colorectal liver metastases yielded a mean response rate of 42%, with a range between 2.4% and 73.0%. The mean interval before disease progession was 8.2 months (range: 4.5–12.5 months) [8]. The variability of response rates is related to several factors, such as vascular access, infusion time, drug plasma concentration, tumor vascularization, and tumor sensitivity to the drug(s) of choice.

The drug selection for regional chemotherapy is usually deduced from effectiveness in systemic chemotherapy. Since chemotherapeutic agents in high concentrations show different response behaviors and histologically identical tumors demonstrate different individual sensitivities to identical drug treatments, we investigated different drugs' effects on colorectal liver metastases and other tumors when administered in high dose intra-arterial chemotherapy (HDIAC). For this purpose, tumor biopsies were tested for their chemosensitivity by means of the Human tumor colony-forming assay (HTCA) according to the method originally described by Hamburger and Salmon [5]. After ascertaining concentration-dependent high toxicity of the drugs tested in the HTCA with 55 tumors, mainly of colorectal origin, we investigated whether drugs active in the HTCA at high concentrations in vitro can be reliably selected for HDIAC of liver tumors. A previous prospective correlative trial in which in vitro chemosensitivity test results in the HTCA were correlated to the clinical outcome of HDIAC proved that clinical response and resistance could be predicted in vitro [12]. Therefore, we designed a pilot study in which liver metastases were treated with drugs proposed by chemosensitivity testing in the HTCA. Initial results are reported in this paper.

[1] Department of General Surgery, University of Ulm, Steinhövelstraße 9, 7900 Ulm, FRG.

H. G. Beger et al. (Eds.), Cancer Therapy

Table 1. Tumors tested in the human tumor colony-forming assay (1985-1986)

Type	n
Colorectal carcinoma (LM)	21
Glioblastoma	6
Melanoma (M)	4
Breast carcinoma (LM)	4
Cerebral tumors (M)	2
Ovarian carcinoma (M)	3
Lung (M)	1
Adenocarcinoma (LM)	3
Carcinoid (LM)	2
Hypernephroma (LM)	1
Gallbladder carcinoma (LM)	2
Colorectal primary/extrahepatic (M)	2
Liposarcoma	1
Schwannoma	1
Small-bowel carcinoma (LM)	1
Hepatocholangiocellular carcinoma	1

LM, liver metastases; *M*, metastases (extrahepatic).

Materials and Methods

Chemosensitivity Profiles

Test Drugs and Tumors

Sensitivity rates of drugs qualifying for regional chemotherapy were determined in the HTCA with a total of 55 tumors (Table 1). The drugs were tested at the concentration of 1 μg/ml and 10 μg/ml (adriamycin (ADM), cisplatin (CDDP), 4-epi-doxorubicin (EPI), mitomycin C (MMC), melphalan (L-PAM), mitoxantrone (NOV). Mafosfamide (MAF), and 5-Fluorouracil (5FU) were tested at 10 μg/ml or 100 μg/ml. The lower concentrations are regarded as representative for drug levels achievable clinically or, in the case of MAF experimentally. Sensitivity profiles based on the sequence of activity of the drugs were generated for colorectal liver metastases ($n=21$) and other solid tumors ($n=34$).

Human Tumor Colony-forming Assay (HTCA)

The HTCA was performed according to the method originally developed by Hamburger and Salmon [5] for drug testing with human material in systemic chemotherapy. The whole procedure has been described extensively elsewhere [12]. In short, tumor material was transported after excision to the laboratory where necrotic and connective nonmalignant tissue was removed, the tumor minced into 1- to 2-mm pieces mechanically, and then digested enzymatically overnight in a solution of 0.03% deoxiribonuclease and 0.14% collagenase. Then the suspension was filtered through sterile gauze, the filtrate pushed through 21-gauge needles to further disrupt the cellular complexes, and then washed twice. A suspension of 3×10^6 viable tumor cells per ml was then adjusted using trypan blue dye exclusion and microscopic cytological examination. Drugs were exposed to 1.5×10^6 viable tumor cells for 1 h at the concentrations indicated. Following incubation, the cells were washed twice and distributed over three 35-mm dishes at each test point in a soft agar, bilayer system. After 2-6 weeks, colonies could be identified. Colony growth of treated cells was calculated as a percentage of an untreated control. If colony growth was $< 50\%$ of the untreated control, a drug at the particular test concentration was regarded as active and the tumor evaluated as sensitive. If colony growth exceeded 50% of the untreated control the tumor colony was evaluated as resistant.

A typical colony of a colorectal carcinoma liver metastasis grown in soft agar is shown in Fig. 1. Figure 2 demonstrates a typical dose-response curve for various

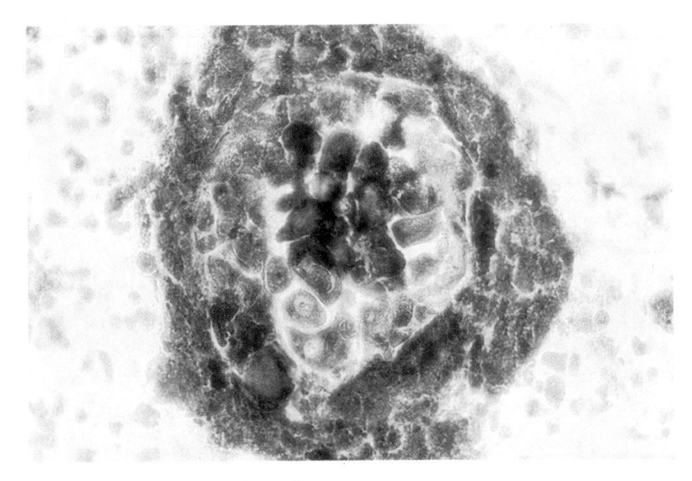

Fig. 1. HE-stained soft agar colony of a colorectal carcinoma

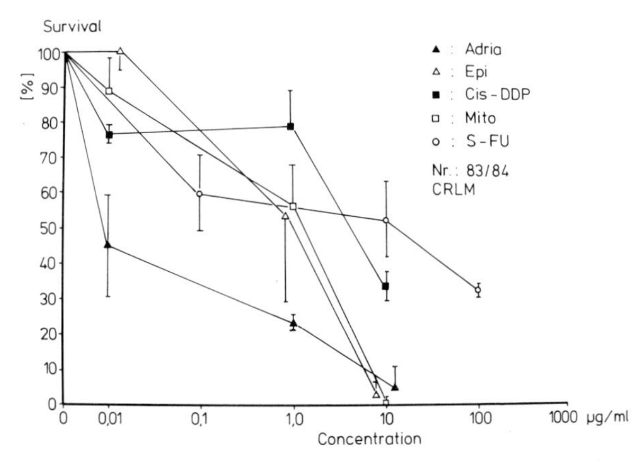

Fig. 2. Dose-response curve of a colorectal carcinoma liver metastasis in the human tumor colony-forming assay

test drugs in a colorectal carcinoma liver metastasis. Here, the five test drugs were exposed to the cell suspension at three concentrations, and colony growth decreased with increasing drug concentrations.

Decision-Aiding Pilot Study

Patients

In patients selected for the decision-aiding trial, drugs tested in the HTCA were chosen according to the priority lists of the chemosensitivity profiles. L-PAM and MAF were excluded owing to a lack of clinical experience in hepatic artery infusion with those drugs. After HTCA evaluation, the patients were treated according to their chemosensitivity in the HTCA, and the in vitro sensitivity/resistance was correlated to the clinical responses in HDIAC.
In the decision-aiding pilot study, nine patients (five male, four female) with a mean age of 60 years (range: 42–72) were included. Eight patients had isolated liver metastases of colorectal cancer (three patients), breast cancer (two patients), carcinoid tumors (two patients), and ovarian carcinoma (one patient), and one patient had a primary hepatocholangiocellular carcinoma. Tumor stages according to Pettavel [14] were I for one patient, II for three patients, and III for five patients (Table 2). Patients were referred to the study if they had either advanced colorectal liver metastases (the alternate standard treatment protocol for patients with colorectal liver metastases was MMC and 5 × 5-FU at 4-week intervals) or less frequent tumor types qualifying for regional chemotherapy but with no existing standard protocol for intra-arterial infusion. One patient had liver metastases of an initially unknown primary tumor (83/86) that later was diagnosed as a previously occult breast carcinoma.

Clinical Treatment

An implantable port catheter (Implantofix, B. Brown Melsungen AG, Melsungen, FRG) was inserted with the tip just reaching into the common hepatic artery via the peripherally ligated gastroduodenal artery. Collaterals and the right gastric artery were ligated, and prophylactic cholecystectomy was performed. Hepatic vascularization was "normal" in eight patients, with the right and the left hepatic artery originating from the proper hepatic artery. One patient (105/85) received an additional catheter into the right hepatic artery, which originated from the superior mesenteric artery. A biopsy was taken for histology, and drug testing in the HTCA. Since chemosensitivity testing usually requires at least 14 days, the patients received the first postoperative regional treatment cycle without HTCA results, unless soft agar growth was sufficient for early evaluation (in patients 71/86 and 83/86). Subsequently, the most active drug(s) (according to in vitro sensitivity testing) were infused, partly in combination with 5-FU. If the tumor turned out to be resistant in vitro, the patient was treated with a standard protocol (37/86) or with the drug most active in the resistant range (57/85). The patients were treated

Table 2. Patient characteristics of the decision-aiding pilot study

Patient number	Age (years)	Tumor type	Stage
87/84	56	Carcinoid LM	III
57/85	55	Hepatocholangiocellular carcinoma	III
102/85	59	Colorectal carcinoma LM	III
105/85	71	Colorectal carcinoma LM	II
34/86	70	Carcinoid LM	II
37/86	63	Colorectal carcinoma LM	III
64/86	64	Breast carcinoma LM	II
71/86	42	Ovarian carcinoma LM	I
83/86	56	Breast carcinoma LM	III

LM, liver metastases.
Lausanne classification according to Pettavel [14].

by hepatic artery infusion for 5–7 cycles. Responses were determined according to reduction of tumor marker serum levels (by more than 50% of the preoperative value) or to axial computed tomography (CT).

Results

Chemosensitivity Profiles

In Table 3, the test results of the various drugs at the test concentrations indicated are shown for colorectal liver metastases, other tumors, and all tumors tested. The sensitivity rates (sensitive tests/total tests; sensitive = inhibition of colony formation by > 50% as compared with an untreated control) served as an indicator for one drug's effect on a particular tumor category. In Table 4, the various drugs are ranked according to degree of drug activity at the two test concentrations used (sensitivity profile). At the concentration of 1 μg/ml, ADM, NOV, and MMC were among the most active drugs in each category. In colorectal carcinoma, CDDP was the third most active drug.

Decision-Aiding Pilot Study

Of the nine patients, seven were sensitive to at least one test drug in the HTCA, and two were resistant at the concentration range achievable by intra-arterial infusion (Table 5).

In seven patients, the in vitro tests results correlated correctly with the predicted clinical responses (six sensitive in vitro/responsive in vivo, one resistant in vitro/resistant in vivo). In two patients, the in vitro/in vivo results did not correlate: one patient (37/86) was predicted to be resistant but actually showed a partial response. This patient received two MMC infusions with a reduction of arterial blood flow before the relevant HTCA result was available. A dose of 1 μg/ml

Table 3. Chemosensitivity test results of colorectal carcinoma liver metastases (LM), other tumors, and all tumors testes

Drug	Dose (μg/ml)	Colorectal LM		Others		Total	
		(Sensitive/ total tested)	Sensitivity (%)	(Sensitive/ total tested)	Sensitivity (%)	(Sensitive/ total tested)	Sensitivity (%)
Adriamycin	1	(7/11)	64	(9/20)	45	(16/31)	52
	10	(9/10)	90	(14/16)	88	(23/26)	88
ASTA Z 7654	10	(2/5)	75	(3/10)	30	(5/15)	33
(Mafosfamid)	100	(3/4)	75	(7/7)	100	(10/11)	91
CDDP	1	(4/7)	57	(6/21)	29	(10/28)	36
	10	(10/14)	71	(5/13)	38	(15/27)	56
Epidoxorubicin	1	(1/5)	20	(3/10)	30	(4/15)	27
	10	(5/6)	83	(7/9)	78	(12/15)	80
5-Fluorouracil	10	(3/6)	50	(1/10)	10	(4/16)	25
	100	(2/4)	50	(0/6)	0	(2/10)	20
Mitomycin C	1	(10/20)	50	(12/28)	43	(22/48)	46
	10	(14/17)	83	(18/24)	75	(32/41)	78
Melphalan	1	(2/4)	50	(4/7)	57	(6/11)	55
	10	(2/3)	67	(5/7)	71	(7/10)	70
Novantron	1	(9/15)	60	(14/24)	58	(23/39)	59
	10	(12/14)	86	(21/24)	88	(33/38)	87

LM, liver metastasis(es).

Table 4. Degree of drug activity in colorectal liver metastases, other tumors, and all tumors at the low and high test concentrations

	Colorectal LM	Others	Total
Low test concentration:	1μg/ml, MAF and 5-FU 10 μg/ml MAF and 10 μg/ml 5FU		
	1. ADM	1. NOV	1. NOV
	2. NOV	2. LPAM	2. LPAM
	3. CDDP	3. ADM	3. ADM
	4. MMC	4. MMC	4. MMC
	5. 5FU	5. MAF	5. CDDP
	6. LPAM	6. EPI	6. MAF
	7. MAF	7. CDDP	7. EPI
	8. EPI	8. 5FU	8. 5FU
High test concentration:	10 μg/ml, MAF and 5-FU 100 μg/ml MAF and 100 μg/ml 5FU		
	1. ADM	1. MAF	1. MAF
	2. NOV	2. ADM	2. ADM
	3. MMC	3. NOV	3. NOV
	4. EPI	4. EPI	4. EPI
	5. MAF	5. MMC	5. MMC
	6. CDDP	6. LPAM	6. LPAM
	7. LPAM	7. CDDP	7. CDDP
	8. 5FU	8. 5FU	8. 5FU

MAF, mafosfamide; *5FU*, 5-fluorouracil; *ADM*, adriamycin; *NOV*, mitoxantrone; *CDDP*, cisplatin; *MMC*, mitomycin C; *LPAM*, melphalan; *EPI*, 4-epidoxorubicin; *LM*, liver metastasis(es).

Table 5. Outcome of the decision-aiding pilot study with correlation of drug test (human tumor colony-forming assay) and treatment (high-dose intra-arterial chemotherapy) results

Patient number	Tumor type	Treatment	HTCA	HDIAC
87/84	Carcinoid LM	A	S	S
57/85	Hepatocholangiocellular carcinoma	E	R	R
102/85	Colorectal carcinoma LM	M, C, F	S	S
105/85	Colorectal carcinoma LM	NO, M	S	S
34/86	Carcinoid LM	E	S	S
37/86	Colorectal carcinoma LM	M, F	R	S
64/86	Breast carcinoma LM	NO, F	S	S
71/86	Ovarian carcinoma LM	NO, F, M	S	R
83/86	Breast carcinoma LM	A, M	S	S

LM, liver metastasis(es); *HTCA*, human tumor colony-forming assay; *HDIAC*, high-dose intra-arterial chemotherapy; *A*, adriamycin; *E*, 4-epidoxorubicin; *M*, mitomycin C; *C*, cisplatin; *F*, 5-fluorouracil; *NO*, mitoxantrone; *S*, sensitive (response in vitro or in vivo); *R*, resistant in vitro, stable or progressive disease in vivo.

MMC was considered to be ineffective in the HTCA (colony survival 115% of the untreated control) but seemed to be active at 10 μg/ml (39% colony survival). The first treatment was performed preoperatively according to the Seldinger technique and the second, intraoperatively with a tourniquet infusion performed by centrally occluding the blood flow of the common hepatic artery. With both techniques, concentrations of about 10 μg/ml can easily be reached, and the serum carcinoembryonic antigen (CEA) dropped from 998 ng/ml to 475 ng/ml after the first and from 475 ng/ml to 105 ng/ml after the second intra-arterial infusion. Subsequently, the patient received five cycles with MMC and 5-FU, and the CT scan showed a response accompanied by a further CEA reduction to 29 ng/ml at the lowest level.

The second noncoincident patient had progressive liver metastases from an ovarian carcinoma. She had been previously treated according to a standard gynecologic protocol with surgery and systemic chemotherapy including CDDP. At the time of referral, the patient had no peritoneal disease and no proven evidence of extrahepatic distant metastases. Colony survival (HTCA) with NOV was 10%; with MMC, 17%; and with ADM, 19%. The patient was treated with NOV and 5-FU and later with NOV and MMC. After initial progression, liver metastases remained stable after the third cycle of intra-arterial chemotherapy.

In Fig. 3a and b, the response of a patient with liver metastasis of breast cancer to intra-arterial infusion of a combination of NOV and 3 × 5-FU can be seen. Figure 3a shows a big metastatic nodule in the right liver lobe that decreased by more than 50% 4 months later (Fig. 3b).

Discussion

The rationale for drug selection in regional chemotherapy is based on the effectiveness in systemic protocols and the dose-response behavior in toxicity for the particular drug. The response behavior of tumor to drugs in high concentrations

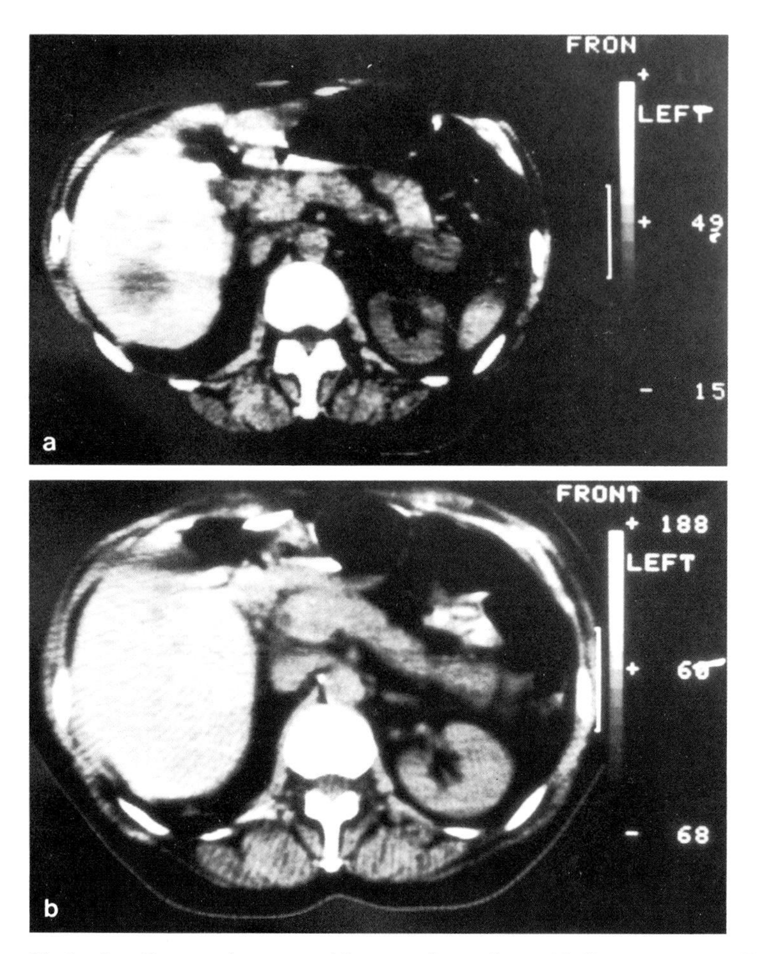

Fig. 3 a, b. Computed tomographic scan of a patient with liver metastases (LM) from a breast cancer before **a** and after **b** regional chemotherapy

differs from the response pattern in low concentrations achievable in systemic chemotherapy experimentally [3] and clinically [10]. Response rates in randomized i.a. vs i.v. studies with continuous infusion of 5-Fluorodeoxyuridine (5-FUDR) via Infusaid pumps for treatment of colorectal carcinoma liver metastases showed significantly higher hepatic response rates after intra-arterial infusion when compared with the systemic i.v. treatment [7, 11]. Overall response rates (2.4%–73%) and durations (4.5–12.5 months) of various protocols using high-dose, short-term or low-dose, continuous intra-arterial treatment for colorectal liver metastases showed a great variability [8]. As selection of the optimal drug is crucial to influence tumor response, we wanted to improve regional chemotherapy by using in vitro drug testing with the HTCA to identify the optimal drug(s) for specific tumor types and to perform regional chemotherapy according to individual chemosensitivity.

Drug testing in systemic chemotherapy showed a coincidence between in vitro and in vivo sensitivity in 64% and resistance in 91% of cases [13]. Therefore, owing to the low predictive accuracy of sensitivity, the HTCA in systemic chemotherapy still seems to be of limited value in drug selection. In a prospective, correlative trial with patients receiving regional chemotherapy for liver metastases whose treatment was not influenced by individual drug testing, we showed higher response rates than those achieved by systemic chemotherapy and produced sufficient evidence for the validity of chemosensitivity-directed drug selection in regional chemotherapy [12]. This study revealed that in 30 patients with liver metastases treated by regional chemotherapy, chemosensitivity in vitro coincided with sensitivity in vivo in 21 patients and resistance in six patients, while three patients predicted to be resistant turned out to be clinically sensitive. (Thus, the predictive accuracy of in vitro sensitivity was 100% and of in vitro resistance was 67%; the overall predictive accuracy was 90%).

Based on these promising results, we tested a variety of drugs for their activity in the concentration range representative for high-dose regional chemotherapy in an in vitro phase II-like study. In colorectal liver metastases ($n=21$), the sequence of activity at 1 μg/ml (for 5-FU and MAF at 10 μg/ml) was: ADM (64% of the tests sensitive in vitro), NOV (60%), CDDP (57%), MMC (50%), 5-FU (50%), L-PAM (50%), MAF (40%), and EPI (20%). Considering all 55 tumors tested, the sequence changed to NOV (59%), L-PAM (55%), ADM (52%), MMC (46%), CDDP (36%), MAF (33%), EPI (27%), and 5-FU (25%). Obviously, the drug activities exceeded those achievable clinically in systemic treatment of colorectal carcinoma [6, 17] and, in most instances, of other solid tumors. In short-term hepatic arterial infusion, intra-arterial drug levels of 1-10 μg/ml can be achieved for MMC [1] or NOV [2], for example, with response rates higher than those reported for systemic chemotherapy or with documented responses of patients previously treated by systemic chemotherapy. Colorectal cancer no longer belong to the category of tumors for which no effective chemotherapy exists [16], as regional chemotherapy with conventional drugs in high concentrations, tested experimentally in the HTCA and clinically in regional chemotherapy has proven effective. Our chemosensitivity profiles can be used to determine the sequence of priority in drug selection for decision-aiding chemosensitivity testing in colorectal liver metastases and other tumors, as the number of drugs to be tested is usually limited by the tumor material sent to the laboratory.

When the drugs were individually selected for regional chemotherapy according to the in vitro sensitivities of the patients' tumors our pilot study confirmed that drug testing in the HTCA is valid not only for in vitro phase II-like studies to determine activity of conventional and new drugs at concentration ranges achievable regionally, but also for individualization of regional chemotherapy. In seven out of nine patients, the in vitro test results correlated correctly with the clinical results, even in some patients where no standard protocol was available. This good correlation between in vitro and in vivo sensitivity encourages continuation of the study of decision-aiding trials and screening of drugs in high concentrations.

References

1. Aigner KR, Link KH, Stemmler F, Warthona M (1985) Intraarterielle Infusion (experimentelle und pharmakokinetische Grundlagen, Klinik). In: Aigner KR (ed) Regionale Chemotherapie der Leber - Isolierte Perfusion, Intraarterielle Infusion und Resektion. Karger, Basel, pp 84-107 (Beiträge zur Onkologie, vol. 21)
2. Aigner KR (1988) Methodische Ansätze zur Optimierung des Konzentrations-Zeit-Faktors in der regionalen Chemotherapie. In Seeber S, Aigner KR, Enghofer E (eds) Die locoregionale Tumortherapie. de Gruyter, Berlin, pp 81-93 (Onkologisches Kolloquium 2)
3. Drewinko B, Patchin M, Yang L, Barlogie B (1981) Differential killing effect of twenty antitumor drugs on proliferating and non-proliferating human tumor cells. Can Res 41: 2328-2333
4. Frei E III, Canellos GP (1980) Dose - A critical factor in cancer chemotherapy. Am J Med 69: 585-594
5. Hamburger AW, Salmon SE (1977) Primary bioassay of human tumor stem cells. Science 19: 461-463
6. Heim ME, Worst P (1986) Neuere Aspekte in der medikamentösen Therapie fortgeschrittener kolorektaler Karzinome. In: Queißer W, Flechtner H (eds) Gastrointestinale Tumoren. Zuckschwerdt, München, p 102 (Aktuelle Onkologie 33)
7. Hohn D, Stagg R, Friedman M, Ignoffo R, Rayner A, Hannigan I, Lewis B (1987) The NCOG randomized trial of intravenous (I.V.) versus hepatic arterial (I.A.) FUDR for colorectal cancer metastases to the liver (abstract). Proc ASCO 6: 85
8. Hottenrott C, Nagel K, Lorenz M (1987) Regionale Chemotherapie der Leber und Extremitäten - Standortbestimmung. Kehrer, Freiburg
9. Howell SB (1984) Intraarterial and intracavitary cancer chemotherapy. Martinus Nijhoff, Boston
10. Huberman MS (1983) Comparison of systemic chemotherapy with hepatic arterial infusion in metastatic colorectal carcinoma. Sem Oncol 10: 238-248
11. Kemeny N, Daly I, Reichman B, Geller N, Botet I, Oderman P (1987) Intrahepatic or systemic infusion of fluorodeoxyuridine in patients with liver metastases from colorectal carcinoma. Ann Intern Med 107: 459-465
12. Link KH, Aigner KR, Kuehn W, Schwemmle K, Kern D (1986) Prospective correlative chemosensitivity testing in high-dose intraarterial chemotherapy for liver metastases. Can Res 46: 4837-4840
13. Nakano H, Saiju N, Sasaki Y, et al. (1987) In vitro drug sensitivity test. Jpn J Can Chemother 14 (5): 1620-1628
14. Pettavel I, Morgenthaler F (1976) Dix ans d'expérience de chimiothérapie artérielle des tumeurs primaires et secondaires du foie. Ann Gastroenterol Hepatol 12: 349-363
15. Schwemmle K, Aigner KR (1983) Vascular perfusion in cancer therapy. Springer, Berlin Heidelberg New York Tokyo (Recent results in cancer research, vol 86)
16. WHO (1985) Essential drugs for cancer chemotherapy: Memorandum from a WHO meeting. Bull WHO 63: 999-1002
17. Wright IC (1986) Update in cancer chemotherapy. Gastrointestinal cancer, colorectal cancer. J Natl Med Assn 78: 295-304

Clinical Development of New Anthracyclines

I. H. KRAKOFF[1]

The development of the anthracyclines began with the isolation, characterization, and development of daunomycin in the early 1960s and continued through the next decade in studies led by Di Marco and his associates [1]. Daunomycin, which is now called daunorubicin, was shown to have a therapeutic effect on human cancer (primarily in acute childhood leukemia) by Tan et al. [2] in 1967. Early in the course of clinical studies, it was recognized that the administration of daunorubicin was accompanied by several kinds of disturbing toxicity. Myelosuppression was not unexpected and was not different from that seen with many previously developed antitumor agents. The occurrence of marked alopecia was not an insurmountable problem. More disturbingly, severe cardiac toxicity presented major obstacles to the administration of this new therapeutic agent. It should be noted that cardiac toxicity was not recognized during the early Phase I studies. Only after patients had received large cumulative doses in the course of Phase II and Phase III studies was this problem defined.

The characterization by Arcamone et al. [3] of a related anthracycline, doxorubicin (Adriamycin), the 14-hydroxy derivative of daunorubicin, provided an agent with superior antitumor activity in both experimental tumors [4] and in human cancer [5]. Unfortunately, doxorubicin exhibited the same spectrum of toxicity as daunorubicin; myelosuppression, alopecia, and cardiac toxicity have been regular complications of its use [6].

Although modifications of the rate and the schedule of administration have modified cardiac toxicity somewhat [7-9], there remains a high likelihood of the development of cardiomyopathy and congestive heart failure in patients who receive cumulative doses in excess of 500 mg/m^2. The search for more effective and less toxic anthracyclines has continued.

Other derivatives were synthesized and studied during the 1970s without obvious therapeutic or toxicologic improvement. Many agents have been studied in attempts to block cardiotoxicity; these efforts, too, have proven ineffective. Recent studies [10] with the bisdioxopiperazine (ICRF-187), however, suggest that it may effectively prevent or modify the cardiac toxicity of doxorubicin.

In the early 1980s, three new derivatives were studied [11-14]. 4-Demethoxydaunorubicin is an orally active compound still in Phase II evaluation; 4′-epidoxorubicin appears to be similar in activity and toxicity to doxorubicin, although it is

[1] University of Texas System Cancer Center, M.D. Anderson Hospital, 1515 Holcombe Boulevard, Houston, TX 77030, USA.

H. G. Beger et al. (Eds.), Cancer Therapy

slightly less potent; 4′-deoxydoxorubicin has not produced sufficient therapeutic activity to warrant large-scale trials.

In 1984, a cyanomorpholinyl derivative of doxorubicin (MRA-CN) was found to be 1000 times as active as doxorubicin, not cross-resistant, and cardiotoxic only at doses equimolar with doxorubicin. This promising compound has not yet entered clinical trial. However, it is one of the most interesting of the anthracyclines presently under development. Since its cardiotoxicity is similar to that of doxorubicin but its potency is approximately 1000 times that of doxorubicin, MRA-CN has, in effect, a therapeutic/toxicologic "window" which renders it, for practical purposes noncardiotoxic. This will presumably also apply to human beings, although tests on humans have not yet been conducted.

A related group of compounds, in which the 3′ substituent is morpholinyl rather than cyano-morpholinyl, has been prepared and studied. One of these, a Japanese compound, 3′-deamino-3′-morpholino-13-deoxo-10-hydroxycarminomycin HCl (MX2) [15-16], has had extensive preclinical evaluation. It has greater therapeutic activity than doxorubicin and is less cardiotoxic and not cross-resistant with doxorubicin. It, too, will be of interest in clinical testing [16].

Another anthracycline of Japanese origin (2″R)-4′-0-tetrahydropyranyladriamycin (THP) was synthesized by Umezawa [17] in 1979 and was demonstrated to be superior to doxorubicin in several murine tumors [18]. Danchev et al. [19] observed less myocardial toxicity and alopecia than with doxorubicin. Phase I [20-21] and early Phase II [22] studies established the tolerated dose and patterns of toxicity in human beings and confirmed the therapeutic effectiveness. In a Phase I study at the M. D. Anderson Hospital [23], granulocytopenia, which appeared at higher dose levels, was the limiting factor. Following the administration of 25 mg/m_3 daily for 5 days, 5 of 19 courses resulted in prolonged granulocytopenia, requiring delay of the third dose. Moderate thrombocytopenia occurred at the highest dose levels but was not limiting.

Nonmyelosuppressive toxicity included mild gastrointestinal complaints seen in four patients, stomatitis in two, and phlebitis at the venous injection site in one. Mild alopecia occurred in only two patients. As noted above, all patients were monitored for cardiac toxicity, but no such toxicity was observed. However, large cumulative doses were not attained in this study [24].

In clinical pharmacokinetic studies [24], THP disappeared from the plasma in a triphasic manner with half lives as follows: α 5.6 ± 0.9 min; β 1.1 ± 0.3 h, and γ 14.3 ± 2.1 h. The plasma clearance rate was 1.7 ± 0.2 L/h per kilogram; that is about twice the clearance rate previously demonstrated with doxorubicin. The volume of distribution was 5.3 ± 1.4 L/kg, suggesting a rapid transfer to the tissue or blood components.

The maximum accumulation of THP in the plasma and formed elements of the blood occurred within 15 min after adminstration. The highest concentration was in polymorphonuclear cells; and this concentration was higher than that previously demonstrated with doxorubicin. Only 9% of the injected dose of THP was excreted in the urine within 72 h. There was no evidence of significant conversion of THP to doxorubicin.

No major therapeutic responses were seen in the course of the Phase I study. However, the demonstrated differences in toxicity between THP and doxorubicin

are sufficient to warrant Phase II trials, which are proposed in several tumor types at a dose of 20 mg/m^2 per week for 3 weeks.
Doxorubicin has become one of the most widely used and important drugs in cancer chemotherapy. The development of additional drugs of this general group can provide us with agents that are more effective and less toxic, extending their value considerably.

References

1. Di Marco A, Gaetani M, Dorigotti L, et al (1964) Daunomycin: a new antibiotic with antitumor activity. Cancer Chemother Rep 38: 31
2. Tan C, Kou-Ping Y, Murphy ML, Karnofsky DA (1967) Daunomycin an antitumor antibiotic, in the treatment of neoplastic disease. Clinical evaluation with special reference to childhood leukemia. Cancer 20: 333
3. Arcamone F, Cassinelli G, Fantini G, et al (1969) Adriamycin, 14-hydroxydaunomycin, a new antitumor antibiotic from *S. peucetius var. caesius*. Biotechnol Bioeng 11: 1101
4. Di Marco A, Gaetani M, Scarpinato B (1969) Adriamycin (NSC-123127): a new antibiotic with antitumor activity. Cancer Chemother Rep 53: 33
5. Carter SK, DiMarco A, Ghione M, Krakoff IH, Mathé G (1972) International symposium on adriamycin. Springer-Verlag
6. Benjamin RS, Weirnik PH, Bachur NR (1974) Adriamycin chemotherapy: efficacy, safety, and pharmacology basis of an intermittent single high-dosage schedule. Cancer 33: 19
7. Weiss AJ, Metter GE, Fletcher WA, et al (1976) Studies on adriamycin using a weekly regimen demonstrating its clinical effectiveness and lack of cardiac toxicity. Cancer Treat Rep 60: 813
8. Hoff D von, Layard MW, Basa P, et al (1979) Risk factors for doxorubicin-induced congestive heart failure. Ann Intern Med 91: 710
9. Benjamin RS, Legha SS, Mackay B, et al (1981) Reduction of adriamycin cardiac toxicity using a prolonged continuous intravenous infusion. Proc Am Assoc Cancer Research 22: 179
10. Green MD, Speyer JL, Stecy P, et al (1987) ICRF-187 (ICRF) Prevents doxorubicin (Dox) cardiotoxicity (Ctox): Results of a randomized clinical trial. Proc Am Soc Clin Oncol 6: 26
11. Arcamone F, Bernadi L, Giardino P, et al (1976) Synthesis and antitumor activity of 4-demethoxy-daunorubicin, 4-demethoxy-7,9-diepi-daunorubicin, and their anomers. Cancer Treat Rep 60: 829-834
12. Casazza AM, Di Marco A, Bertazzoli C, et al (1978) Antitumor activity, toxicity and pharmacological properties of 4'epiadriamycin. Curr Chemother 2: 1257-1260
13. Di Marco A, Casazza AM, Pratesi G (1977) Antitumor activity of 4-demethoxy-daunorubicin administered orally. Cancer Treat Rep 61: 893-894
14. Bonadonna G, Bonfanti V (1982) Clinical evaluation of 4'-epi doxorubicin and 4-demethoxy-daunorubicin. In: Muggia FM, Young CW, Carter SK (eds) Anthracycline antibiotics and cancer therapy. Martinus Nijhoff, The Hague
15. Takahashi Y, Kinoshita M, Masuda T, et al (1982) 3'-Deamino-3'-morpholino derivatives of daunomycin, adriamycin, and carminomycin. J Antibiot 35: 117
16. Fukushima H, Uchida T (1987) Antitumor activities of MX2, a new morpholino anthracycline. Japanese-French Conference on Antibiotics in Tumor Pharmacology, 1987 (Abstract)
17. Umezawa H, Takahashi Y, Kinoshita M, Naganawa H, Ishizuka M, Takeuchi T (1979) Tetrahydropyranyl derivatives of daunomycin and adriamycin. J Antibiot 32: 1082
18. Usuruo T, Lida H, Tsukagoshi S, Sakurai Y (1982) 4'-0-Tetrahydropyranyl adriamycin as a potential new antitumor agent. Cancer Res 42: 1462
19. Danchev D, Painstrand M, Hayat M, Bourut C, Mathe G (1979) Low heart and skin toxicity of a tetrahydropyranyl derivative of adriamycin (THP-ADM) as observed by electron and light microscopy. J Antibiot 32: 1085
20. Ogawa M, Miyamoto H, Inagaki J, Horikoshi M, Ezaki K, Inoue K, Ikeda K, Usui N, Nakada H (1983) Phase I clinical trial of a new anthracycline: 4'-0-tetrahydropyanyl adriamycin. Invest New Drugs 1: 169

21. Majima H (1983) Exploratory clinical study of 4′-0-tetrahydropyranyl Doxorubicin (THP-ADM)-Phase I-(in Japanese). Jpn J Cancer Chemother 10: 134
22. Yamada K, Shirikawa S, Ohno R, Yamada H, Hirota Y, Ohara K, Yamagata K, Kobayashi M, Hirano M, Ikeda Y, Oguri T, Mitomo Y, Mizuno H, Yoshikawa S, Shiku H, Kimura K (1987) A Phase II study of (2″R)-4′-0-tetrahydropyranyladriamycin (THP) in hematological malignancies. Invest New Drugs 5: 299
23. Raber M, Legha S, Gorski C, Krakoff IH (1987) Phase I clinical trial of tetradropyranyl adriamycin (THP-Adria). Proc AACR 28: 223
24. Lu K, Raber M, Krakoff IH, Newman RA (1987) Phase I clinical trial of tetrahydropyranyl adriamycin (THP-Adria). Proc AACR 28: 223

First Clinical Experience with Cytorhodin S – The First Compound of a New Class of Anthracyclines

J. VERWEIJ,[1] E. SALEWSKI,[2] and G. STOTER[1]

Introduction

The widespread use of doxorubicin in cancer treatment has prompted studies of compounds with similar structures. Preferably, such new compounds should retain or exceed the activity of doxorubicin but have fever of its toxic side effects. Activity in doxorubicin-resistant tumors has also stimulated further research of such compounds.
Rodorubicin (Cytorhodin S) is the first compound of a group of tetraglycosidic anthracycline derivatives [1]. The drug was found to be a strong intercalator and to act by blocking the synthesis of nucleic acids. Its structural formula is shown in Fig. 1. Cytorhodin S is easily soluble in water and in normal saline solution. In the usual prescreen, it is only active in vitro in L 1210 leukemia and in vivo in B 16 melanoma. However, in vitro in the human tumor stem-cell assay and in vivo in the xenograft, Cytorhodin S proved to be active in a wide variety of tumors [1], including anthracycline-sensitive and anthracycline-resistant tumors. The drug showed considerable activity against transplanted gastric, colonic and pancreatic tumors. Animal toxicology studies revealed glomerular and tubular renal toxicity after long-term daily administration and reversible cardiotoxicity at the highest studied dose level. No myelosuppression was observed. The lethal dose for 10% of the population (LD_{10}) in mice was 2610 μg/m^2; therefore, the starting dose for human studies in 260 μg/m^2.
A phase I study of Cytorhodin S was carried out at the Rotterdam Cancer Institute with three objectives:

1. To determine the maximally tolerated dose of Cytorhodin S administered intravenously as a short-term (30 min) infusion once every 3 weeks
2. To determine and quantitate the clinical toxicities of Cytorhodin S
3. To document preliminary evidence of the antitumor effects of Cytorhodin S in patients with advanced cancers

[1] Oncology and Biologic, Hoechst-Roussel Pharmaceutical Inc., Summerville, NJ 08876, USA.
[2] Clinical Research, Behringwerke AG Marburg, P.O. Box 1140, 3550 Marburg 1, FRG.

H. G. Beger et al. (Eds.), Cancer Therapy

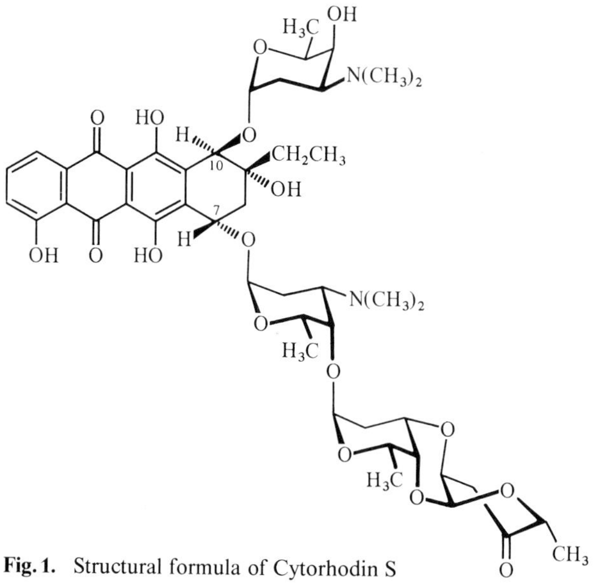

Fig. 1. Structural formula of Cytorhodin S

Materials and Methods

Eligibility and Follow-up

The study protocol was in accordance with European Organization for Research and Treatment of Cancer (EORTC) guidelines for phase I trials with single agents [2]. Eligibility criteria for entry into the study included histological confirmation of cancer, resistance to conventional therapy, proven progressive disease, a life expectancy of at least 2 months, a performance score of WHO 2 or better, age 18–75 years, no chemotherapy or radiotherapy for at least 4 weeks before entry (for mitomycin C, nitrosourea, and extensive radiotherapy, 6 weeks), recovery from toxic effects of prior treatment, white blood count (WBC) $\geq 4 \times 10^9$/L, platelet count $\geq 100 \times 10^9$/L, normal liver function tests (unless abnormalities could be attributed to metastatic disease; bilirubin still had to be normal), and normal renal function (serum creatinine ≤ 125 μmol/L or creatinine clearance ≥ 60 ml/min). Patients with impaired central nervous system functions, brain metastases, cardiac and/or pulmonary dysfunction requiring treatment, or with concomitant steroid treatment were considered ineligible. All patients gave written informed consent prior to therapy. Before entry, all patients underwent a complete physical examination, and a thorough medical history was obtained. Height, weight, performance status, and tumor measurements were recorded. Initial laboratory data obtained included a complete blood count (CBC), differential WBC count, platelet count, serum electrolytes, blood urea nitrogen (BUN), creatinine, glucose, total protein, albumin, alkaline phosphatase, total bilirubin, gamma-glutamyl transferase (γ-GTP), aspartate aminotransferase (ASAT), alanine aminotransferase (ALAT), and serum lactic dehydrogenase (SLDH). Urinalysis, including creatinine clearance, chest X-ray films, gated cardiac blood pool scan and ECG were also performed before the start of the study. All blood tests and urinalyses were repeated weekly while the patients were on study; the other parameters were repeated prior to each scheduled cycle.

Drug Formulation and Dosage

Cytorhodin S was supplied by Behringwerke AG Marburg, Federal Rerpublic of Germany. The salt of Cytorhodin S together with D-gluconic acid is a deep orange amorphous powder, well soluble in water and in normal saline solution. The drug was available in vials containing 1000 μg Cytorhodin S-D-gluconate, 400 mg mannitol, and 25 mg sodium chloride, to be reconstituted in 10 ml water for injection. The prescribed dose was further diluted with 0.9% NaCl solution to a total of 100 ml for administration as a 30-min infusion. In later stages of the study, greater amounts of fluids and longer infusion times were also used. In aqueous solution, Cytorhodin S is stable over 24 h, but because of minor degradation under the influence of light, care was taken to administer the solution protected from light directly after dissolution. The starting dose was 260 $\mu g/m^2$, which represents 1/10 of the LD_{10} in mice [3]. Dose escalation was done according to the modified Fibonacci scheme. At least three patients were studied at each dose level, and there was no dose escalation with a single patient. Cycles were repeated every 3 weeks.

Results

Twenty-one patients were entered on study and received a total of 51 cycles. All patients were evaluable for at least one treatment cycle. Patient characteristics are given in Table 1. All patients except two had received prior chemotherapy; three patients had been pretreated with radiotherapy. There were no drug-related deaths. The dose levels studied were 260, 520, 860, 1290, and 1700 $\mu g/m^2$.
No patients had leukocytopenia, thrombocytopenia or hair-loss. The dose-limiting side effects of Cytorhodin S were proteinuria and phlebitis. Proteinuria was first

Table 1. Patient characteristics

Number of patients entered	21
Male/female (*n*)	11/10
Age in years: median (range)	53 (45-72)
Primary tumor (*n*)	
Renal cancer	9
Colonic cancer	4
Unknown primary	2
Lung cancer	2
Soft-tissue sarcoma	1
Malignant melanoma	1
Gastric cancer	1
Breast cancer	1

noted at the dose level of 860 μg/m² (Table 2). None of the patients studied at lower dose levels had proteinuria even at cumulative doses of up to 2860 μg/m² (Fig. 2). At the dose levels of 860 and 1290 μg/m², proteinuria usually appeared after the second treatment cycle, reaching a plateau level of 5-8 g/L. At a dose of 1700 μg/m², proteinuria occurred after the first cycle of treatment. By increasing the administered amount of fluid to 500 or 1000 ml and by prolonging the infusion time to 3 or 6 h, proteinuria could be delayed (Fig. 2) but not prevented. Proteinuria merely consisted of albuminuria with no concomitant increase in β_2-microglobulin. In those patients whose urinary protein loss could be monitored after discontinuation of Cytorhodin S, proteinuria completely disappeared within 3-6 weeks. Serum creatinine increases were only observed in one patient. This patient was treated with a dose of 1700 μg/m² as a 3-h infusion. Shortly after the third cycle, at

Table 2. Proteinuria

Dose (μg/m²)	Infusion time (min)	Patients (*n*)	(Cycles) (*n*)	Tumor responses (*n*) (WHO grade)				
				0	1	2	3	4
260	30	3	13	13	0	0	0	0
520	30	3	7	7	0	0	0	0
860	30	3	9	4	0	5	0	0
1290	30	3	6	3	1	2	0	0
1700	30	4	6	1	1	4	0	0
1700	180	3	6	0	2	4	0	0
1700	360	2	4	1	1	2	0	0

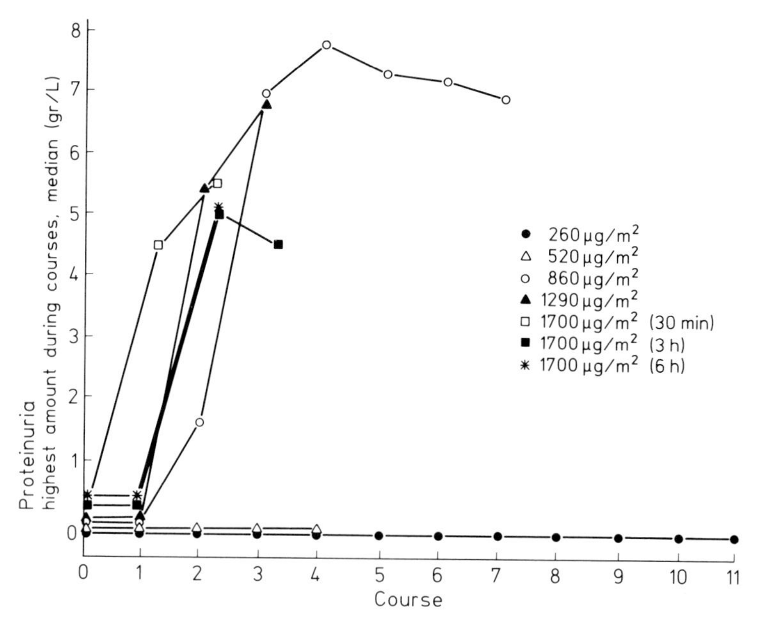

Fig. 2. Cytorhodin S-induced proteinuria related to cumulative dose

a cumulative dose of 5100 μg/m², oliguric renal failure developed, which appeared to be reversible in the following 3 weeks with complete recovery of renal function.

Phlebitis of the infusion vein was first observed at a dosage of 1290 μg/m² (Table 3). It worsened with increasing dosage and with longer infusion times. Some of the patients showed initials signs of phlebitis 7–10 days after the infusion of Cytorhodin S. There was no recall phlebitis. In one patient, there was even a retrograde phlebitis, reaching up to the occiput and far into the external jugular vein. In five instances, phlebitis caused a reversible contracture of the affected arm.

Nausea and vomiting were mild to moderate and mainly present at the highest studied dose level (Table 4). By prolonging the infusion time, a tendency towards more severe and more frequent nausea and vomiting was noticed.

In three patients, a decrease in left vetricular ejection fraction (LVEF) was observed, reaching abnormal levels (normal ≥ 50%). In all three patients, the abnormal LVEF was found after three or more treatment cycles (Table 5). In two patients, the decreased LVEF did not cause symptoms but was reason to discontinue treatment. In both patients, LVEF recovered to normal after 6–8 months. A third patient developed an abnormal LVEF during a period of renal insufficiency. Un-

Table 3. Phlebitis

Dose (μg/m²)	Infusion time (min)	Patients (*n*)	Cycles (*n*)	Reactions (*n*) Grade				
				0	1	2	3	4
260	30	3	13	13	0	0	0	0
520	30	3	7	7	0	0	0	0
860	30	3	9	9	0	0	0	0
1290	30	3	6	3	3	0	0	0
1700	30	4	6	2	4	0	0	0
1700	180	3	6	3	2	1	0	0
1700	360	2	4	0	0	0	4	0

Grade 1: pain; grade 2: inflammation; grade 3: reversible contracture; grade 4: irreversible contracture

Table 4. Nausea and vomiting

Dose (μg/m²)	Infusion time (min)	Patients (*n*)	Cycles (*n*)	Reactions (*n*) WHO grade				
				0	1	2	3	4
260	30	3	13	12	1	0	0	0
520	30	3	7	7	0	0	0	0
860	30	3	9	9	0	0	0	0
1290	30	3	6	6	0	0	0	0
1700	30	4	6	5	1	0	0	0
1700	180	3	6	3	0	1	2	0
1700	360	2	4	0	3	1	0	0

Table 5. Cardiotoxicity

Patients (n)	Dose per course (μg/m²)	Cumulative dose (μg/m²)	Final LVEF (%)
1	860	6020	43
1	1290	3870	35
1	1700	5100	34

fortunately, LVEF could not be followed up in this patient. Finally, a feeling of fatigue was noted in several patients treated at 1700 μg/m², which subsided after treatment discontinuation.

Tumor responses according to WHO criteria were not observed. Two patients experienced brief (<4 weeks) tumor regressions of less than 50%.

Discussion

Cytorhodin S is an interesting new anthracycline antitumor agent with a toxicity profile different from other anthracyclines.

This phase I study has shown that the dose-limiting toxicities of Cytorhodin S administered once every 3 weeks are phlebitis and proteinuria. Phlebitis appeared 1–10 days after infusion, with a retrograde phlebitis in one patient. Changing the infusion time and volume could not prevent phlebitis. Phlebitis is also a minor problem with other anthracyclines [4] but has never been dose limiting. The reason for the delayed appearance of venous irritation remains unclear. There was no increase in the severity of phlebitis with increasing cumulative doses, so at the level of 1290 μg/m², this side effect is tolerable for repeated administrations.

The proteinuria induced by Cytorhodin S appears to be related to the amount of drug per administration as well as to the cumulative dose. Proteinuria leveled off at values of 5–8 g/l and never induced a nephrotic syndrome. The fact that proteinuria was merely albuminuria suggests a glomerular disorder. Whether this has any relation to the single case of reversible renal failure that was observed remains an open question. Proteinuria could be delayed but not prevented by prolonging the infusion time and increasing the infused volume. Also, proteinuria was found to be reversible after discontinuation of treatment, even after relatively high cumulative doses. These data coincide with the animal data and, to our knowledge, Cytorhodin S is the first anthracycline that causes proteinuria in man. For doxorubicin, proteinuria has been reported in animals, but this drug is not nephrotoxic in humans. The cardiotoxic potential of Cytorhodin S should be further investigated because the limited number of patients in the present phase I study does not permit definitive conclusions. We only suggest that Cytorhodin S may be cardiotoxic. Nausea and vomiting were mild to moderate. Myelotoxicity and hair loss were completely absent, and in combination with the observed toxicities, this suggests that Cytorhodin S is, indeed, a different anthracycline when compared to previously tested compounds. The two patients showing minor signs of tumor regression had both previously failed to react to doxorubicin treatment. Here again, we cannot draw definitive conclusions, but this observation suggests that Cytorhodin S is not cross resistant with doxorubicin, which would confirm preclinical data. Further Phase I trials with multiple divided dosages should be performed.

Conclusion

Cytorhodin S is the first of a new class of anthracyclines. It has a different toxicity profile compared to other anthracyclines. Cytorhodin S is not myelotoxic and does not cause alopecia. Based on a limited number of patients, we cannot exclude a cardiotoxic potential. The dose-limiting side effects of Cytorhodin S, given once every 3 weeks, are proteinuria and phlebitis. Prolonging infusion time slightly delayed the appearance of proteinuria but increased the occurrence of nausea and vomiting and, more importantly, worsened phlebitis. Besides, one case of reversible renal failure was observed after three courses of a 3-h infusion at a dosage of 1700 $\mu g/m^2$. The maximum tolerated dose of Cytorhodin S once every three weeks is 1700 $\mu g/m^2$. Although the study will be extended, it is expected that a dose of 1290 $\mu g/m^2$ in a 30-min infusion every 3 weeks should be the recommended dose for phase II trials. In such trials, renal and cardiac function should be monitored very closely.

References

1. Kraemer HP, Berscheid HG, Ronneberger H, Zilg H, Sedlacek HH (1987) Preclinical evaluation of Cytorhodin S. A new anthracycline with activity in a human tumor based screening system. Invest New Drugs
2. EORTC New Drug Development Commitee (1985) EORTC guidelines for phase I trials with single agents in adults. Eur J Cancer Clin Oncol 21: 1005–1007
3. Cytorhodin S, Investigators' brochure
4. Brown TD, Donehower RC, Grochow LB, Rice AP, Ettinger DS (1987) A phase I study of Menogaril in patients with advanced cancer. J Clin Oncol 5: 92–99

Pirarubicin: A New Drug in the Treatment of Malignant Diseases

B. GREIFENBERG[1]

Introduction

Doxorubicin (ADM) has become one of the most frequently used and important drugs in the treatment of solid tumors. However, its usefulness is limited by its well-known side effects [1-3]. Besides myelosuppression, which represents the dose-limiting, acute toxicity, alopecia is a common side effect. Furthermore, severe nausea and vomiting may cause patients significant distress.

Cardiac toxicity represents an important obstacle to the use of ADM as well. There are two aspects of this toxicity: An acute syndrome (supraventricular arrhythmia, heart block, ventricular tachycardia, and a significant drop in the ejection fraction) can be seen hours to days after administration of ADM and sometimes causes congestive heart failure. The other aspect is the cumulative, dose-dependent cardiomyopathy that appears in 1%-10% of the patients receiving a total dose of 550 mg/m^2 of ADM.

To decrease toxicity of ADM while preserving its antitumor activity, new anthracycline analogues have recently been developed by altering the chemical structure of ADM. Pirarubicin (4'-*0*-tetrahydropyranyl-doxorubicin, THP) is one of these derivates of doxorubicin and was first synthesized by Umezawa [4] in 1979.

Chemistry, Pharmacology, and Antineoplastic Effects of Pirarubicin

Regarding its chemical structure, THP is a new compound possessing a tetrahydropyranyl group at the 4-0 position of ADM (Fig. 1). This structural difference between THP and ADM, leads to differences in the pharmacology and the mode of action. Initial comparative pharmacokinetic studies in rabbits showed that cells take up THP (K_{12}: 52.84 h^{-1}) much faster than ADM (K_{12}: 3.91 h^{-1}). Furthermore, studies have revealed that the distribution volume of THP is much greater than that of ADM. In dogs, the distribution volume of THP is 42.6 L/kg, whereas that of ADM is 6.4 L/kg. The two substances differ significantly in their tissue distribution. THP attains high concentrations in the spleen, lung, and thymus, whereas ADM becomes highly concentrated in the heart muscle and bile [5, 6].

Regarding the antineoplastic effects, fluorescence spectroscopic analysis has shown that tumor cells (L518 Y) adsorb THP 170 times faster than ADM. In in

[1] Clinical Research, Behringwerke AG Marburg, P.O. Box 1140, 3550 Marburg 1, FRG.

H. G. Beger et al. (Eds.), Cancer Therapy

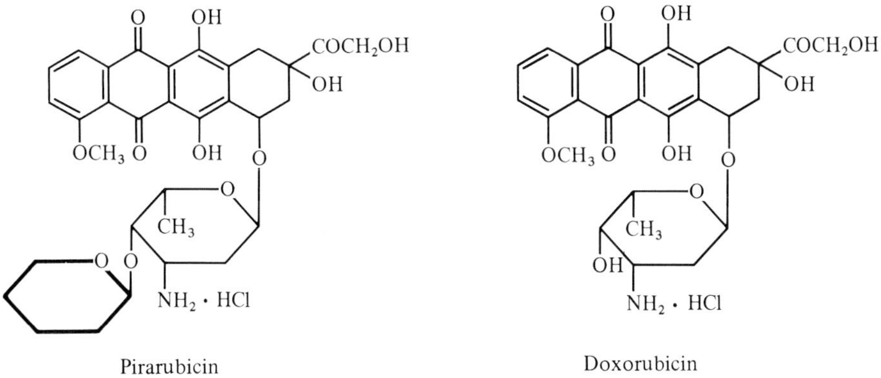

Pirarubicin Doxorubicin

Fig. 1. Chemical structure of pirarubicin (THP) and of doxorubicin (ADM)

Table 1. Cytotoxic doses of different cytostatic compounds in Friend leukemia cells [8]

	Cytotoxic dose (IC_{50}, ng/ml)	
	Sensitive (FLC)	ReM-RFLC3)
THP	1.7	500
ADM	1.8	1700
Mitoxantrone	2.8	1000
Epi-Doxirubicin	4.6	3800
Daunorubicin	11.0	3950

ADM, doxorubicin; *FLC*, Friend leukemic cells; *THP*, pirarubicin.

vitro experiments, Tapiero et al. [7] analyzed the uptake, storage, and cytotoxicity of THP. They found that more than 50% of the THP administered was taken up by Friend leukemia cells within 2 min; 80 min were necessary for epirubicin to achieve the same effect, and ADM took more than 4 h. It is noticeable that there was a direct correlation between the rapid uptake of the anthracyclines and their cytostatic effects [8]. Further in vitro experiments confirm the high antitumor activity of THP.

In the proliferation assay (cell line: L 1210), THP was significantly (nearly 100 times) more cytostatic than ADM, even when equally toxic doses were administered. The drug is also active in the clonogenic assay with L 1210 leukemia cells using continuous (7-day), as well as short-term (1-h) incubation periods [9]. Tapiero et al. [8] have compared the cytotoxic doses (IC_{50}) of different cytostatics in ADM-sensitive and ADM-resistant Friend leukemia cells (ADM-RFLC3). Their results show that THP has a cytotoxic effect in both cell types at a dose which is relatively low compared with epirubicin, daunorubicin and mitoxantrone (Table 1). In vivo tests also confirm that the antineoplastic effect of THP is at least comparable to that of ADM.

In experiments using cell lines of B 16 melanoma (s.c. application), colon adenocarcinoma 26 (i.p. application), and colon adenocarcinoma 38 (s.c. application),

THP exhibited an antitumor activity equal to or higher than that of ADM. Furthermore, THP is more effective than ADM in the inhibition of lung metastases caused by Lewis lung carcinoma [10].

Clinical Development

Owing to the encouraging preclinical results with THP, clinical trials were first conducted in Japan in 1981. Later, European countries and the USA participated in the clinical development. In addition to ongoing studies in Austria, results are already available from Japanese, French, German, and American studies.

Japan

In Japan, 49 patients with different tumors were treated with THP in a cooperative phase I trial. Different dosages were used; the maximum single dose was 100 mg per body and the maximum total dose was 840 mg per body. The maximum tolerable single dose was 66 mg/m^2. Single-dose administration of THP led to leukocytopenia, which reached the lowest levels around day 13. The value fell in some cases below 3000 leukocytes per mm^3 and returned to normal after about 8 days. Thrombocytopenia also occurred and reached the lowest levels around day 10. The values recovered to normal within 7 days. At a dosage of 45 mg/m^2, the thrombocyte count fell to below 10000 per mm^3 in five of eight patients (range, 95000-44000 thrombocytes). No signs of cardiotoxicity were detectable. The liver, lungs, kidneys, and CNS showed no signs of toxic effects. Only slight alopecia resulted from the THP therapy. The dosage recommendation for the phase II studies was 35-45 mg/m^2 every 3 weeks or i.v. bolus doses of 40-50 mg/m^2 every 3 weeks [11-13].

In Japan, extensive phase II studies have been conducted on THP in solid tumors, leukemia, and lymphomas. One study involving 162 patients yielded the following response rates for leukemia and lymphoma: in acute lymphatic leukemia (ALL), the rates complete remissions and partial remissions (CR + PR) were 44.4%, in acute myeloid lymphoma, 27.3%; in Hodgkin's lymphomas, 75.0%; and in non-Hodgkin's lymphomas, 48.5% [14].

In another phase II study in which 499 patients were treated for solid tumors with THP only, good response rates were achieved, especially in the following carcinomas: head and neck tumors, 18.8%; stomach carcinoma, 13.1%; breast carcinoma, 21.4%; renal carcinoma, 22.2%; ovarian carcinoma, 26.8%; uterine carcinoma, 24.2%; vaginal carcinoma, 50.0%; and sarcomas, 12.5%. Seventy-nine of these 499 patients (15.8%) had previously been treated with anthracyclines [15]. The side effects observed in this study can be seen in Table 2.

In a randomized, controlled study of 64 patients with advanced breast cancer, the efficacy and compatibility of therapy with a combination of cyclophosphamide, ADM, and 5-fluorouracil (CAF), were compared with a combination of cyclophosphamide, THP, and 5-fluorouracil [16]. The dosages employed were: THP and ADM, 30 mg/m^2 i.v. on days 1 and 8; 5-fluorouracil, 500 mg/m^2 i.v. on

Table 2. Side effects of therapy with pirarubicin (THP) (558 patients, phase II, Japan) [15]

Side effects	WHO grade			
	1	2	3	4
	Incidence (%)			
Nausea/vomiting	18	9	2	0
Stomatitis	4	1	0	0
Alopecia	5	4	1	0
Leukocytopenia (1000/mm^3)	14.5	28.0	24.6	6.5
Thrombocytopenia (1000/mm^3)	4.9	3.8	4.0	2.7
Incidence (%)				
Fever			7.2	
Changes in ECG			2.8	

days 1 and 8; cyclophosphamide, 100 mg per person p.o. daily from day 3 to day 16. The schedule was repeated every 28 days. Generally, three cycles were given. Response rates of 30% (8/27 patients) and 35% (13/27 patients) were obtained for the ADM and THP combination, respectively. In the group treated with THP, the rate of side effects, i.e., anorexia and alopecia, was significantly lower than in the group that received the regimen containing ADM ($P<0.1$ and $P<0.01$ respectively) [16].

The antineoplastic effect and toxicity of ADM and THP were compared in combination with vincristine (VCR) and nimustin (ACNU) in a randomized phase III trial on 42 patients with previously untreated small-cell lung cancer. Here, the following schedule was employed: ADM, 25 mg/m^2 i.v. on days 2 and 3; VCR, 2 mg per body on day 1 and 1 mg per body on days 8, 15, and 22 i.v.; and ACNU, 100 mg/m^2 on day 10. The regimen of THP/VRC/ACNU consisted of THP at a dose of 30 mg/m^2 i.v. on days 2 and 3, and VCR and ACNU administered as described above. No significant difference was observed in patient characteristics between the two groups. In the ADM-containing regimen, a partial response was observed in 11 out of 20 patients (55%). One CR and 14 PR among 22 patients (overall response rate: 68%) were observed in the THP-containing regimen. The incidence of alopecia tended to be higher in the ADM regimen [17].

France

At the Paul Brousse Hospital (Villejuif, France), 39 patients were administered 20–30 mg/m^2 THP for 3 consecutive days every weeks. In each case, the dose was increased in several dose steps. Leukopenia was a dose-limiting factor. No cardiac abnormality was observed. One CR and 10 PR were seen, with reductions in tumor volume greater than 50%. The CR and seven of the PR occurred in the 18 patients who had not previously received ADM. The total response rate for the whole group of 39 patients was thus 28% but was 44% in the 18 patients who had not previously been treated with ADM [20].

At the same hospital, 48 patients with metastatic breast carcinoma received combinations of THP (15–20 mg/m^2 i.v. for 3 days) and vindesin (31 patients); 5-fluorouracil (48 patients) potentiated by folic acid (36 patients) or cyclophosphamide (29 patients); or thiotepa (13 patients). Five CR were observed (10.4%) and 18 PR (47.5%). Here the total response rate was 47.9%. In the 22 patients with no prior chemotherapy, the overall response rate was 59%, and the rate of CR was 18%. Deaths due to toxic effects occurred in none of the regimens or drug combinations. Hematologic toxicity was usually a dose-limiting factor [27].

Germany

An examination of the Japanese dosage recommendation in the course of a phase I trial in Germany showed that no dose-limiting toxicity occurs with a dosage of 50 mg/m^2 pirarubicin. The maximum tolerable dosage was found to be 70 mg/m^2. Leukocytopenia (nadir: day 14, recovery within 7 days) was a dose-limiting factor. The study showed that, up to a cumulative dose of 700 mg/m^2, no cardiotoxicity occurs and the incidence of alopecia and nausea remains low. No WHO grade 1 and 4 cases of alopecia occurred, and WHO grade 2 and 3 alopecia occurred in 3 out of 19 patients. Out of 19 patients with nausea and vomiting, there were 5 with grade 1 and 2 symptoms but no cases of grade 3 and 4 reactions [18, 19].

Kaukel et al. investigated the effectiveness of THP in patients with pleuramesotheliomas who had not previously been treated with chemotherapeutic agents. At doses of 65–74 mg/m^2 (median: 69 mg/m^2), 4 out of 25 patients achieved PR. In 16 out of 25 patients, the progress of the disease was halted, and in 5 patients, the disease remained unaffected [22, 23]. The course of treatment with THP was well tolerated. Table 3 lists the side effects that occurred in this study.

A further study was performed in elderly patients (median age: 74 years) suffering from advanced small-cell lung cancer. In most of the patients, the performance status did not permit conventional aggressive combination chemotherapy. These patients were treated with 70 mg/m^2 THP i.v. on day 1 every 21 days. Preliminary results were published recently [24]. In ten patients who were evaluable for re-

Table 3. Side effects of therapy with pirarubicin (THP) 28 patients, phase II, Federal Republic of Germany [23]

Side effects	WHO grade			
	1	2	3	4
Cycles (n=121)				
Leukocytopenia	18	14	9	1
Thrombocytopenia	2	0	0	0
Cycles (n=117)				
Alopecia	28	29	4	0
Nausea/vomiting	44	14	0	0
Infection	2	0	0	0
Stomatitis	0	1	0	0

sponse, one CR and five PR could be achieved. Besides leukopenia, no other significant toxic side effects were observed. The clinical investigators statet that the subjective tolerance of the treatment was excellent. The trial is still being conducted, and further results should be available soon.
Twenty-three patients with advanced head and neck cancer (age: 34–78 years) were palliatively treated with THP (70 mg/m^2 i.v. on day 1 at 3-week intervals). For all patients, pretreatment included surgery, local irradiation, and chemotherapy with cisplatin but without anthracyclines. The remission rate in 16 evaluable patients was: 2 CR (5 months and 6 months), 5 PR, 6 failures to respond, and 3 cases of disease progression. The overall response rate was 44%. The main side effect of treatment was leukocytopenia (WHO grades 3 and 4 in 17, two cycles respectively of a total of 58 cycles). Further side effects were minimal: Nausea and vomiting and alopecia (WHO grade 4) occurred in no cycles, while grade 3 (both side effects) was observed in two cycles [25].

USA

In a phase I study at the M.D. Anderson Hospital (Houston, Texas, USA) 5, 15, 20, or 25 mg/m^2 THP were given weekly for 3 weeks. Myelosuppression was the dose-limiting factor, with nadirs as follows:

Dose (mg/m^2 per week)	Granulocytes (1000/mm^3 per day)	Platelets (1000/mm^3 per day)
15	1.3 (24)	223 (23)
20	1.1 (23)	155 (18)
25	0.7 (21)	161 (21)

No major therapeutic responses were seen. However, the group consisted of patients who had previously received extensive chemotherapy. The investigators recommend further phase II studies with a dosage of 20 mg/m^2 per week for 3 weeks [26].

Cardiotoxicity of THP

The main problem of ADM cardiotoxicity has already been mentioned. Extensive studies were performed with THP to get more information about its potential cardiotoxicity. Comparative electron microscope investigations of the effect of different anthracyclines on the heart of the golden hamster have shown that pirarubicin is less cardiotoxic than mitoxantrone, epirubicin, ADM, and daunorubicin. The measurements were performed with equitoxic dosages of each anthracycline [16].
Human neutrophils exposed to 10^{-4} *M* ADM and the derivates epirubicin and THP revealed a different intracellular penetration and distribution pattern. While ADM was found to be a potent inducer of superoxide generation from resting

cells, epirubicin was less effective. In contrast, THP did not show any superoxide-inducing effect. Anthracycline-stimulated superoxide production seems to correlate with the cardiotoxic effects [21]. Considering the favorable preclinical data, the correlation to the later clinical findings seem noteworthy.

In two separate Japanese phase I studies, ten patients received a cumulative dose of between 900 and 1000 mg/m^2 THP and revealed no signs or symptoms of cardiac failure. Two cases received higher total doses of 1920 mg per body (1390 mg/m^2) and 1860 mg per body (1410 mg/m^2). The first patient did not reveal any signs or symptoms of cardiac toxicity. The second patient, however, developed irreversible cardiac failure. The Japanese investigators concluded that THP is not cardiotoxic up to a cumulative dose of 900 mg/m^2 and that toxic cardiac effects begin to occur with a total dose of between 900 mg/m^2 and 1400 mg/m^2 [28].

Extensive investigations were additionally conducted in Japan to measure the acute cardiotoxicity of anthracyclines by using long-term continuous ECG (Holter ECG). Seven patients in each group were treated with ADM and THP. No effect on the specialized conduction system was observed with either ADM or THP. However, the ventricular premature beat tended to increase after ADM administration, and the mode of appearance of the ventricular extrasystole was dangerous and life threatening in one patient [29].

In France, 38 patients with various malignancies were evaluated for cardiotoxicity after having received more than 500 mg/m^2 anthracyclines (maximum: 1650 mg/m^2). The total dose of THP in these cases ranged from 90 mg/m^2 to 1125 mg/m^2 and was usually given after relapse following pretreatment with ADM. Clinical congestive heart failure was observed in two patients. One of them first received the cumulative dose of 525 mg/m^2 ADM and then 1125 mg/m^2 THP (total anthracycline dose: 1650 mg/m^2). The other patient received 805 mg/m^2 THP. In both cases, the congestive heart failure disappeared after discontinuation of treatment. In two further patients with cumulative anthracycline doses of 937 mg/m^2 and 1103 mg/m^2, the treatment had to be discontinued owing to a significant decrease in ventricular function as measured by ultrasound or muga scan. However, these patients developed no heart failure [30].

To compare the cardiotoxicity of new drugs with those of ADM, one should not only focus on the different cumulative doses but also on the dose in the individual cycle that is necessary to achieve an antitumor effect. In the above-mentioned trials, the dose of THP was equal to or lower than the dose one could expect with ADM. Taking into consideration that Japanese investigators stated the maximal cumulative dose of THP to be around 900 mg/m^2 in patients who had not previously been treated with anthracyclines [31], THP appears to have a lower chronic cardiotoxicity than ADM. One should however keep in mind that the number of patients who received high cumulative doses (> 550 mg/m^2) of THP is small and, therefore, the significance of the results regarding cardiotoxicity is limited. Further results, that means, more patients under study, are necessary to validate the available data.

Open Questions and Perspectives

THP has shown significant anticancer activity in several solid tumors. Especially in breast cancer but also in small-cell lung cancer, the results with THP are comparable to those of ADM. Administration of ADM for head and neck tumors has achieved an overall response rate or around 23% [32], THP has shown remarkable and unexpectedly high response rates in these tumors. All available data with THP confirm that its main side effect is leukocytopenia and that the drug is subjective well tolerated.
However, sufficient experience with THP is available for only a small number of tumors, whereas in many tumors in which ADM has proven effective, the number of patients treated with THP is too small to compare antitumor activity of both drugs. Furthermore, it is still unclear whether THP has the same tumor spectrum as ADM. The preliminary results (e.g., response in head and neck cancer) underline the importance of screening further THP sensitive tumors.
In the tumors in which THP has already shown antitumor activity, further extensive studies of combination therapy have to be initiated. They should investigate whether THP really provides a benefit in the treatment of advanced malignant disease – prolonging the survival time and improving the quality of life.

References

1. DeVita VT, Hellman S, Rosenberg S (1985) Cancer – principles and practice of oncology, 2nd edn. Lippincott, Philadelphia
2. Benjamin RS, Weirik PH, Bachur NR (1974) Adriamycin chemotherapy: Efficacy, safety, and pharmacology basis of an intermittent single high-dosage schedule. Cancer 33: 19
3. von Hoff DD, Layard MW, Basa P, Davis HL, von Hoff AL, Rosenzweig M, Muggia F (1979) Risk factors for doxorubicin-induced congestive heart failure. Ann Intern Med 91: 710
4. Umezawa H, Takahasi Y, Kinoshita M, Naganawa H, Matsuda T, Ishizuka M, Tatsuta K, Takeuchi T (1979) Tetrahydropyranyl derivatives of daunomycin and adriamycin. J Antibiot, pp 1082–1084
5. Fuijita H, Ogawa K, Tone H, Iguchi H, Shomura T, Murata SS (1986) Pharmacokinetics of doxorubicin (2″R)-4-*0*-tetrahydropyranyl-adriamycin and aclarubicin. Jpn J Antibiot 39 (5): 1321–1336
6. Dantchev D, Bourut C, Maral R, Mathe G (1983) Cardiotoxicity and alopecia of 12 different anthracyclines and 1 anthracycline in the golden hamster model. In: Spitzy KH, Karrer K (eds) Proceedings of the 13th international congress of chemotherapy, 28 August–2 September 1983, Vienna, part 211, pp 15–19
7. Tapiero H, Munck JN, Fourcade A (1986) Relationship between the intracellular accumulation of anthracyclines and effectiveness in vitro and in vivo. Drugs Expl Clin Res XII (1/2/3): 257–264
8. Tapiero H, Fourcade A, Munck JN, Zwingelstein G, Lampidis TJ (1986) Cellular pharmacology of anthracycline resistance and its circumvention. Drugs Expl Clin Res XII (1/2/3): 265–273
9. Kraemer HP, Sedlacek HH (1984) Modified screening system to select new cytostatic drugs, Behring Inst Mitt No 74. Research Laboratories of Behringwerke, Marburg, pp 301–28
10. Tsuruo T, Iida H, Tsukagoshi S, Sakurai Y (1982) 4′-*0*-tetrahydropyranyl-Adriamycin as a potential new antitumor agent. Cancer Res 42: 1462–67
11. Majima H (1983) Phase I and preliminary phase II clinical study of 4′-*0*-tetrahydropyranyl-doxorubicin (THP-ADM). In: Spitzy KH, Karrer K (eds) Proceedings of the 13th international congress of chemotherapy, 28 August–2 September 1983, Vienna, part 260, pp 28–31

12. Wakui A, Yokoyam M, Konno K, Nagai Y, Sakano T, Koyama Y, Imamura Y, Nakajima O, Niijima T, Akaza H, Kimura I, Ohnishi T, Saito T (1986) Phase I trial of 4'-0-tetrahydropyranyl-doxorubicin (THP) - a multiinstitutional cooperative study. In: Lapis K, Eckhardt S (eds) 14th international cancer congress, Budapest, 21-27 Aug 1986, Abstract No 1737
13. Majima H (1986) Clinical (phase I and II) and clinical pharmacologic studies of 4'-0-tetrahydropyranyl-doxorubicin (THP-ADM). 14th international cancer congress, Budapest, 21-27 Aug 1986, Abstract No 1738
14. Kimura K (1986) A phase II study of (2''R)-4'-O-tetrahydropyranyl-Adriamycin (THP) in patients with hematological malignancies. Jpn J Cancer Chemother 13 (2): 368-375
15. Saito T, Kasai Y, Wakui A, Furue H, Majima H, Niitani H, Niijima T, Takeda C, Abe O, Koyama Y, Nakao I, Ogawa M, Kimura K, Ohta K, Yamada K, Taguchi T, Kimura I, Hattori T, Inokuchi K, Kato T (1986) Phase II study of (2''R)-4'-0-tetrahydropyranyl-Adriamycin (THP) in patients with solid tumors. Jpn J Cancer Chemother 13: 1060-1069
16. Abe O, Tominaga T, Enomoto K, Abe R, Iino Y, Koyama H, Fujimoto M, Nomura Y, Tanaka T (1986) A randomized controlled study on (2''R)-4'-0-tetrahydropyranyl-Adriamycin and Adriamycin in combination with cyclophosphamide and 5-fluorouracil in the treatment of advanced and recurrent breast cancer. Jpn J Cancer Chemother 13 (3-1): 578-585
17. Nittani H, Kurane S, Hino M, Shibuya M, Shimabukuro Z, Kawachi S, Yoshimura A (1987) A randomized phase II study of THP and ADM combined with VCR and ACNU for small cell lung cancer. In: Berkada B, Kuemmerle HP (eds) 15th international congress of chemotherapy, Istanbul, 22-24 July 1987, abstract No W-12. ecomed, Munich
18. Kleeberg UR, Richter-von-Arnauld HP, Miller AA, Seeber S (1985) Phase I study of a new anthracycline derivative: Theprubicin in patients with disseminated cancer. Abstract, 14th international congress of chemotherapy, Kyoto, Japan, 23-28 June 1985
19. Miller AA, Kleeberg UR, Seeber S, Schmidt CGA (1988) Phase I-II study of pirarubicin. J Cancer Res Clin Oncol 114: 91-94
20. Mathe G, Brienza S, Umezawa H, Tapiero H, de Vassal F, Misset JK, Ribaud P, Musset M, Despax R, Burki F, Goldschmidt E (1987) Oriented phase II trial in advanced breast cancer of 4'-0-tetrahydropyranyl-Adriamycin (THP-ADM). In: Berkada B, Kuemmerle HP (eds) 15th international congress of chemotherapy, Istanbul, 22-24 July 1987, abstract no W-12. ecomed, Munich
21. Schinetti ML, Rossini D, Bertelli A (1987) Interaction of anthracycline antibiotics with human neutraphils: superoxide production, free radical formation and intracellular penetration. J Cancer Res Clin Oncol 113: 15-19
22. Kaukel E, Koschel G, Gatzemeier U, Heckmayr M, Hartmann W (1987) Phase II study of pirarubicin in patients with pleuramesotheliomas. In: Berkada B, Kuemmerle HP (eds) 15th international congress of chemotherapy, Istanbul, 22-24 July 1987, abstract no W-12 ecomed, Munich
23. Gatzemeier U, Calvrezos A, Kaukel E, Koschel G, Magnussen H, Radenbach D (1986) The new anthracycline THP-ADM (4'-0-tetrahydropyranyl-Adramycin) in the treatment of malignant pleuramesotheliomas. J Cancer Res Clin Oncol 111 [Suppl] 6: 66 (abstract No Lun 13)
24. Henss H, Arnold H, Fiebig HH, Löhr GW (1987) Phase II study with THP-doxorubicin in small cell bronchogenic carcinoma. Blut 55: 205 (abstract no 144)
25. Schroeder M, Purea H, Westerhausen M (1988) Clinical experience with pirarubicin in the treatment of patients with pretreated head and neck cancer. In: Nagel GA, Kornhuber B (eds) Proceedings 19th national cancer congress of the German cancer society, 28 February - 5 March 1988, abstract no 4/27-M-010. J Cancer Res Clin Oncol [Suppl] 114
26. Krakoff IH, Raber MN, Newman RA (1987) Clinical and clinical pharmacologic studies of 4'-0-tetrahydropyranyl-Adriamycin (THP-ADM). In: Berkada kB, Kuemmerle HP (eds) 15th international congress of chemotherapy, Istanbul 22-24 July 1987, abstract no W-12. ecomed, Munich
27. Mathe G, Brienza S, Misset JL, deVassal F, Muset M, Goldschmidt E, Despax R, Ribaud P, Gastiaburu J, Ecstein E (1987) THP-ADM combined to alkylating agents (cyclophosphamide or thiotepa), vindesin and fluorouracil in metastatic breast cancer. In: Berkada B, Kuemmerle HP (eds) 15th international congress of chemotherapy, Istanbul, 22-24 July 1987, abstract no W-12. ecomed, Munich

28. Majima H (1987) Clinical phase I and pharmacokinetic studies on (2″R)-4-tetrahydropyranyl-Adriamycin (THP-ADM). In: Berkada kB, Kuemmerle HP (eds) 15th international congress of chemotherapy, Istanbul, 22–24 July 1987, abstract no W-12. ecomed, Munich
29. Okuma K, Furuta I, Ota K (1984) Acute cardiotoxicity of antracyclines – analysis by using holter ECG. Jpn J Cancer Chemother 11: 901–911
30. Marino JP, Brienza D, Dantchev JL, Musset M, DeVassal F, Goldschmidt E, Ribaud P, Levi F, Despax R, Mathe G (1987) Reduced cardiotoxicity of THP-Adriamycin in cancer patients. Biennial conference (Bicon) on chemotheapy of infectious diseases and malignancies, Munich, 26–29 April 1987, abstract no 325. Paul Ehrlich Society for Chemotherapy
31. Morikawa K, Takada T, Imura H, Itoh N, Shirakawa S, Sobue R, Maruyama F, Kojima H, Ono Y, Matsui T, Ino T, Ezaki K, Hirano M (1987) Assessment of anthracycline cardiotoxicity with radionuclide angiocardiography. Jpn J Clin Hematol 28: 213–219
32. Monfardini S, Brunner K, Crowther D, Eckhardt S, Olive D, Tanneberger S, Veronesi A, Whitehouse JMA, Wittes R (eds) (1987) Manual of adult and pediatric medical oncology (UICC). Springer-Verlag, Berlin Heidelberg New York Tokyo

Pirarubicin – A New Anthracycline with High Activity in Untreated Patients with Small-Cell Cancer of the Lung

H.-H. FIEBIG,[1] H. HENSS,[1] and H. ARNOLD[1]

Introduction

A phase II study was carried out with 16 elderly patients with small-cell cancers of the lung who had received no prior chemo- or radiotherapy. The new anthracycline, pirarubicin (formerly Theprubicin or 4′-(R)-*0*-tetrahydropyranyl-adriamycin-hydrochlorid), was administered at a dose of 70 mg/m^2 i.v. every 3 weeks. Among 16 evaluable patients (one tumor-related early death was excluded), one patient achieved a complete remission (CR), seven had a partial remission (PR), three showed initially no change, and four had disease progression. The median time from the beginning of therapy to progression was 12 months for the patient in CR and 4 months for the patients in PR (range, 2–7 months). The median survival time was 13 months for patients with CR and PR (range, 3–15+ months) and 4 months for patients with initially no change or disease progression (range, 1–8 months). The dose-limiting toxicity consisted of leukopenia; WHO grades III and IV were observed in 16% of all treatment cycles. The subjective tolerance was good; vomiting, alopecia, and stomatitis were observed in a few cases. No cardiac, hepatic, renal, or CNS toxicity was encountered. Pirarubicin is a new anthracycline, which was initially developed in Japan [1]. The structure is shown in Fig. 1. It was selected for clinical development because it showed greater or similar activity in experimental tumor models when compared with other anthracyclines [2–4]. Preclinical studies showed that pirarubicin was less cardiotoxic than adriamycin. Pirarubicin showed a different organ distribution from adriamycin, with higher

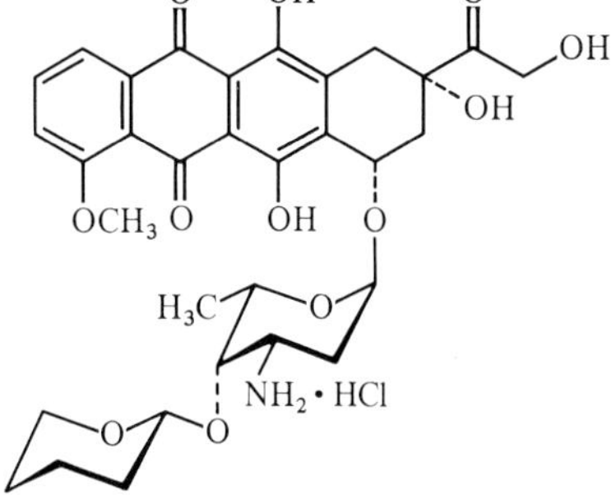

Fig. 1. Structure of 4′-(R)-*0*-tetrahydropyranyl-adriamycin-hydrochloride

[1] Department of Internal Medicine, University Clinic Freiburg, Hugstetter Straße 55, 7800 Freiburg 1, FRG.

H. G. Beger et al. (Eds.), Cancer Therapy

concentrations found in the lungs, spleen, and thymus and lower concentrations found in the heart and gallbladder [5]. Previous clinical phase II studies have been performed in several countries. Pirarubicin showed definite activity in acute lymphoblastic leukemia, lymphomas, and in carcinomas of the ovary, uterus, cervix, and breast [6, 7]. Leukopenia has been reported to be the major toxicity.
We performed a phase II study on untreated patients with small-cell cancers of the lung. To evaluate the therapeutic potential of this new anthracycline, the study was conducted on untreated patients because pretreated patients usually show a markedly lower response rate. For ethical reasons, only a subgroup of patients with no chance of cure with the standard combination chemotherapy were treated. They included elderly patients over 65 years of age, the majority presenting with extensive disease [8, 9].

Patients and Methods

Patient eligibility criteria included histologic proof of a small-cell cancer of the lung, measurable tumor lesions, no prior chemo- or radiotherapy, age of more than 65 years, a good performance status of at least 60% on the Karnofsky scale, normal bone marrow (leukocytes $>4000/mm^3$, thrombocytes $>100000/mm^3$), normal liver and renal function ($<125\%$ of normal values), no brain metastasis or cardiac disease, and informed consent. Pirarubicin was administered at a dosage

Table 1. Patient characteristics

n: to 16[a]		
Sex: male: 14 female: 2		
Age in years: Median: 74		
Range: 65–86		
Stage (no. of patients):		
Extensive: 14		
Limited: 2		
Performance status (Karnofsky scale):		
Median: 65		
Range: 60–90		
Prior chemo- or radiotherapy (no. of patients):		0
Sites of metastases		
	Liver	7
	Lymph nodes	2
	Lung nodes	2
	Bone marrow	2
	Other	4
No. of cycles applied		
Median 3		
Range 1–8		

[a] Sixteen patients were eligible; 1 early death due to tumor progression was excluded from evaluation of efficacy.
[b] Efficacy and toxicity were evaluated according to WHO criteria.

Table 2. Efficacy of pirarubicin in untreated small-cell carcinoma of the lung ($n=16$)

Complete remission	1	6%	Duration	12 months
Partial remission	7	50%	Median duration	4 months (range 2–7)
No change[a]	3	19%		
Progression	4	25%		
Median survival time in months				
Complete and partial remission		13	(range: 3+–13)	
No change and disease progression		4	(range: 1–>8)	
Overall		5		

[a] For ≥2 months.

of 70 mg/mm^2 as an i.v. injection every 3 weeks. Therapy was delayed for 1–2 weeks if the leukocytes were below 4000/mm^3. The subsequent dose was reduced to 75% if the nadir reached WHO grade III and to 50% if the nadir of the leukocytes was WHO grade IV.

Patients' characteristics are shown in Table 1. Of the 16 eligible patients, one was excluded because of early death due to tumor progression. The therapeutic efficacy and toxicity were evaluated according to WHO criteria [10].

Results and Discussion

Efficacy

Of 15 evaluable patients, one achieved a complete remission, seven had a partial remission, three initially showed no change, and four had disease progression (Table 2). The median time from the start of treatment until tumor progression was 12 months for the patient in CR and 4 months for the patients in PR. The median survival time was 13 months for patients in CR or PR and 4 months for patients with no change or progression. The overall survival time was 5 months.

Side Effects

The side effects are shown in Table 3). The dose-limiting toxicity was leukopenia. A leukocyte count below 2000/mm^3 was observed in 16% of all cycles. The median nadir of leukopenia occurred after 15 days, with recovery after 7 days. Only one case of pneumonia was seen in the 56 treatment cycles. Vomiting, alopecia, and stomatitis were observed in a few cases. No patient developed cardiovascular, hepatic, renal, or CNS toxicity.

Pirarubicin has definite activity in small-cell cancer of the lung. Its therapeutic activity appears to be superior to adriamycin, which has shown a response rate of approximately 35%–45% in several studies [11]. However, most of these patients were pretreated. The low incidence of side effects and the very good subjective tolerance in this group of elderly patients indicate the need for further clinical studies, especially in combination chemotherapy.

Table 3. Side effects in 16 patients treated with pirarubicin

Toxicity	WHO grade	First course (n=16)	All cycles (n=56)
Leukocytes	4	2	3
	3	4 (38%)	6 (16%)
	2	2	18
	1	0 (62%)	12 (84%)
	0	8	17
Thrombocytes	4+3	0	0
	2	1	1
	1	2	4
	0	13	51
Gastrointestinal complaint			
Vomiting	2+3	3	
Nausea	1	1	
	0	12	
Alopecia	3		1
	2		2
	1		0
	0		13
Stomatitis	2	1	
	1	0	
	0	15	

References

1. Umezawa H, Takahashi Y, Kinoshita M, Naganawa H, Matsuda T, Ishizuka M, Tatsuta K, Takeuchi T (1979) Tetrahydropyranyl derivates of daunomycin and adriamycin. J Antibiot 32: 1082-84
2. Tsurus T, Iida H, Tsukagoshi S, Sakurai Y (1982) 4′-*0*-tetrahydropyranyladriamycin as a potential new antitumor agent. Cancer Res 42: 1462-67
3. Kraemer HP, Sedlacek HH (1984) A modified screening system to select new cytostatic drugs. Research Laboratories of Behring-Werke, Behring Inst Mitt No 74, pp 301-28
4. Leder G, Fiebig HH, Henss H, Löhr GW (1988) Activity of theprubicin - a new anthracycline - in vitro and in vivo. J Cancer Res Clin Oncol [suppl] 114: 152
5. Fujita H, Fujita Y, Ogawa K, Shomura T, Murata S, Iguchi H, Tone H (1984) Comparative studies on the pharmacokinetics of adriamycin, 4′-*0*-tetrahydropyranyladriamycin and aclacinomycin. Department of Bacteriology, Tsurumi University, Central Research Laboratories, Meiji Seika Kaish; Central Research Laboratories, Sanraku-Ocean, Japan
6. Majima H (1983) Phase I and preliminary phase II clinical study 4′-*0*-tetrahydropyranyladriamycin doxorubicin (THP-ADM). In: Spitzy KH, Karrer K (eds) Proceedings of the 13th international congress of chemotheapy, Vienna. Egermann, Vienna, pp 28-31
7. Ogawa M, Inagaki J, Horikoshi N, Inoue K (1983) Clinical study of 4′-*0*-tetrahydropyranyladriamycin (THP-adriamycin).
8. Pallares C, Bastus R, Lopez JJ, de Andres L (1987) Long-term survival in small cell carcinoma of the lung. Eur J Cancer Oncol 23: 541-544 Invest New Drug 1: 169
9. Wolf M, Havemann K, Holle R, Drings P, Hans K, Schroeder M (1987) Rezidivhäufigkeit und Langzeit-Überleben beim kleinzelligen Bronchialkarzinom. Onkologie 10: 357-366
10. Miller AB, Hoogstraten B, Staquet M, Winkler A (1979) Reporting results in cancer treatment. Cancer 47: 207-214
11. Monfardini S, Brunner K, Crowther D, Eckardt S, Olive D, Tannenberger S, Veronesi A, Whitehouse JMA, Wittes R (eds) (1987) Manual of adult and paediatric medical oncology. Springer-Verlag, Berlin Heidelberg New York Tokyo, p 217

New Approaches in the Hormonal Therapy of Breast Cancer

K. HÖFFKEN[1]

Introduction

Hormonal therapy plays a central role in the overall treatment strategy of sex-specific cancer. Long before the detection of hormones and hormone receptors, ablation of sex hormone glands became part of the treatment of breast and prostate cancer because, in spite of malignancy, the cell growth retained hormone dependence. Moreover, the demonstration of estrogen and/or progesterone receptors as a predictor for the effectiveness of hormonal manipulations in two-thirds to three-fourths of all breast cancers warranted further research in this field.
Following the accepted principle that treatment of advanced breast cancer and prostate cancer can only be of a palliative nature, new approaches to hormone therapy were developed to attempt reduction of treatment-related morbidity. Surgical ablative procedures were gradually replaced by the specific manipulation of hormonal feedback mechanisms.
As shown in Fig. 1, the main source of sex steroids in premenopausal women is the ovary, whereas, in postmenopausal women, estrogen is produced by aromatization of adrenal androgens. It is the purpose of this review to outline recent successes in suppressing ovarian function by agonists of the luteinizing hormone-releasing hormone (LHRH) and in the interference with the aromatase enzyme system. The first approach mimics ovarian ablation, the second one, adrenalectomy.

Agonists of the Luteinizing-Hormone-Releasing Hormone

Ovarian ablation has a long-standing history in the treatment of metastatic breast cancer. At the end of the last century, Schinzinger [35] and Beatson [1] independently reported on the beneficial effect of surgical removal of the ovaries in premenopausal women with advanced breast cancer. Subsequently, this treatment became the standard systemic hormonal therapy in such patients. In a random premenopausal patient population, oophorectomy produces an average 33% objective response rate [15]. Thus, this treatment has the disadvantage that only a minority of patients respond, while the remainder suffer unnecessary treatment morbidity.

[1] University Clinic of Internal Medicine (Tumor Research), West German Tumor Center, Hufelandstraße 55, 4300 Essen 1, FRG.

H. G. Beger et al. (Eds.), Cancer Therapy

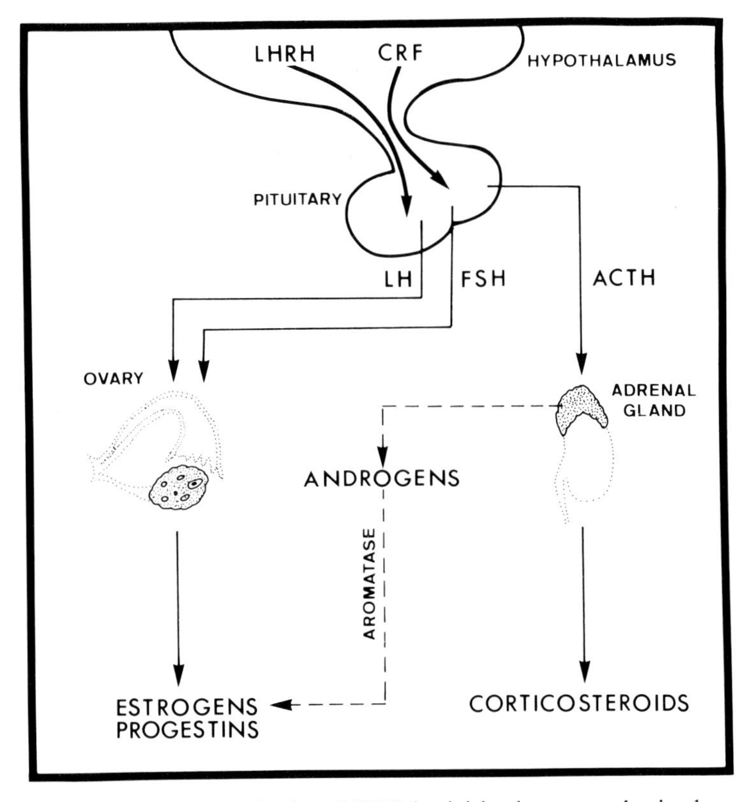

Fig. 1. Mechanisms of female hormone production. *LHRH*, luteinizing-hormone-releasing hormone; *CRF*, corticotropin-releasing factor; *LH*, luteinizing hormone; *FSH*, follicle-stimulating hormone; *ACTH*, adrenocorticotropic hormone

Since its introduction, hormone receptor determinations have assisted prediction of hormonal therapy effectiveness. This has resulted in nearly 70% response rates in patients with hormone receptor-positive tumors. However, there still remain patients who are oophorectomized unnecessarily (about one-third) and patients with receptor-negative tumors, who might respond to hormonal ablation therapy (about one-tenth).

For these reasons, less invasive methods of attaining a response to hormonal treatment in advanced breast cancer have been sought. Initially, this was attempted by treating premenopausal patients with high doses of an anti-estrogen. Results of this approach, however, are still controversial, both in terms of response rates and with regard to whether it is a reliable tool for predicting the effectiveness of subsequent ovarian ablation therapy [20, 21, 31].

Soon after the introduction of LHRH agonists designed for the treatment of primary sterility or endometriosis, it became apparent that these substances induced a down-regulation of pituitary receptors, thus leading to sustained hypogonadotropic ovarian insufficiency. Subsequent preclinical studies showed that LHRH agonists were effective in a variety of hormone-dependent tumors, including dimethylbenzanthracene (DMBA)-induced mammary tumors in female rats [29, 34].

During the last 5 years, analogues of LHRH have been investigated in pre- and postmenopausal women. Encouraging results have been obtained in premenopausal patients with metastatic breast cancer [13, 14, 22-25, 38, 39]. Presently, treatment with LHRH agonists of about 150 premenopausal patients with breast cancer has been reported. About 40% of these women experienced an objective (complete or partial) remission lasting for 3-54 months. Treatment failed in approximately 50% of the patients; the remainder benefited from LHRH agonists, as evidenced by stabilization of previously progressive tumor growth. Considering prognostic subgroups, patients with positive hormone receptors of the primary or secondary tumor, those with a long relapse-free interval between mastectomy and the first manifestation of metastases, and patients with locoregional relapses only benefited more from the LHRH agonist treatment than their respective counterparts [19, 24, 25].

Side effects of the treatment consisted of menopausal symptoms. Rarely, local irritations at the subcutaneous injection site were observed. In spite of the theoretical conception that the initial rise in ovarian hormones could induce a tumor flare up, no such event has been reported unequivocally.

In summary, treatment with LHRH agonists of premenopausal patients with advanced breast cancer has yielded results similar to those of surgical ovarian ablation. However, no prospectively randomized trial has been conducted yet, so it cannot be concluded that "chemical castration" with LHRH agonists replaces oophorectomy. On the one hand, patients responded to surgical ovarian ablation after the failure of LHRH agonists to suppress ovarian function effectively [39]; on the other, LHRH agonist treatment always yielded slightly higher remission rates than the surgical procedure, suggesting that the direct antitumor effect of these substances [7, 8] may contribute to the clinical effectiveness. This could also account for the occasionally reported tumor responses in postmenopausal patients [30, 38]. Obviously, this question should be addressed more systematically in future trials.

With the recent availability of depot forms of LHRH agonists administered only every 4-8 weeks, it remains to be seen whether this "medical oophorectomy" may ultimately be substituted for the surgical procedure or whether it will serve as a predictor of the efficacy of irreversible ovarian failure induced by other therapeutic means.

Aromatase Inhibition

In earlier years, adrenalectomy was performed on patients with hormone-responsive, advanced breast cancer to remove the source of estrogens in women with artificial (following oophorectomy) or natural menopause [15].

Aminoglutethimide

Aminoglutethimide was originally introduced as an anticonvulsant drug but was withdrawn after it was reported to induce adrenal insufficiency [4]. Subsequent investigations suggested that aminoglutethimide inhibits several steps in the synthesis of adrenal steroids [5] and the aromatase enzyme-mediated peripheral conversion of adrenal androgens into estrone [32]. This indicated that aminoglutethimide may be useful as an antiestrogen in the treatment of breast cancer, and a number of clinical trials have shown that aminoglutethimide is effective in the treatment of advanced postmenopausal breast cancer. In these trials, objective response rates of 30%-50% were achieved, which are similar to those obtained by surgical adrenalectomy or tamoxifen [9, 10, 12, 16, 33, 36].

Considering prognostic subgroups, patients with positive estrogen hormone receptors in the primary or secondary tumor and those with predominantly bone metastases responded best to the aminoglutethimide treatment. Pretreatment with other hormonal measures did not preclude responses to aminoglutethimide.

Side effects of standard-dose treatment (1 g/day) with aminoglutethimide are considerable and consist of central nervous, gastrointestinal, and cutaneous symptoms. In about 10%, treatment had to be discontinued owing to the severity of side effects. With regard to toxicity, two issues have repeatedly been the subject of controversy. First, the question arose as to whether a reduction in the dose of aminoglutethimide would result in less toxicity while sustaining efficacy. Second, interference with adrenal steroid biosynthesis led to the question of whether cortisol replacement was mandatory during aminoglutethimide treatment.

The first issue has been solved. It is now generally acknowledged that a decrease in the dose (500 mg/day) of aminoglutethimide maintains clinical efficacy in postmenopausal patients with advanced breast cancer [2, 11, 17, 28. 37]. Evidence suggests that even lower doses (250 mg/day) yield tumor responses. The observation that the addition of cortisol reduces the side effects of aminoglutethimide has not been substantiated [37]. We were able to reduce the toxicity notably by a decrease in the dose of aminoglutethimide without the addition of cortisol [17]. Most probably, this was the result of lower plasma aminoglutethimide levels during the first 6 weeks of treatment with 500 mg aminoglutethimide per day [26]. This coincides with the period of time when side effects are most likely to occur and then spontaneously subside. The rate and degree of side effects of both dose levels were comparable to those observed in studies using the respective doses of aminoglutethimide together with cortisol replacement [16, 17].

The second issue still remains a topic of controversy. There is general agreement that aminoglutethimide blocks the aromatase enzyme system, thus acting as an anti-estrogenic drug. The degree of inhibition of enzymes of the adrenal steroid biosynthesis (20,22-desmolase; 21-hydroxylase; 11β-hydroxylase) has been estimated differently by various authors.

We observed that inhibition of the enzymes was counteracted by a reactive rise in adrenocorticotropic hormone (ACTH) that resulted in an increase in precursor levels, thus keeping the serum level of cortisol constant [16]. Even more important, ACTH provocation tests yielded adequate cortisol responses [16, 27], thus supporting the concept that hydrocortisone supplementation appears not to be mandatory, either for an increase in efficacy or for a decrease in side effects of the treatment. It should be noted, however, that individual differences in acetylation of aminoglutethimide may result in drug concentrations that could also block, rather than inhibit, 11β-hydroxylase. This would explain the adrenal insufficiencies developing occasionally in both epileptic children [4] and in patients with breast can-

cer even after low-dose treatment [28]. Therefore, the omission of hydrocortisone supplementation should be paralleled by the regular determination of serum cortisol levels.
In summary, aminoglutethimide has proved to be an effective anti-estrogenic drug via aromatase inhibition. In view of its toxicity even with low doses, it is recommended for hormonal treatment following tamoxifen in patients with artificial or natural menopause suffering from advanced breast cancer. General rules of indication for hormonal treatment must be acknowledged.

4-Hydroxyandrostenedione

Soon after elucidation of the general mechanism of action of aminoglutethimide in estrogen deprivation, compounds have been studied that could be candidates for replacing aminoglutethimide in that they (a) inhibit aromatase, (b) do not interfere with adrenal steroid biosynthesis, and (c) have no side effects. Among several steroidal compounds, 4-hydroxylated native androstenedione has proved to compete with the natural substrates, androstenedione and testosterone, for the aromatase. This substance is being tested in clinical studies [3]. Presently, some 200 postmenopausal patients with advanced breast cancer have been treated by an English group [6] and by our group [18]. Several doses, dose schedules, and routes of administration have been used. Available data indicate that about 30% of the patients achieved objective (complete or partial) remissions, whereas 40% failed to benefit from treatment with 4-hydroxyandrostenedione. The remainder of the women experienced stabilization of previously progressive disease. Side effects were unspecific and consisted mostly of local pain and/or sterile abscesses at the intramuscular injection site in a dose-dependent fashion. Oral treatment may overcome this problem. Considering prognostic subgroups, patients with estrogen receptor-positive tumors and those with bone metastases responded best.
In summary, 4-hydroxyandrostenedione is an effective aromatase inhibitor, yielding clinical results in breast cancer comparable to those achieved by aminoglutethimide. The optimal dose schedule and administration route remains to be clarified.

Other Aromatase Inhibitors

Among other potential candidates, CGS 16 949A (Ciba Geigy), a nonsteroidal aromatase inhibitor, has entered phase I clinical trials. Presently, estradiol reduction has been confirmed in postmenopausal patients with far advanced breast cancer. Occasionally, objective tumor responses have already been observed (Höffken et al., unpublished work). Further results are being awaited with interest.

Concluding Remarks

Hormonal therapy of malignant diseases, e.g., prostate and breast cancer, has come of age after its first tentative efforts at the turn of this century. Novel approaches have followed outstanding investigations that were awarded the Nobel prize (e.g., Huggins for androgen ablation in prostate cancer; Schally for the synthesis of LHRH). It is, therefore, not astonishing that the intriguing story of hormonal manipulation serves as a paradigm for attempts to interfere predictively with natural feedback mechanisms in order to reverse the deregulated balance between proliferation and differentiation of malignant cell growth. Epithelial growth factors or hemopoetic differentiation factors are already called "cell hormones," supporting the concept that regulatory factors exist that can be exploited for the treatment of malignancies.

In parallel, the increase in knowledge of the endocrine systems directly benefited the patients, making it no longer necessary to perform mutilating surgical procedures, which often necessitated a life-long substitution of essential hormones. In this way, new approaches to the hormonal therapy of cancer gave way to a remarkable reduction in treatment-related morbidity.

Acknowledgements. The cooperation of the following persons in obtaining the above-mentioned data is gratefully acknowledged: C.U. Anders, E. Aulbert, R. Becher, R. Callies, C. Doberauer, P. Faber, B. Hoffmann, W. Jonat, H. Kempf, H.K. Kley, M. Kölbel, E. Kurschel, A.A. Miller, B. Miller, C. Oesterdickhoff, K. Possinger, M.E. Scheulen, and C.G. Schmidt. We also thank F. Bosse and G. Coenenberg for their help in the preparation of the manuscript. Aminoglutethimide, 4-hydroxyandrostenedione, and CGS 16 949A were provided by Ciba-Geigy GmbH, Wehr/Baden, FRG; Buserelin and Depot-Buserelin were provided by the Behringwerke AG, Marburg, FRG.

References

1. Beatson GT (1896) On the treatment of inoperable cases of carcinoma of the mamma: suggestions for a new method of treatment with illustrative cases. Lancet 2: 104-107, 162-165
2. Bonneterre J, Coppens H, Mauriac L, Metz M, Rouesse J, Armand JP, Fargeot P, Mathieu M, Tubiana M, Cappelaere P (1985) Aminoglutethimide in advanced breast cancer: Clinical results of a French multicenter randomized trial comparing 500 mg and 1 g/day. Europ J Cancer Clin Oncol 21: 1153-1158
3. Brodie AMH, Garrett WM, Tsai-Morris CH, Wink LC (1984) Aromatase inhibition: a new perspective in the treatment of breast cancer. In: Nagel GA, Santen RJ (eds) Aminoglutethimide as an aromatase inhibitor in the treatment of cancer. 13th International Congress of Chemotherapy, Vienna, Hans Huber, Berne, pp 11-23
4. Camacho AM, Brough AJ, Cash R, Wilroy RS (1966) Adrenal toxicity associated with the administration of an anticonvulsant drug. J Pediatr 68: 852-853
5. Cash R, Brough AJ, Cohen MNP, Satoh PS (1967) Aminoglutethimide as an inhibitor of adrenal steroidgenesis: mechanism of action and therapeutic trial. J Clin Endocrinol Metab 27: 1239-1248
6. Coombes RC, Goss PE, Dowsett M, Hutchinson G, Cunningham D, Jarman M, Brodie AMH (1987) 4-Hydroxyandrostenedione treatment for postmenopausal patients with advanced breast cancer. Tumor Diag Ther 8: 271-273
7. Foekens JA, Henkelmann MS, Fukkink JF, Blankenstein MA, Klijn JGM (1986) Direct effects of LHRH analogs on tumor cells. Eur J Cancer (abstr III-s) 22: 725
8. Foekens JA, Henkelmann MS, Bolt-de Vries J, Portengen H, Fukkink JF, Blankenstein MA, van Steenbrugge GJ, Mulder E, Klijn JGM (1987) Direct effects of LHRH analogs on breast and prostatic tumor cells. In: Klijn JGM, Paridaens R, Foekens JA (eds) Hormonal manipulation of cancer: peptides, growth factors, and new (anti) steroidal agents. Raven, New York,

pp 369–380 (Monograph series of the european organization for research on treatment of cancer [EORTC], vol 18)

9. Gale KE (1982) Treatment of advanced breast cancer with aminoglutethimide. A 14-year experience. Cancer Res [suppl] 42: 3389s–3396s
10. Griffiths CT, Hall TC, Saba Z, Barlow JJ, Nevinny HB (1973) Preliminary trial of aminoglutethimide in breast cancer. Cancer 32: 31–37
11. Harris AL, Dowsett M, Smith IE, Jeffcoate SL (1983) Endocrine effects of low-dose aminoglutethimide alone in advanced postmenopausal breast cancer. Br J Cancer 47: 621–627
12. Harris AL, Powles TJ, Smith IE, Coombes RC, Ford HT, Gazet JC, Harmer CL, Morgan M, White M, Parsons CA, McKinna JA (1983) Aminoglutethimide for the treatment of advanced postmenopausal breast cancer. Eur J Cancer Clin Oncol 29: 11–17
13. Harvey HA, Lipton A, Santen RJ, Escher GC, Hardy MA, Glode LM, Sealoff A, Landau RL, Schneir H, Max DT (1981) Phase II study of a gonadotropin-releasing hormone analogue (Leuprolide) in postmenopausal advanced breast cancer patients. Proc Am Ass Cancer Res Am Soc Clin Oncol (Abstract C-436) 22: 444
14. Harvey HA, Lipton A, Max DT, Pearlman OHG, Diaz-Perches R, de la Garza J (1984) Effective medical castration produced by the GnRH analog Leuprolide in metastatic breast cancer. Proc Am Soc Clin Oncol (abstr C-435) 3: 111
15. Henderson IC, Cannelos GP (1980) Cancer of the breast. The past decade: Part 1. New Engl J Med 302: 17–30
16. Höffken K, Kempf H, Miller AA, Miller B, Schmidt CG, Faber P, Kley HK (1986) Aminoglutethimide without hydrocortisone in the treatment of postmenopausal patients with advanced breast cancer. Cancer Treat Rep 70: 1153–1157
17. Höffken K, Miller AA, Miller B, Becher R, Aulbert E, Hoffmann B, Anders CU, Callies R, Schmidt CG (1986) Niedrigdosierte Aminoglutethimid-Therapie ohne Cortisolsubstitution beim metastasierenden Mammakarzinom in der Postmenopause. Med Klin 81: 638–642
18. Höffken K, Jonat W, Possinger K, Kölbel M, Kunz T, Becher R, Callies R (1988) Aromatase inhibition with 4-hydroxyandrostenedione (4-OHA) in treatment of postmenopausal advanced breast cancer (BC). Verh Dtsch Krebsgesellschaft (to be published)
19. Höffken K, Oesterdickhoff C, Becher R, Callies R, Kurschel E, Anders CU, Scheulen ME, Schmidt CG (1989) LH-RH agonist treatment with Buserilin in premenopausal patients with advanced breast cancer: a phase II study. Cancer Ther Contr 1: (in press)
20. Hoogstraten B, Gad-el-Mawla N, Maloney TR, Fletcher WS, Vaughn CB, Tranum BL, Athens JW, Costanzi JJ, Foulkes M (1984) Combined modality therapy for first recurrence of breast cancer. A Southwest Oncology Group Study. Cancer 54: 2248–2256
21. Ingle JN, Krook JE, Green SJ, Kubista TP, Everson LK, Ahmann DL, Chang MN, Bisel HF, Windschitl HE, Twito DI, Pfeifle DM (1986) Randomized trial of bilateral oophorectomy versus tamoxifen in premenopausal women with metastatic breast cancer. J Clin Oncol 4: 178–185
22. Klijn JGM, de Jong FH (1982) Treatment with a luteinising hormone-releasing hormone analogue (Buserelin) in premenopausal patients with metastatic breast cancer. Lancet 1: 1213–1216
23. Klijn JGM, de Jong FH, Lamberts SWJ, Blankenstein MA (1985) LHRH-agonist treatment in clinical and experimental human breast cancer. J Steroid Biochem 23: 867–873
24. Klijn JGM, Paridaens R, Foekens JA (eds) (1987) Hormonal manipulation of cancer: peptides, growth factors, and new (anti) steroidal agents. Raven, New York, (Monograph series of the european organization for research on treatment of cancer [EORTC]. vol 18)
25. Klijn JGM, de Jong FH (1987) Long-term LHRH-agonist (Buserelin) treatment in metastatic premenopausal breast cancer. In: Klijn JGM, Paridaens R, Foekens JA (eds) Hormonal manipulation of cancer: peptides, growth factors, and new (anti) steroidal agents. Raven, New York, pp 343–352 (Monograph series of the european organization for research on treatment of cancer [EORTC], vol 18)
26. Miller AA, Miller BE, Höffken K, Schmidt CG (1987) Clinical pharmacology of aminoglutethimide in patients with metastatic breast cancer. Cancer Chemother Pharmacol 20: 337–341
27. Miller AA, Miller BE, Höffken K, Schmidt CG (1987) Conventional-dose aminoglutethimide without hydrocortisone replacement in patients with postmenopausal breast cancer: serum cortisol levels and response to ACTH stimulation. J Exp Clin Cancer Res 16: 135–138

28. Murray R, Pitt P (1985) Low-dose aminoglutethimide without steroid replacement in the treatment of postmenopausal women with advanced breast cancer. Eur J Cancer Clin Oncol 21: 19–22
29. Nicholson RI, Maynard PV (1979) Anti-tumour activity of ICI 118630, a new potent luteinizing hormone-releasing hormone agonist. Br J Cancer 39: 268–273
30. Plowman PN, Nicholson RI, Walker KJ (1986) Remissions of metastatic breast cancer in postmenopausal women with luteinising hormone releasing hormone (ICI 118630) therapy. Eur J Cancer (abstract III-18) 22: 746
31. Pritchard KI, Thomson DB, Myers RE, Sutherland DJA, Mobb BG, Meakin JW (1980) Tamoxifen therapy in premenopausal patients with metastatic breast cancer. Cancer Treat Rep 64: 787–796
32. Santen RJ, Santner S, Davis B (1978) Aminoglutethimide inhibits extraglandular estrogen production in postmenopausal women with breast carcinoma. J Clin Endocrinol Metab 47: 1257–1265
33. Santen RJ, Worgul TJ, Samojlike E, Interrante A, Boucher AE, Lipton A, Harvey HA, White DS, Smart E, Cox C, Wells SA (1981) A randomized trial comparing surgical adrenalectomy with aminoglutethimide plus hydrocortisone in women with advanced breast cancer. N Engl J Med 305: 545–551
34. Schally AV, Redding TW, Comaru-Schally AM (1984) Potential use of analogs of luteinizing hormone-releasing hormones in the treatment of hormone-sensitive neoplasms. Cancer Treat Rep 68: 281–289
35. Schinzinger AS (1889) Über Carcinoma mammae. Zentralbl Chir [Suppl] 16: 55–56
36. Stuart-Harris RC, Smith IE (1984) Aminoglutethimide in the treatment of advanced breast cancer. Cancer Treat Rev 11: 189–204
37. Stuart-Harris RC, Dowsett M, Bozek T, McKinna JA, Gazet JC, Jeffcoate SL, Kurkure A, Carr L, Smith IE (1984) Low-dose aminoglutethimide in treatment of advanced breast cancer. Lancet 2: 604–607
38. Waxman JH, Harland SJ, Coombes RC, Wrigley PFM, Malpas JS, Powles T, Lister TA (1985) The treatment of postmenopausal women with advanced breast cancer with Buserelin. Cancer Chemother Pharmacol 15: 171–173
39. Williams MR, Walker KJ, Turkes A, Blamey RW, Nicholson RI (1986) The use of an LH-RH agonist (ICI 118630, Zoladex) in advanced premenopausal breast cancer. Br J Cancer 53: 629–636

Reproductive Toxicity with and Without Administration of Luteinizing-Hormone-Releasing Hormone Agonist During Adjuvant Chemotherapy in Patients with Germ Cell Tumors*

E. D. KREUSER,[1] W. D. HETZEL,[2] F. PORZSOLT,[1] and R. HAUTMANN[3]

Introduction

Since the introduction of aggressive chemotherapy, irradiation, and bone marrow transplantation, long-lasting remissions and cures have been achieved in patients with certain types of neoplastic diseases. With this therapeutic success, late side effects may become clinically significant in long-term survivors. It has been shown that all patients treated for germ cell tumors have severe and long lasting reproductive failure after curative chemotherapy consisting of four to six courses [1-7]. In contrast, the degree and duration of reproductive impairment after two courses of adjuvant chemotherapy are not known.

Since dividing cells are more sensitive to cytotoxic drugs than are cells at rest, it has been assumed that interruption of the pituitary-gonadal axis by luteinizing-hormone-releasing hormone agonist ($LHRH_A$) treatment may induce proliferation arrest of germ cells, thereby rendering them less susceptible to chemotherapeutic agents [8-13, 22-24]. Using animal models, several investigators have suggested that $LHRH_A$-induced arrest of spermatogenesis during exposure to cytotoxic drugs may reduce reproductive toxicity [9-13]. Since protection of gonadal functions in patients with testicular cancer by $LHRH_A$ treatment during chemotherapy has not been studied so far, we undertook this prospective study to investigate drug-induced gonadal toxicity with and without $LHRH_A$ protection during adjuvant chemotherapy.

Materials and Methods

Patients

Fourteen men with germ cell tumors were prospectively studied. All patients had a unilateral orchiectomy and unilateral retroperitoneal lymph node dissection prior to two courses of adjuvant chemotherapy. Therefore, all patients had ejaculatory

* Supported in part by a grant from the Deutsche Krebshilfe Contract No. M 16/86.

[1] Department of Internal Medicine III (Hematology/Oncology), University Clinic Ulm, Oberer Eselsberg, Robert-Koch-Straße, 7900 Ulm, FRG.

[2] Department of Internal Medicine I (Endocrinology), University of Ulm, Steinhövelstraße 9, 7900 Ulm, FRG.

[3] Department of Urology, University of Ulm, Steinhövelstraße 9, 7900 Ulm, FRG.

H. G. Beger et al. (Eds.), Cancer Therapy

Table 1. Patient characteristics

	With $LHRH_A$	Without $LHRH_A$
Number	6	8
Age (years)		
Median	26	29
Range	19-34	17-48
Stage II disease	6	8
Surgery		
Unilateral orchiectomy	6	8
Unilateral RLND	6	8
Follow-up (months)		
Median	24	28
Range	22-29	24-32

RLND, retroperitoneal lymph node dissection; *$LHRH_A$*, luteinizing-hormone-releasing hormone agonist.

capacity after surgery. Six patients were treated with and eight patients without $LHRH_A$. The latter served as controls. Further patient characteristics are summarized in Table 1.

Hormone Determination

Baseline levels of testosterone, luteinizing hormone (LH), and follicle-stimulating hormone (FSH) were obtained before therapy. Hormone determinations were performed by radioimmunoassays using kits from Serono (Freiburg) and Laboserv (Gießen). During administration of $LHRH_A$ and chemotherapy, blood samples were tested for FSH, LH, and testosterone twice a week and after cessation of treatment at 3-month intervals. The normal range of hormone levels in men in our laboratory was: FSH, 175-700 ng/ml; LH, 25-100 ng/ml, and testosterone, 300-1000 ng/100 ml.

Semen Analysis

Semen analyses were performed on freshly produced specimens after a suggested 5-day abstinence before treatment and at 3-month intervals thereafter. The samples were analyzed for sperm density, morphology, and motility. Normal parameters in our laboratory were: density $>20 \times 10^6$/ml, normal morphology $>60\%$, normal motility $>60\%$.

Treatment

All 14 patients were treated with two courses of PVB regimen, consisting of cisplatin 20 mg/m^2 i.v. on days 1-5, vinblastine 6 mg/m^2 i.v. on days 1+2, and ble-

Table 2. Treatment schedule of *d*-Ser(TBU)^6-LHRH ethylamide, buserelin (Suprefact)

Before chemotherapy:
(day 14–0): 3 × 0.5 mg subcutaneously
During chemotherapy:
(day 1–33): 3 × 0.4 mg intranasally
After chemotherapy:
(day 33–48): 3 × 0.4 mg intranasally

omycin 12 mg/m^2 on days 1–5. The courses were repeated at 4-week intervals. No patient received maintenance therapy.
The treatment schedule with *d*-Ser(TBU)^6 LHRH ethylamide, buserelin (Suprefact), is outlined in Table 2. Six patients were treated with buserelin. Before chemotherapy, $LHRH_A$ was administered subcutaneously 3 × 0.5 mg at a daily dose of 1.5 mg. During chemotherapy and during the interval between the courses, patients were treated with $LHRH_A$ 3 × 0.4 mg intranasally. The protocol for this study was reviewed and approved by the Ethics Committee of the University of Ulm. Written informed consent was obtained by all patients treated with $LHRH_A$.

Statistics

To compare hormone levels after chemotherapy in the protected and unprotected group, we used the Mann-Whitney *U* test, with $P < 0.05$ being considered significant.

Results

Patients with $LHRH_A$ Administration

Before therapy, plasma testosterone levels (median, 475; range, 410–890 ng/100 ml), LH values (median 52; range, 28–86 ng/ml) and FSH serum levels (median, 481 ng/ml; range 215–677 ng/ml) were normal in all patients. Semen analyses showed normozoospermia in two of six, oligozoospermia in two of six and azoospermia in two of six patients before therapy. Testosterone and LH serum levels were effectively suppressed during pretreatment therapy with $LHRH_A$ within 14 days. Serum values of FSH remained below normal throughout the duration of $LHRH_A$ therapy (by intranasal application) in all men. Testosterone and LH serum levels normalized in six of six patients within 4 weeks after $LHRH_A$ treatment was discontinued owing to intact Leydig cell function. In contrast, FSH serum levels rose and reached a maximum 6 months after cessation of chemotherapy in all six protected patients owing to germ cell loss and subsequent azoospermia. However, FSH levels normalized in all six men 16–23 months (median, 17 months) after completion of chemotherapy, indicating recovery of spermatogenesis (Figs. 1, 2). All men showed recovery of sperm density within 14–22 (median, 17)

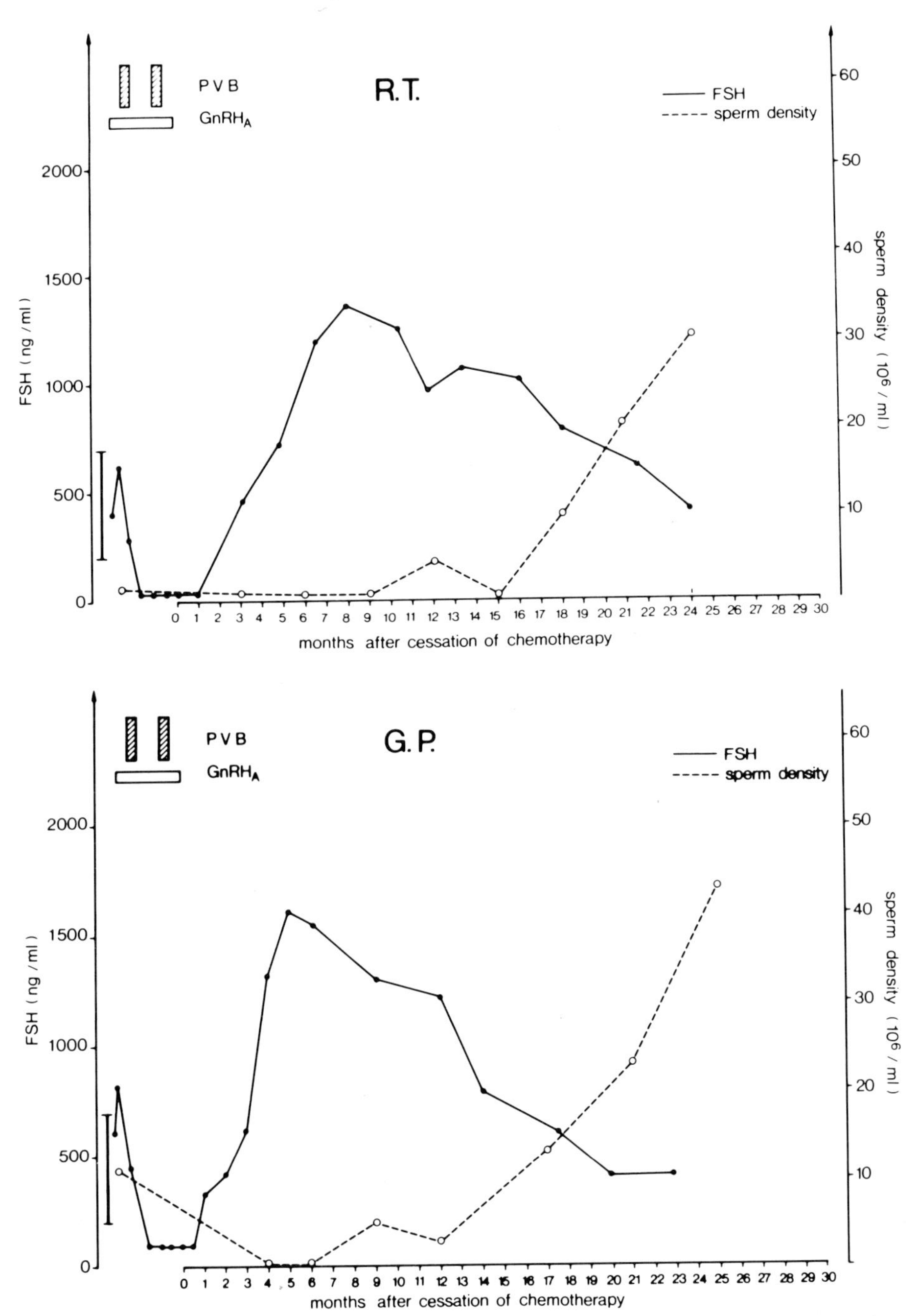

Fig. 1. FSH levels (———) and sperm densities (- - -) in three patients (R.T., G.P., H.M.) before, during, and after $GnRH_A$ treatment and two cycles of PVB chemotherapy. The normal range of FSH is denoted by the *bar* at the *y*-axis. *FSH*, follicle-stimulating hormone; *$LHRH_A$*, luteinizing hormone-releasing hormone agonist; *PVB*, cisplatin/vinblastine/bleomycin regimen

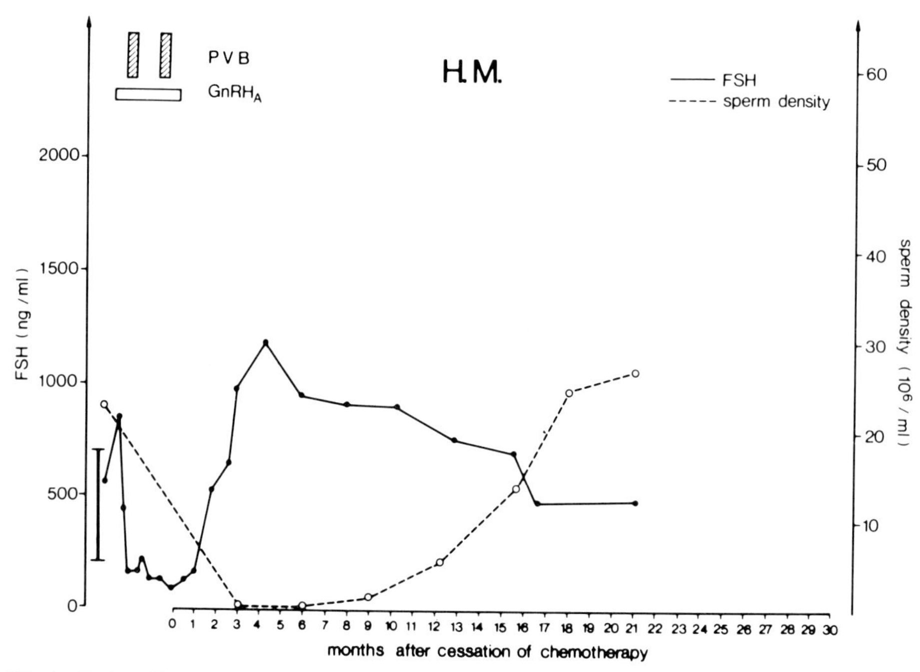

Fig. 1. Patient H. M. Legend see p. 295

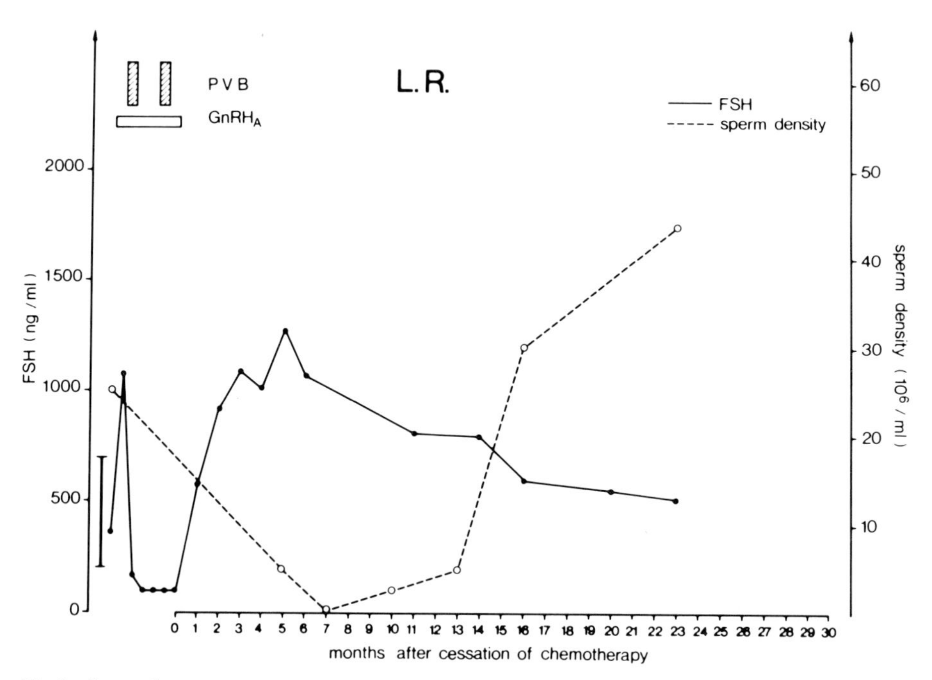

Fig. 2. Legend see next page

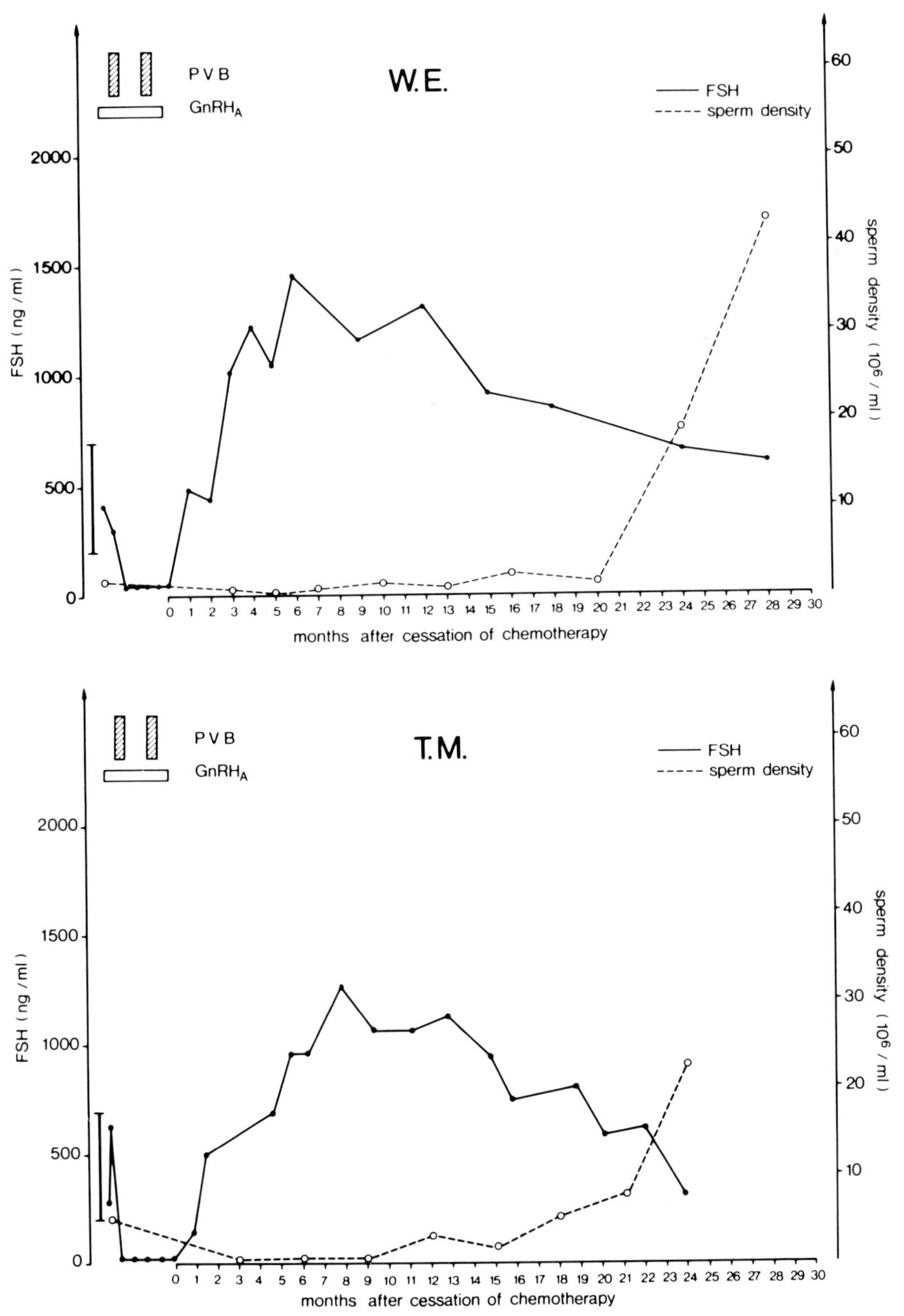

Fig. 2. FSH levels (———) and sperm densities (- - -) in three patients before, during, and after $LHRH_A$ treatment and two cycles of PVB chemotherapy. The normal range of FSH is denoted by the *bar* at the *y*-axis. For definition of abbreviations, see Fig. 1

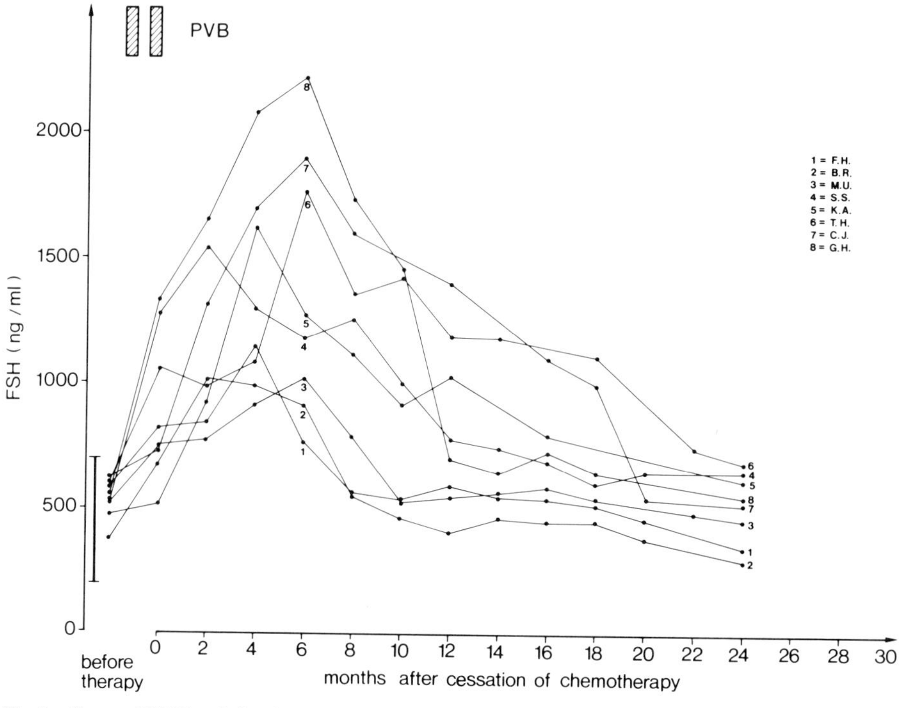

Fig. 3. Serum FSH levels in eight patients with germ cell tumors before, during, and after two cycles of PVB chemotherapy without $GnRH_A$ serving as controls. The normal range of FSH is denoted by the *bar* at the *y*-axis. *PVB*, cisplatin/vinblastine/bleomycin regime

months after cessation of chemotherapy. Side effects attributable to $LHRH_A$ were minimal: All men complained of impotence within 4 weeks after starting $LHRH_A$. However, all had normal sexual functions within 4 weeks after completing $LHRH_A$ treatment. None complained of local irritation at the site of the $LHRH_A$ injection.

Patients Without $LHRH_A$ Administration

In eight of eight patients, FSH, testosterone, and LH serum levels were within normal limits before, during, and after chemotherapy. In all eight patients, FSH levels rose and reached a maximum 6 months after cessation of chemotherapy (Fig. 3). All patients showed azoospermia after chemotherapy (Fig. 4). However, FSH levels and sperm densities normalized spontaneously 8–24 (median, 16) months after completion of chemotherapy in all eight patients treated (Fig. 3). In all eight patients, serum levels of testosterone and LH were within normal limits during and after chemotherapy. Comparing recovery time of spermatogenesis in the $LHRH_A$ and the control group, there was no significant difference (18 vs 16 months). Comparison of serum FSH levels 6 months after cessation of chemotherapy in the pro-

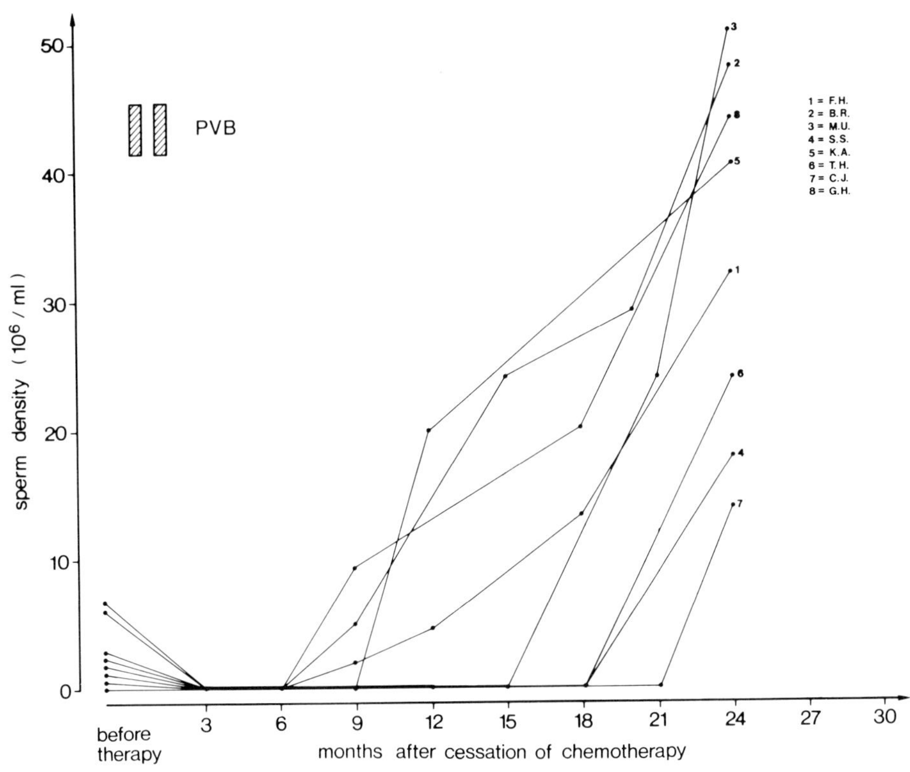

Fig. 4. Sperm densities in eight patients with germ cell tumors before and after two cycles of PVB chemotherapy without $GnRH_A$ serving as controls. *PVB*, cisplatin/vincristinelbleomycin regimen

tected (1293 ± 260; $\bar{x} \pm SD$) and unprotected group (1324 ± 370; $\bar{x} \pm SD$) revealed no statistically significant difference ($P < 0.05$).

Discussion

Pulsatile secretion of luteinizing-hormone-releasing hormone (LHRH) is a prerequisite of normal gonadal functions in men and women. Nonpulsatile treatment with $LHRH_A$ results in a dose-dependent suppression of FSH and LH release from the pituitary. This phenomenon has been called desensitization, which may be defined as a modulation of a target organ's responsiveness to a hormone by previous exposure of the target gland to the hormone [14].

In addition, administration of $LHRH_A$ may produce changes at the gonadal level [18]. Low FSH and LH levels induce reversible inhibition of gonadal steroidogenesis and spermatogenesis in human beings [14–17], as well as in animal models [18–21]. In the present study, $LHRH_A$ was administered three times daily. This nonpulsatile treatment schedule has been proved to interrupt the pituitary gonadal axis effectively [14, 15].

All 14 patients treated with two courses of the PVB regimen with and without $LHRH_A$ became azoospermic and showed elevated FSH levels, indicating severe germ and gonial stem cell loss. Comparing elevated FSH levels in the protected and unprotected group, there was no significant difference, suggesting no difference in acute reproductive toxicity in both groups.
In all patients, reversibility of reproductive impairment was complete. All patients with and without $LHRH_A$ protection regained normal sperm density and normal FSH levels after adjuvant chemotherapy. Moreover, median recovery time of spermatogenesis did not differ significantly between the LHRH-protected and the unprotected group (18 vs 16 months). Therefore, our data suggest that $LHRH_A$ application during two courses of adjuvant chemotherapy has no protective effect on acute and chronic reproductive toxicity in patients with germ cell tumors.
Our data are consistent with other reports, suggesting no ultimate reduction of reproductive toxicity by simultaneous application of $LHRH_A$ and cytotoxic drugs. No improvement of reproductive failure could be demonstrated in men treated for lymphoma with MOPP-chemotherapy (mechlorethamine, vincristine, procarbazine, and prednisone) after a median follow-up period of 52 weeks [23]. Recently, it has been reported that $LHRH_A$ treatment during the MVPP regimen (mechlorethamine, vinblastine, procarbazine, and prednisone) was ineffective in conserving reproductive capacity in both male and female patients with Hodgkin's disease [24].
Several reasons might be given for the lack of efficacy of $LHRH_A$ treatment. Patients generally receive multidrug chemotherapy, inducing more profound toxicity than single drugs, which are mostly given in animal trials [9-12, 22]. Moreover, PVB chemotherapy is known to induce profound germ cell and stem cell depletion [2-7]. Therefore, it seems evident that proliferation arrest of gonadal stem cells by $LHRH_A$ cannot prevent their depletion by cytotoxic drugs.
We and others have shown that serum FSH levels are a feasible marker to assess the degree and duration of reproductive toxicity after chemotherapy, while LH levels are indicative of endocrine gonadal toxicity [2, 3, 5, 6, 25, 26]. Germ and stem cell depletion induced by cytotoxic drugs cause azoospermia and diminished inhibin secretion, resulting in an increased FSH secretion by the pituitary. Considerable evidence suggests that Sertoli cells are capable of producing inhibin [27] and that inhibin is a physiologically important modulator of FSH secretion [28]. Moreover, a significant inverse correlation has been demonstrated between the depletion of germ cells and elevated serum FSH levels [29-31]. Therefore, in the present study we investigated whether serum FSH levels may be a marker to define acute and chronic reproductive toxicity. In all patients, FSH levels were elevated, indicating azoospermia or severe oligozoospermia ($> 10 \times 10^6$/ml). Normalization of FSH levels were associated with normalized sperm densities in patients with or without $LHRH_A$ treatment. We defined, therefore, the recovery time of reproductive function as the interval between the beginning of chemotherapy and the normalization of FSH levels. Since multiple sperm analyses during and after chemotherapy are often not possible, sequential FSH determinations seem to be a reliable method to assess the duration of chronic reproductive toxicity in patients after chemotherapy.

During $LHRH_A$ treatment, testosterone and LH were suppressed due to an interruption of the pituitary-gonadal axis. There was no evidence of impaired gonadal steroid synthesis after cessation of therapy in either the $LHRH_A$ or the control group. Intact Leydig cell function after chemotherapy has also been reported in patients treated for acute leukemia [20], Hodgkin's disease [27], and for germ cell tumors [2-7]. This resistance to cytotoxic drugs may be due to their extremely low mitotic rate.

In conclusion, our data suggest completely reversible reproductive toxicity after two courses of adjuvant chemotherapy in all patients. It seems that $LHRH_A$ treatment during chemotherapy has no protective effects on germ cells since acute reproductive toxicity occurred in all patients with $LHRH_A$ protection and recovery time did not differ significantly between the $LHRH_A$-protected and the unprotected group (18 vs 16 months). Sequential FSH determinations after chemotherapy is a feasible method to determine the degree and duration of reproductive toxicity caused by cytotoxic drugs.

References

1. Lange PH, Narayan P, Vogelzang NJ, Shafer RB, Kennedy BJ, Fraley EE (1983) Return of fertility after treatment for nonseminomatous testicular cancer: changing concepts. J Urol 129: 1131-1135
2. Drasga RE, Einhorn LH, Williams SD, Patel DN, Stevens EE (1983) Fertility after chemotherapy for testicular cancer. J Clin Oncol 1: 179-183
3. Fossa SD, Ons S, Abyholm T, Norman N, Leob M (1985) Posttreatment fertility in patients with testicular cancer. Cancer 57: 210-214
4. Johnson DH, Hainsworth JD, Linde RB, Greco A (1984) Testicular function following combination chemotherapy with cis-platin, vinblastine, and bleomycin. Med Pediat Oncol 12: 233-238
5. Kreuser ED, Harsch U, Hetzel WD, Schreml W (1986) Chronic gonadal toxicity in patients with testicular cancer after chemotherapy. Eur J Cancer Clin Oncol 22: 289-294
6. Nijman JM, Schraffordt Koops H, Kremer J, Sleijfer DT (1987) Gonadal function after surgery and chemotherapy in men with stage II and III nonseminomatous testicular tumors. J Clin Oncol 5: 651-663
7. Leitner SP, Bosl GJ, Bajorunas D (1986) Gonadal dysfunction in patients treated for metastatic germ cell tumors. J Clin Oncol 4: 1500-1505
8. Chapman RM, Sutcliffe SB (1981) Protection of ovarian function by oral contraceptives in women receiving chemotherapy for Hodgkin's disease. Blood 58: 849-851
9. Glode LM, Robinson J, Gould SF (1981) Protection from cyclophosphamide-induced testicular damage with an analogue of gonadotropin-releasing hormone. Lancet I: 1132-1134
10. Goodpasture JE, Bergstrom K, Waller DP, Vickery BH (1984) Interactions between a LHRH analogue and cancer chemotherapeutic agents at the testicular level. In: Labrie F, Belanger A, Dupont A (eds) LHRH and its analogues. Elsevier, Amsterdam, pp 156-172
11. Lewis RW, Dowling KJ, Schally AV (1985) D-Trp-6 analog of luteinizing-hormone-releasing hormone as a protective agent against testicular damage caused by cyclophosphamide in baboons. Proc Natl Acad Sci USA 82: 2975-2979
12. Nesyo UO, Huben RP, Klioze SS, Pontes JE (1985) Protection of germinal epithelium with luteinizing-hormone-releasing hormone analogue. J Urol 34: 187-190
13. Vickery BH, Goodpasture JC, Waller DP (1984) Interactions between an LHRH analogue and cancer chemotherapeutic agents at the testicular level. J Steroid Biochem 20: 1370
14. Linde R, Doelle GC, Alexander N, Kirchner F, Vale W, Rivier J, Rabin D (1981) Reversible inhibition of testicular steroidogenesis and spermatogenesis by a potent gonadotropin-releasing hormone agonist in normal men. N Engl J Med 305: 663

15. Doelle GC, Alexander AN, Evans RM, Linde R, Rivier J, Vale W, Rabin D (1983) Combined treatment with an LHRH agonist and testosterone in man. Reversible oligozoospermia without impotence. J Androl 4: 298-302
16. Faure N, Labrie F, Lemay A, Bélanger A, Gourdeau Y, Laroche B, Robert G (1982) Inhibition of serum androgen levels by chronic intranasal and subcutaneous administration of a potent luteinizing-hormone-releasing hormone (LHRH) agonist in adult men. Fertil Steril 37: 416-424
17. Schürmeyer T, Knuth UA, Freischem CW, Sandow J, Akhtar FB, Nieschlag E (1984) Suppression of pituitary and testicular function in normal men by constant gonadotropin-releasing hormone agonist infusion. J Clin Endocrinol Metab 59: 19-24
18. Hsueh AJW, Jones PhBC (1981) Extrapituitary actions of gonadotropin-releasing hormone. Endocr Rev 2: 437-461
19. Mann DR, Gould KG, Collins DC (1984) Influence of continuous gonadotropin-releasing hormone (GnRH) agonist treatment on luteinizing hormone and testosterone secretion, the response to GnRH, and the testicular response to human chorionic gonadotropin in male rhesus monkeys. J Clin Endocrinol Metab 58: 262-267
20. Vickery BH, McRae GI, Briones W, Worden A, Seidenberg R, Schaubacher BD, Falro R (1984) Effects of an LHRH agonist analog upon sexual function in male dogs. Suppression, reversibility, and effects of testosterone replacement. J Androl 5: 28-41
21. Clayton RN, Katikineni M, Chan V, Dufau ML, Catt KJ (1980) Direct inhibition of testicular function by gonadotropin-releasing hormone: Mediation by specific gonadotropin-releasing hormone receptors in interstitial cells. Proc Natl Acad Sci 77: 459-463
22. Glode LM, Robinson J, Gould SF, Nett TM, Mervill D (1982) Protection of spermatogenesis during chemotherapy. Drug Exp Clin Res 8: 367
23. Johnson DH, Linde R, Hainworth JD, Vale W, Rivier J, Stein R, Flexner J, van Welch R, Greco A (1985) Effect of a luteinizing-hormone-releasing hormone agonist given during combination chemotherapy on post-therapy fertility in male patients with lymphoma: preliminary observations. Blood 65: 832-836
24. Waxman JH, Ahmed R, Smith D, Wrigley PFM, Gregory W, Shalet S, Crowther D, Rees LH, Besser GM, Malpas JS, Lister TA (1987) Failure to preserve fertility in patients with Hodgkin's disease. Cancer Chemother Pharmacol 19: 159-162
25. Kreuser ED, Xiros N, Hetzel WD, Heimpel H (1987) Reproductive and endocrine gonadal capacity in patients treated with COPP-chemotherapy for Hodgkin's disease. J Cancer Res Clin Oncol 113: 260-266
26. Kreuser ED, Hetzel WD, Heit W, Hoelzer D, Kurrle E, Xiros N, Heimpel H (1988) Reproductive and endocrine gonadal functions in adults following multidrug chemotherapy for acute lymphoblastic or undifferentiated leukemia. J Clin Oncol 19: 316-324
27. Steinberger E, Steinberger A (1975) Spermatogenetic function of the testis. In: Greep RO, Astwood EB (eds) Handbook of physiology, Sect 7, Endocrinology, American Physiological Society, Washington, DC, pp 1-20
28. Scott RS, Burger HG (1980) An inverse relationship exists between seminal plasma inhibin and serum follicle-stimulating hormone in man. J Clin Endocrinol Metab 52: 796-803
29. Kretser de DM, Burger GH, Bremner WJ (1983) Control of FSH and LH secretion. Monogr Endocrinol 35: 12-43
30. Kretser de DM, Burger HG, Hudson B (1974) The relationship between germinal cells and serum FSH levels in males with infertility. J Clin Endocrinol Metab 38: 787-793
31. Schütte B (1984) Hodenbiopsie bei Subfertilität. In: Schirren C, Holstein AF (eds) Fortschritte der Andrologie. G. Grosse, Berlin, pp 166-167

Subject Index

ACNU 273
actinomycin D 7
ADCC (antibody-dependent cellular cytotoxicity) 32, 42, 109
-, augmentation 49
-, in vitro 36
adenocarcinoma, colon 26, 38, 229, 271
-, small-bowel 105
ADM (adriamycin) 250, 257, 263, 270
adrenal androgens, aromatization 284
adrenalectomy 284
ALL (acute lymphoblastic leukemia) 96, 272
allogenic tumor cells 133
alopecia 272
alpha-IFN's 115
aminoglutethimide 286
anal cancer 158, 159, 161
anemia, refractory (RA) 91
anthracycline 263, 280
antibody accumulation 231
- therapy 34
- transport 230
antibody-dependent cellular cytotoxicity 32, 42, 109
anti-CEA monoclonal antibodies 20
antimouse antibodies 46
antineoplastic effects 270
antitumor activity 277
aromatase inhibition 286
- enzyme system 284
arterial cannulation 192
assay, blocking 11
-, clonogenic 243, 271
-, pretherapeutic 244
-, proliferation 271
athymic mice 6
AUA1 20
autoradiography 224

B16 melanoma 271
BCNU 98
biliary sclerosis 149
biliodigestive bypass 155
binding kinetics of the MAB 223
biodistribution of MAB 223
biological response modifiers 109, 150
biomodulators 85
biotherapy 143
bleomycin 3
blocking assay 11
blotting agents, Western 11
BMT (bone marrow transplantation) 96, 99
-, autologous 96
bone marrow 106
- - insufficiency 96
brain metastasis 88
breast cancer 158, 161, 252, 272, 284
- -, hormonal therapy 284

CA19-9 35
cancer/carcinoma (s. a. tumors), breast 158, 161, 252, 272, 284
-, colorectal/anal/rectal 18, 42, 105, 132, 146, 156, 158, 159, 161, 176, 195
-, esophageal 158, 159, 161
-, gastrointestinal 56, 144, 145, 155
-, hepatocellular 105
-, hepatocholangiocellular 252
-, lung 272
-, ovarian 18, 19, 252, 272
-, pancreatic 32, 56, 154
-, peritoneal 146
-, prostate 284
-, renal 272
-, sex-specific 284
-, small-cell lung 273, 280
-, stomach 272
-, thyroid, papillary 156
-, uterine 272
-, vaginal 272
cannulation, arterial 192
- of the inferior vena cava 191
carcinoid disease 165, 252
carcinomas (s. a. cancer)
cardiac toxicity 270
cardiomyopathy 270
catheter, perfusion 192
-, port- 252

catheter, port-implantable 166
CDDP (cisplatin) 250
CEA (carcinoembryonic antigen) 10, 18, 35
- antibody C1P83 224
-, cell-bound 15
-, circulation 15
chemoembolization 201, 205
chemoimmunoconjugates 3
chemoimmunotherapy 3
chemosensitivity 249
-, individual 256
- profiles 250, 252, 253
- testing, HTCA 249
chemotherapy 56, 96, 158, 243
-, adjuvant 292
-, drug testing 257
-, intra-arterial 190
-, intraperitoneal 148
-, intraportal 146
-, regional 163, 190, 249, 255, 256
-, -, liver metastases 148
-, systemic 148, 249
chlorambucil 3
cholecystojejunostomy 155
cisplatin 98
clonogenic assay 243, 271
CMML (chronic myelomonocyte leukemia) 91
collagen, submucosal 220
colon adenocarcinoma 229, 271
colony growth 251
colony-stimulating factors 40
colorectal cancer/carcinoma 18, 42, 105, 132, 146, 156, 158, 159, 161, 176, 195
- -, metastases 195
- -, recurrences 146
-, systemic treatment 257
- liver metastases 249, 256
- surgery 144
colostomy 158
conditioning 98
CSF (colony-stimulating factor) 90, 103
-, granulocyte-macrophage 103
CY (cyclophosphamide) 85
cyano-morpholino doxorubicin 6
cyclophosphamide 98, 272
-, low-dose 76
cytokines 56, 124
-, cancer treatment 73
cytolytic T-lymphocytes 87
cytorhodin S (rodorubicin) 263
cytostatic polychemotherapy 133
cytotoxicity 109, 271
-, antibody-dependent cellular 109
-, monocyte-mediated 109

daunomycin 3
daunorubicin 271
dearterialization of ther liver 201
2′-deoxycoformycin 112
distribution of monoclonal antibodies 223
-, volume 270
doxorubicin (ADM) 3, 257, 263, 270
drug activity 253
- carriers 7
- combinations 247
- concentration 246
- infusion pump, totally implantable 148
- selection 249, 255
- testing 250, 252, 257
- - in systemic chemotherapy 257
- - in vitro 256
dye laser 219

EGF (epidermal growth factor) 7
EGFR1 (epidermal growth factor receptors) 19, 20
ejection fraction, left ventricular (LVEF) 267
endosonography 156
EORTC (European Organization for Research and Treatment of Cancer) 264
EPI (4-epidoxorubicin) 250
epirubicin 275
esophageal cancer 158, 159, 161
estrogen 284
ex vivo human tumor perfusion 223
extracorporeal circulation 193
extrahepatic metastases 197, 199
extremity perfusion, isolated 158

folic acid 274
Friend leukemia cells 271
5-FU (5-fluorouracil) 194, 250, 257, 272
FUDR (fluorodeoxyuridine) 148
fungi imperfectii 7

gamma-IFN's 115, 124
ganglioside antibodies, treatment of tumor patients 51
gangliosides 51
gastrectomy, total 144, 145, 156
gastrointestinal cancer 56, 144, 145, 155, 158
- -, early 158
GD3-ganglioside antibody, intrathecal application 52
germ cell tumors 292
gliomas 18, 19
GM-CSF (granulocyte-macrophage colony-stimulating factor) 49, 62, 76, 79, 90, 96, 103
granulocyte colony-stimulating factor 80
granulocyte-macrophage colony-stimulating factor 49, 62, 76, 79, 90, 103

granulocytes 99
granulocytopenia 96
granulopoiesis 94
growth factor, epidermal (EGF) 7
– – receptors, epidermal (EGFR1) 19, 20
–, regulation of tumor 131

H17E2 19, 20
hairy cell leukemia 112, 124
HAMA (human antimouse antibody) 35, 38, 39
–, pharmacokinetics 36
HCL (hairy cell leukemia) 124
HD (s.a. Hodgkin's disease) 96
head and neck tumors 272
hematologic toxicity 274
hematopoiesis 96
hepatic artery occlusion 166
– – infusion 150, 165, 253, 257
– – –, short-term 257
– dearterialization 165
– metastases 20
hepatocellular carcinoma 105
hepatocholangiocellular carcinoma 252
high-dose therapy 198
HMFG1/HMFG2 20
Hodgkins's diseases 96
– lymphomas 272
Holter ECG 276
hormon receptors 284
hormonal- and chemotherapy 233ff.
– feedback mechanisms 284
– therapy 288
– –, breast cancer 284
HpD (haematoporphyrin derivate) 217
HTCA 256, 257
–, chemosensitivity testing 249
human colon adenocarcinoma 229
– tumor perfusion, ex vivo 223
4-hydroxyandrostenedione 288
hyperthermia 150, 193, 198
–, interstitial 216

IFN's (interferons) 112
–, alpha- 115
–, gamma- 115, 124
–, receptors 115
IL2 (interleukin 2) 40, 49, 62, 75, 85
immune reactivity 47
immuno response modifiers 40
immunochemotherapy 3
immunoconjugates 3
immunohistochemical investigations 34
immunohistochemistry 35
immunohistology 228
immunologic effector mechanism 51
immunomodulators 40
immunoperoxidase staining 21
immunoscintigraphy 10, 34, 35, 226
immunotherapy of malignant melanomes 51
– of pancreatic cancer with monoclonal antibody 32
–, side effects 37
implantable drug infusion pump 148
– port catheter 166
– pumps 164
in vitro drug testing 256
– – phase II-like studies 257
– – resistance 257
– – test system 245
– – tests 253
injection 96, 274
– complications 96
–, hepatic artery 165, 253, 257
–, – –, short-term 257
–, intraperitoneal 163
–, long-term 164
–, portovenous 163
– pump, totally implantable 148
–, short-term 164
interferon action, mechanism 124
interstitial hyperthermia 216
intra-arterial and intra-venous therapy 176
– chemotherapy 190
– treatment 256
intransit metastases 158
intraoperative radiotherapy 147, 148
intraperitoneal chemotherapy 148
– infusion 163
intraportal chemotherapy 146
intrathecal application of GD3-ganglioside antibody 52
intratumoral administration 65
irradiation, total-body 96
isolated extremity perfusion 158
– liver perfusion 190
– regional liver perfusion 193

LAK (lymphokine-activated killer) 75, 85
– of bone marrow transplantation 99
– cells 56, 57
laser 216, 217, 219
–, dye 219
– therapy 150
leucocytopenia 272
leukemia, acute lymphatic (ALL) 272
– cells, Friend- 271
– –, L1210 271
–, chronic myelomonocyte (CMML) 91
Lewis lung carcinoma 272
LHRH (luteinizing hormone-releasing hormone) 284, 292
liver 201
– metastases 158, 176, 190, 249, 252

liver, metastases, colorectal 249, 256
- -, regional chemotherapy 148
- perfusion, isolated 190
- -, regional, isolated 193
- tumors 201, 249
long-term infusion 164
lung cancer, small-cell 273, 280
- -, Lewis 272
LVEF (left ventricular ejection fraction) 267
lymph node dissection, radical 145, 146
- - metastases 156
lymphoblastic leukemia, acute (ALL) 96
lymphoid malignancies 96
lymphoma, acute myeloid 272
-, Hodgkin's 272
-, non-Hodgkin's (NHL) 96, 272

MAb (monoclonal antibodies) 3, 4, 10, 18, 40, 56
-, 9.2.27 4, 7
-, 14G2A 6
-, 17-1A 42, 45, 56
- -, survival 48
-, 90Y-labelled 19
-, anti-CEA 20
-, binding kinetics 223
-, biodistribution 223
-, distribution 223
-, immunotherapy 32
-, LM609 7
-, NRML-0,5 7
-, radiolabelled 18
MAF (mafosfamide) 250, 257
maintenance therapy 85
malignant melanoma 75, 154, 158, 159
- -, immunotherapy 51
maximum single dose 272
- tolerable single dose 272
M-CSF (monocyte colony-stimulating factor) 49
MDS (myelodysplastic syndromes) 90
melanoma 3, 4, 53, 85, 105
-, B16 271
melphalan 98, 250
metastases, breast cancer 284
-, colorectal carcinomas 195
-, extrahepatic 197, 199
-, hepatic 20
-, intransit 158
-, liver 158, 176, 190, 249, 252
-, treatment 146
methotrexate 3
mice, athymic 6
-, nude 57
microspheres 205
mitoxantrone 250, 271
MMC (mitomycin C) 64, 148, 194, 250
monoclonal antibodies (s. MAb)
monocyte-mediated cytotoxicity 109
mycotoxins 7
myeloid cell proliferation 108
- lymphoma, acute 272
myeloma, multiple 116
myelomonocyte leukemia, (CMML) 91
myelosuppression 108
myosarcoma 27

NCA (nonspecific cross-reacting antigens) 10
necroses, tumor 199
necrosis factor, tumor (TNF) 77, 109, 124
neodymium YAG 217
neuraminidase (VCN) 133
neuroblastoma 5, 53, 96
neutropenia 96
NHL (non-Hodgkin's lymphoma) 96, 272
nimustin 273
NK (natural killer cell) 88
no-touch technique 146
nude mice 57

oophorectomy 284
operative procedures, extension of standard 145
- -, standard 144
osteosarcoma 161
ovarian ablation 284
- cancer 18, 19, 252, 272
- function 284

pancreatectomy 154
-, regional 145
pancreatic carcinoma 56, 145, 154
- -, immunotherapy 32
pancreaticosplenectomy 145
papillary thyroid cancer 156, 159
PDT (photodynamic therapy) 216, 217
perfusion catheter 192
- circuit 193
peritoneal carcinosis 146
pharmacokinetic studies 194, 270
-, HAMA 36
-, serum 45, 47
phase I study 263
- II studies 272
- II-like studies, in vitro 257
- III 273
phlebitis 265
phthalocyanines 218
pirarubicin (4'-0-tetrahydropyranyl-doxorubicin, THP) 270
pirarubin 280
pleuramesotheliomas 274
port catheter 252
portovenous infusion 163

postembolization syndrome 209
postmenopause 284
premenopausal patient 284
pretherapeutic assay 244
- sensitivity tests 56
progesteron receptors 284
proliferation assay 271
- tumor cells 131
prostate cancer 284
proteinuria 265
pumps, implantable 164

quality of life 154, 277

radiation 161
radical lymph node dissection 145, 146
radioimmunodetection 27
radioimmunotherapy 18, 27
radiolabelled monoclonal antibodies 18
radiolabelling 21
radionuclides 20
radiotherapy 158
-, intraoperative 147, 148
rectal carcinoma 156
regional chemotherapy 163, 190, 249, 255, 256
- therapy 201
regression 166
regulation of tumor growth 131
renal carcinoma 272
- cell cancer 75
reproductive toxicity 292
resection, anterior 144
resistance, in vitro 257
rhGM-CSF (recombinant human granulocyte-macrophage colony stimulating factor) 96
rHuGM-CSF 104
rIFN-gamma 56
rodorubicin (Cytorhodin S) 263
rTNF-alpha 56

sarcomas 272
-, soft-tissue 158, 161
sensitivity, assay 244
- profiles 250
- rates 253
- tests, pretherapeutic 56
-, in vitro 257
sensitivity/resistance, in vitro 252
serum pharmacokinetics 45, 47
sex-specific cancer 284
short-term infusion 164
side effects 101
- -, immunotherapy 37
skin rash 101
small-bowel adenocarcinoma 105
small-cell cancer, lung 273, 280
soft-tissue sarcomas 158, 161
specificity, assay 244
stomach carcinoma 272
stomatitis 274
submucosal collagen 220
superoxideinducing effect 276
systemic chemotherapy 249

TAA (tumor-associated antigens) 42
-, CO17-1A 42
targeting, tumor 231
test drugs 250, 252
-, predictive 246
-, pretherapeutic sensitivity 56
- system, in vitro 245, 253
testicular tumors 20
4′-0-tetrahydropyranyl-doxorubicin (THP) 270
therapy/treatment, adjuvant 138
-, bio- 143
-, cancer 79
-, chemo- and hormonal 233ff.
-, colorectal carcinoma, systemic 257
-, combined modality 158
- cytokines 73
-, ganglioside antibodies 51
-, high-dose 198
-, hormonal 288
-, intra-arterial 256
-, intra-arterial and intra-venous 176
-, laser 150
-, maintenance 85
- metastases 146
-, regional 201
thiotepa 274
THP (4′-0-tetrahydropyranyl-doxorubicin) 270
thrombocytopenia 272, 274
thyroid cancer, papillary 156, 159
thyroidectomy 156
T-lymphocytes, cytolytic 87
TNF (tumor necrosis factor) 109, 124
Torekow 166
total gastrectomy 144, 145, 156
total-body irradiation 96
toxicity 87, 165
-, hematologic 274
-, reproductive 292
-, systemic 148
transport of antibodies 230
trichothecenes 7
tumor, calcification 166
-, carcinoid 252
- cells, allogenic 133
- -, proliferation 131
- destruction, local 217
-, germ cell 292
- growth, regulation 131
-, head and neck 272
-, liver 201, 249

tumor necroses 199
- necrosis factor 77
- perfusion, human, ex vivo 223
- - system 224
- targeting 231
-, testicular 20
- vaccination 132
tumor-associated antigens 3
two-port concept 166, 167

uterine carcinoma 272

vaccination, tumor 132
vaginal carcinoma 272
VCN (neuraminidase) 133
VCR (vincristine) 273
vena cava, cannulation 191
verrucarin A 7
vindesin 274
VP-16 98
VRC 273

Western blotting agents 11
Whipple operation 144
- procedure 155

90Y-labelled monoclonal antibodies 19
YAG, neodymium 217
yttrium 21